Social Well-Being, Development, and Multiple Modernities in Asia

Jaeyeol Yee · Hiroo Harada · Masayuki Kanai
Editors

Social Well-Being, Development, and Multiple Modernities in Asia

Springer

Editors
Jaeyeol Yee
Department of Sociology
Seoul National University
Seoul, Republic of Korea

Hiroo Harada
Senshu University
Kawasaki, Japan

Masayuki Kanai
School of Human Sciences
Senshu University
Kawasaki, Japan

ISBN 978-981-97-3865-6 ISBN 978-981-97-3866-3 (eBook)
https://doi.org/10.1007/978-981-97-3866-3

This Springer imprint is published by the registered company Springer Nature Singapore Pte Ltd.
The registered company address is: 152 Beach Road, #21-01/04 Gateway East, Singapore 189721, Singapore

Preface

The book *Social Well-Being, Development, and Multiple Modernities in Asia* provides insight into the complex nature of well-being in diverse societies, where long-standing traditions coexist with rapid progress. In Asia, social well-being is an important pursuit that is shared across borders.

This explores the complexities of eight distinct Asian societies: Indonesia, Japan, Korea, Mongolia, the Philippines, Thailand, Taiwan, and Vietnam. The book provides a comprehensive analysis of each society's historical trajectory, socio-cultural nuances, and institutional frameworks. From the bustling streets of Tokyo to the serene temples of Yogyakarta, and from the vibrant markets of Bangkok to the tranquil villages of the Mekong Delta, a variety of dimensions of well-being are experienced.

Why do some societies thrive while others grapple with persistent challenges? How do cultural norms, economic structures, and governance systems intersect to shape the well-being of individuals and communities? These questions form the heart of our exploration. We seek to unravel the conundrums that perplex policymakers, scholars, and citizens alike.

Our journey begins by identifying unique and common factors that shape the well-being of individuals and communities. Through the collection of survey data from eight societies and a comparative analysis, we have endeavored to uncover any unexpected connections.

The second part, *Development and Social Well-Being*, explores possible explanations for conundrums related to social well-being by revealing and interpreting unique and common factors from the context of social well-being in different Asian societies.

The third part, *Diverse Mechanisms of Social Well-Being*, is a crucial section of our inquiry that examines the various mechanisms that contribute to social well-being. Each chapter thoroughly analyzes these mechanisms in relation to diverse issues affecting the determinants of social well-being, using rigorous quantitative analyses of original cross-national survey data.

The concept of well-being is a multifaceted one that extends beyond economic prosperity or physical health. It encompasses social connections, psychological resilience, and environmental harmony. In this analysis, we aim to explore the unique characteristics of each society and interpret them using comparative data analysis.

As we explore the complexities of well-being, we recognize its intimate connection with development. Our investigation delves into the effects of progress on happiness and whether economic growth and globalization can harmonize with life satisfaction and communal solidarity. To accomplish this, we must achieve a nuanced equilibrium between individual and societal well-being.

As we embark on this intellectual journey, we acknowledge the intricacies involved. Our guide is curiosity, empathy, and a commitment to rigorous scholarship. We cordially invite readers to join us in deciphering the intricate patterns that underlie well-being in Asia. Whether you are an experienced researcher, a policymaker, or simply a curious individual, this book encourages you to explore, question, and engage.

As we navigate the crossroads of tradition and progress, we can work together to find pathways towards a more harmonious and flourishing Asia.

The completion of this book project was made possible thanks to the support of various institutions and individuals. For several years, the Japanese Ministry of Education, Culture, Sports, Science and Technology (MEXT) [S1491003], the Japan Society for the Promotion of Science (JSPS) [19H01570], and the Joint Support-Center for Data Science Research at Research Organization of Information and Systems (ROIS-DS) [002RP2017, 003RP2018, 022RP2019, 028RP2020, 014RP2021, 014RP2022, 059RP2023] have generously provided funding to enable scholars from different Asian countries to collaborate, share data, and present their findings. The Social Well-Being Survey in Asia (SoWSA) data was collected through the MEXT Supported Program for the Strategic Research Foundation at Private Universities titled "Forming a Social Well-being Research Consortium in Asia" from 2014 to 2018. The data was harmonized with the financial support of ROIS-DS and the expertise of Korea Social Science Data Archive (KOSSDA). Presently, the SoWSA data is available to all researchers (https://kossda.snu.ac.kr/handle/20.500.12236/23941). The final meeting for manuscript presentation and discussion was supported by the National Research Foundation of Korea (NRF-2020S1A5A2A03045598).

This book is the result of a genuine international collaboration. We would like to extend our sincere appreciation to all members of the International Consortium for Social Well-Being Studies and the Center for Social Well-Being Studies, Institute for the Development of Social Intelligence at Senshu University.

Although COVID-19 caused a delay in publication and coordination difficulties arose among researchers from eight different countries, we were able to overcome these obstacles. We appreciate Springer's patience and are confident that the final product will be worth the wait.

Seoul, Republic of Korea — Jaeyeol Yee
Kawasaki, Japan — Hiroo Harada
Kawasaki, Japan — Masayuki Kanai

Contents

Editors and Contributors

About the Editors

Jaeyeol Yee is a professor of sociology at Seoul National University and an international project member of the Center for Social Well-being Studies, Institute for the Development of Social Intelligence, Senshu University. He has contributed to the harmonization of social well-being surveys in Asia as director of the Korea Social Science Data Archives. His research interests include social quality, social well-being, social capital, disaster and safety issues, and sociological theory construction.

Hiroo Harada is an adjunct research fellow of the Center for Social Well-being Studies, Institute for the Development of Social Intelligence, and a professor emeritus of Economics at Senshu University. He was the chairs of the MEXT-Supported Program for the Strategic Research Foundation at Private Universities entitled "Exploring Social Capital towards Sustanable Development in East Asia" from 2009 to 2013 and "Forming a Social Well-being Research Consortium in Asia" from 2014 to 2018. His research interests are in the fields of public finance, taxation, regional economy, public choice, and social capital/well-being.

Masayuki Kanai is a research fellow of the Center for Social Well-being Studies, Institute for the Development of Social Intelligence, and a professor of sociology at the School of Human Sciences, Senshu University. He was the secretary-general of the MEXT-Supported Program for the Strategic Research Foundation at Private Universities entitled "Forming a Social Well-being Research Consortium in Asia" from 2014 to 2018. His research interests include subjective well-being, social capital, and social inequality in comparative perspectives.

Contributors

Dolgion Aldar Independent Research Institute of Mongolia, Ulaanbaatar, Mongolia

Liang-Wei Chen Research Center for Humanities and Social Sciences, Academia Sinica, Taipei, Taiwan

Yi-Fu Chen Department of Sociology, National Taipei University, New Taipei City, Taiwan

Muhammad R. Damm Department of Sociology, Universitas Indonesia, Depok, Indonesia

Ruzaki Hamda Department of Sociology, Universitas Indonesia, Depok, Indonesia

Hiroo Harada Senshu University, Kawasaki, Japan

Hye-ok Heo Korea Social Science Data Archive, Seoul National University, Seoul, Republic of Korea

Carola Hommerich Sophia University, Tokyo, Japan

Dong-Kyun Im Department of Sociology, Seoul National University, Seoul, Republic of Korea

Masayuki Kanai School of Human Sciences, Senshu University, Kawasaki, Japan

Jun Kobayashi Department of Contemporary Societies, Seikei University, Tokyo, Japan

Hearan Koo Institute for Social Development and Policy Research, Seoul National University, Seoul, Republic of Korea;
Korea Social Science Data Archive, Seoul National University, Seoul, Republic of Korea

Tselmegsaikhan Lkhagva Independent Research Institute of Mongolia, Ulaanbaatar, Mongolia

Dashzeveg Lkhagvanorov Independent Research Institute of Mongolia, Ulaanbaatar, Mongolia

Tadahiko Maeda Center for Social Data Structuring, Joint Support-Center for Data Science Research, Research Organization of Information and Systems, Tokyo, Japan

Sang-Hee Park Division of Social Sciences, Sungkonghoe University, Seoul, Republic of Korea

Indera Ratna Irawati Pattinasarany Department of Sociology, Universitas Indonesia, Depok, Indonesia

Emma Porio Department of Sociology and Anthropology, Ateneo de Manila University, Quezon City, Philippines;
Manila Observatory, Quezon City, Philippines

Francisia S. S. E. Seda Department of Sociology, Universitas Indonesia, Depok, Indonesia

Justin See Anthropology and Development Studies, The University of Melbourne, Parkville, Victoria, Australia

Lugina Setyawati Department of Sociology, Universitas Indonesia, Depok, Indonesia

Kiyohisa Shibai Joint Support-Center for Data Science Research (ROIS-DS), The Institute of Statistical Mathematics, Tokyo, Japan

Eiji Sumi College of Economics, Nihon University, Tokyo, Japan

Ming-Chang Tsai Research Center for Humanities and Social Sciences, Academia Sinica, Taipei, Taiwan

Batsugar Tsedendamba Independent Research Institute of Mongolia, Ulaanbaatar, Mongolia

Bold Tsevegdorj National University of Mongolia, Ulaanbaatar, Mongolia

Byambasuren Yadmaa National Academy of Governance, Ulaanbaatar, Mongolia

Keitaro Yazaki Department of Fine Arts, Tainan University of Technology, Tainan City, Taiwan

Jaeyeol Yee Department of Sociology, Seoul National University, Seoul, Republic of Korea

Introduction

Development, Culture, and Diverse Mechanisms of Social Well-Being in Asia

Jaeyeol Yee

Abstract There is a growing controversy regarding whether economic growth has led to better development and an improved quality of life. To determine what constitutes a good society, it is essential to examine various dimensions of social well-being. This chapter explores two aspects of social well-being: individual and societal. Individual and societal well-being are two distinct concepts. Individual well-being aims to improve quality of life and opportunities, while societal well-being is concerned with the happiness of the community, which is determined by structural flexibility and social quality. This chapter argues that multidimensional well-being includes physical, mental, relational, and social aspects. To compare and explain well-being in Southeast Asia and East Asia, it is necessary to analyze important variables such as value orientation and institutional quality. This chapter discusses three dimensions: embeddedness and individualism, hierarchy and egalitarianism, and mastery and harmony. Countries can be categorized as clan-based, transitional, or individualist societies. Southeast Asian culture is based on clans and traditional human relationships and is strongly influenced by religion. In contrast, Japan, Korea, and Taiwan are developed countries that have achieved significant industrialization, economic growth, and democratization. Due to the influence of digital transformation, they are quickly becoming part of an individualistic society. However, in Southeast Asia, which is a clan-based society, the level of well-being is generally higher than in East Asia. It is an intriguing question whether this level of well-being will persist as economic growth and democratization continue in the future. The creation of social well-being mechanisms in different cultural contexts raises questions about the convergence model, which suggests that convergence can occur through growth. Each country must find a development model that suits its own circumstances.

Keywords Social well-being · Cultural value orientation · Social quality · Clan-based society · Transitional society · Individualist society

---

J. Yee (✉)
Department of Sociology, Seoul National University, Seoul, Republic of Korea
e-mail: jyyee@snu.ac.kr

J. Yee et al. (eds.), *Social Well-Being, Development, and Multiple Modernities in Asia*,
https://doi.org/10.1007/978-981-97-3866-3_1

1 What Is a Good Society: Development and Modernization

What constitutes a "good society" is controversial. Despite rapid economic growth and democratization, polarization in developed Asian societies is severe and social conflicts are constant. The question of the "good society" is not only conceptual, but also a value-laden and normative. It is necessary to make a definition of "good society" through active debate at the theoretical level, and it is also desirable to achieve such a good society through practical programs and policy efforts. In the field of sociology, the issue of "good society" has been best described in development theory. In existing sociological theories, "social change toward a good society" was defined as development. Modernization theory was popular in the 1960s and 1970s, but dependency theory and world systems theory challenged the notion of development based on historical and macroscopic comparative analysis and criticized modernization theory as a conservative viewpoint subordinated to the Western concept of modernity.

The roots of modernization theory go back to Durkheim and Tönnies. After distinguishing between "mechanical" and "organic" solidarity, Durkheim explained the change from the former to the latter as modernization. Similarly, Tönnies juxtaposed Gemeinschaft and Gesellschaft and then classified the former as traditional and the latter as modern. Both explored the psychological, organizational, and social-structural features that can distinguish modernity from tradition. Modernization theorists have been criticized for attributing various structural problems to culture and individual psychology.

Originally, modernization was a term referring to the macrosocial changes in Western Europe since the eighteenth century. Because the historical change originated in the West, it took the developed country of the West as a reference for underdeveloped countries. And it is based on the value judgment that the advanced nations of the West will help the laggards, and that all humanity will benefit from economic growth, the spread of democracy, and the development of science and industry. This equation of modernization with development is based on the belief in enlightened progress, that the advancement of science and technology can stimulate the development of society. There is enormous variation in growth across countries, and it is relatively clear what causes this variation. Inkeles and Smith (1974) concluded that critical deficiencies or shortages in key factors such as market structure, technology, human and physical capital, and beliefs and attitudes are very important factors in explaining the success of modernization.

However, the historical experience of many underdeveloped countries has been different from the predictions of modernization theory. The expansion of transactions with developed countries sometimes reversed material growth and left negative effects on national autonomy or independence. Thus, dependency theory paid more attention to the external effects that operate within the context of the world system in which the country is located than to factors within each individual country. For example, the underdevelopment of Latin American countries is not due to internal factors, but rather to the unequal position of their relations with Europe (Wallerstein, 1974).

The determining factors in the two paradigms are extremely different, but the common limitation of both modernization and dependency theories is that economic growth is seen as the ultimate measure of development. Therefore, both sides can be criticized as an economy-centered model, arguing that economic growth will lead to a "good society". Recently, the importance of non-economic factors such as institutions and culture in explaining development has been increasingly discussed. North (1990, p. 3) defines institutions as "the rules of the game in a society or, more formally, the humanly devised constraints that shape human interaction". While economic institutions, e.g., property rights, entry barriers, shape economic incentives, contracting opportunities, and distribution, political institutions, e.g., form of government, constraints on politicians, shape political incentives and distribution of political power. Kim (2017) defines modernization as a "tilted acculturation from the historically advanced specific mode of modernity". In this process, he emphasizes the active role of host countries, exercised through political and cultural selectivity. His argument about modernization naturally resonates with the idea of multiple modernities. Modernization is an adaptive change, not necessarily a smooth transition from traditional to modern society, and often results in political conflict and moral disorder.

Easterlin raised questions about the economy-centered idea of development. He pointed out that since the end of World War II, per capita income in the United States has steadily increased, but the percentage of people who feel happy is only about 30%, and that the ratio has remained almost unchanged (Easterlin, 1974). Such a trend is called the Easterlin paradox. Of course, looking only at the relationship between economic growth at the national average of people's happiness can lead to "ecological fallacy", as income and happiness at the individual level are still very highly correlated. However, the paradox leads us to reconsider the conventional belief that growth-oriented national policies are legitimate if people's happiness does not increase with continued economic growth.

Among the East Asian countries, Japan, Korea, and Taiwan all experienced rapid economic growth. Japan's per capita income was $610 in 1962, but exceeded $20,000 in 1988. Korea's per capita income was only about $100 in the 1960s, but it has exceeded $20,000 since the mid-2000s, making it an advanced country. By 2023, GDP per capita in Japan, Korea, and Taiwan are higher than $30,000. According to several objective criteria, such as average income, life expectancy, literacy rates, and higher school enrollment rates, Japan, Korea, and Taiwan are advanced, and Japan and Korea are members of the OECD. However, "development" is still a hot topic in Korean politics, and the majority of Koreans feel that their country is not yet developed.

Looking at the comparison at the country level, we find a transitional zone in the relationship between economic growth and people's happiness. In countries below $10,000, there is a strong correlation between national income and happiness. But above $10,000, the correlation becomes weaker (Inglehart & Klingemann, 2000). A compelling interpretation was provided by Hirsch (1976). He distinguished between material and positional goods. A material good is a substance necessary to meet basic survival needs, such as food, shelter, and clothing. Positional goods are products and services whose value is largely (if not exclusively) a function of their ranking in desirability by others relative to substitutes. The extent to which the value of a good depends on such a ranking is called its positionality. Typical examples are high social status, exclusive real estate, a degree from a prestigious university, a reservation at the "hottest" new restaurant, and fame. Competition for material goods can be mitigated by increasing the supply of material goods. But because relative positioning is always important, competition for positional goods is always a zero-sum game, at least in the short run. Positional goods entail economic rents and quasi-rents.

Looking back, Koreans enjoyed the expansion of material goods during the high-growth period. The impact of economic growth was strong for those who suffered from hunger and poverty after the Korean War. The benefit of improved living standards was most appreciated by the least fortunate. All members of society enjoyed the rising tide and believed that tomorrow would be better than today. However, the marginal effect of economic growth has diminished, and competition for a limited number of positions, such as a good neighborhood, a decent job, and a diploma from a prestigious university, has gradually intensified. Looking back at the development process of Korean society over the past six decades, serious problems have arisen after the demand for these material goods has been satisfied and the path to the positional goods has become overcrowded. Let's take the example of higher education in Korea. Compared with 30 years ago, the college enrollment rate of high school graduates has increased from 25 to 85%. Such a drastic increase in the college enrollment rate is unprecedented. At the same time, competition for college admission has become more intense than ever. Moreover, as college graduates are mass-produced, competition for decent jobs has become even more intense. Therefore, the oversupply of college graduates without the expansion of good jobs led to serious youth unemployment. On the other hand, low-skilled workers are hard to find, so the constant shortage is filled by foreign workers. Housing is another example. Despite the nationwide housing penetration rate of 110%, it is extremely difficult for young people to buy their own homes in the Seoul metropolitan area.[1]

It is the paradox of prosperity: despite rapid economic growth and democratization, Koreans are not happy, they do not trust institutions, and social conflict has become more prevalent. One sociologist summarized that after four decades of rapid economic growth and democratization, the hungry society has become an angry society (Jeon, 2008). The symptoms of anger are expressed in various ways. Social anger deepens when people perceive their relative position to be poor. For example,

[1] Hirsch (1976) identifies two types of social scarcity: direct scarcity, which occurs when goods or services are unavailable, and contingent scarcity, which occurs when one person's satisfaction is affected by the number of others who benefit from the goods or services. Social congestion, like traffic congestion, indicates excessive competition for good jobs or admission to prestigious colleges. To prevent a rapid decline in society's quality, it is necessary to reduce competition. This can be achieved through various alternatives, such as increased screening. Only individuals with specific qualifications can enter the privileged zone, intensifying competition for certification. Another option to weaken competition is to impose congestion taxes on those approaching restricted status.

the proportion of low-wage workers in Korea is 25.7%, which is much higher than the OECD average of 16.3%, and the difference between regular and irregular workers is not limited to differences in working hours, but amounts to serious discrimination. The elderly poverty rate is 45.1%, much higher than the OECD average of 13.5%, and the suicide rate per 100,000 people is 31, almost three times the OECD average of 13.

2 Dimensions of Social Well-Being

Contrary to historical modernization, development is a generic and trans-historical process; therefore, it can and must be measured by core developmental values at both the personal and community levels. Personal well-being, which is conditioned by quality of life and life chances, reveals the level of self-fulfillment. Societal well-being, which is conditioned by cultural-moral flourishing, can be measured by structural flexibility and social quality (Table 1).

If the paradox of affluence is true and economic growth reduces people's happiness, it is important to consider what constitutes development. Kim (2002: 92–94) suggests that a good society can be measured by the "core value of development", which cannot be achieved through economic growth alone. It is worth noting that modernization and development have many differences. Modernization is a historical process that involves international acculturation and selective adaptation initiated by the modern Western transformation. On the other hand, development is a trans-historical process that values core developmental values and structural flexibility. It can be facilitated or hindered by modernization.

This book conceptualizes social well-being as a concept that includes both personal and societal well-being. To understand social well-being, it is important to discuss well-being competence. It is necessary to assume that an individual's well-being reflects their health capacity, which consists of multiple dimensions. Well-being can be understood as a multidimensional capacity. Wigglesworth (2014) distinguishes deep intelligence into four categories: physical, cognitive, emotional, and spiritual intelligence. According to Wigglesworth, these four intelligences must be balanced. These four intelligences correspond to body, mind, relationship, and

Table 1 Core development values as life values (Kim, 2002: 92–94)

Dimensions	Individual person		Societal collectivity	
Ultimate goal	Happy person		Happy community	
Consummate values	Self-fulfillment		Cultural-moral flourishing	
Instrumental values	Improved life quality	Expanded life chances	Increased structural flexibility	Enhanced social quality

inner value, respectively. The body needs physical intelligence (competence), and through this it becomes possible to manage the body in a healthy way. The mind needs cognitive ability, and the higher the cognitive ability, the higher the power of thought and analysis. In relation to others, emotional competence is needed, and through this, empathy and communication with others can be achieved. At the community level, it is important to possess a spiritual capacity that provides meaning and value to society (Table 2).

The social well-being can be reconstructed through a framework of the social world that integrates macroscopic, microscopic, objective, and subjective dimensions (Ritzer, 1975, 1981). The framework separates the objective from the constitutive (subjective) dimension and the relational/social/public dimension from the personal/private dimension. The four domains are formed at the intersection of these two axes. Each area corresponds to a domain of social well-being: the body (objective-individual), the mind (subjective-personal), relationships (objective-social), and inner values (subjective-social).

Physical well-being is closely related to the body. The ability to recognize and use your body is known as physical intelligence. Maslow proposed a hierarchy of human needs, with the most basic being satisfied through physical activities such as eating and sleeping, to fulfill higher-level existential needs. When there is no discomfort in physical activity, we can say that we are physically well.

The mind is closely linked to mental well-being. By means of education, one can enhance cognitive competence and understand high levels of cognitive complexity by improving analytical, reasoning, abstraction, language, imagination, and comprehension skills. Mental well-being is a concept that reflects the state of the mind, which can be either stable and positive or negative and unstable.

A healthy relationship (emotional heart) is linked to emotional well-being, including social sensitivity, empathy, and effective communication. It is important to assess whether an individual has appropriate relationships with others, engages in various social activities, and participates in mutual assistance activities to aid those in need. A healthy relationship is closely related to perceptions of fairness and transparency, social support networks, participation in organizations and meetings, donation activities, and volunteering.

Table 2 Dimensions of social well-being and capabilities

Dimension	Well-being	Intelligence: capacity
Body	Physical well-being	Physical intelligence: physical capacity
Mind	Mental well-being	Mental intelligence: analysis, thinking, abstraction, language, imagination, comprehension
Heart	Relational well-being	Emotional intelligence: social sensitivity, empathy and communication ability
Spirit	Societal well-being	Spiritual intelligence: meaning, the ultimate, group pride, value orientation

Inner value, also known as spiritual well-being, is related to one's sense of meaning, purpose, collective pride, and value orientation in life. It is distinct from religiosity, although it may be related to it. This concept encompasses aspects beyond faith or belief in a transcendent existence. For instance, it includes self-esteem and a sense of belonging to a community or nation. Strong social cohesion is achieved when individuals have a strong sense of belonging, a clear internal standard of success, a sense of purpose in life, and trust in one another. Social cohesion is the foundation of community perception and social trust.

It is useful to discuss Aron Antonovsky's concept of salutogenesis in medical sociology. Antonovsky argued that while medicine focuses on uncovering the pathogenesis of diseases caused by bacteria or viruses, sociology should focus on the origin of health. This creates a contrast between pathogenesis and salutogenesis. Salutogenesis is a combination of the Latin word for health, "salus", and the Greek word for origin, "genesis". Antonovsky developed this concept while studying how people cope with stress and maintain their health. Stress is a ubiquitous phenomenon, but not all individuals who experience it become unhealthy. Therefore, it is important to identify common factors among those who maintain good health despite exposure to stress. Antonovsky coined the term "generalized resistance" to describe the positive adaptation of women who survived the Jewish concentration camps under the Nazis by maintaining a positive emotional well-being and coping effectively with the stressful environment. In situations where individuals fail to cope with mild stress, they may suffer from a "general resource deficiency". The capacity to resist stress successfully appears to rely on an individual's sense of coherence or health capacity. Competence in perceiving, managing, controlling, and responding to the current situation comprises three components: meaning, control, and understanding. In stressful situations, it is important to understand the meaning of one's life, maintain control, and have faith in predictability. The ability to think and react positively in such situations can be considered a sense of coherence.

Antonovsky's theory of health (Antonovsky, 1979, 1987, 1993) emphasizes that health and illness are not categorically distinct phenomena, but rather lie on the same continuum. Extreme illness, possibly leading to death, is at the left end of the continuum, while the healthiest state is at the right end. Ordinary people fall somewhere in between. The group includes individuals who perceive themselves as healthy despite having minor illnesses, as well as those who perceive themselves as sick despite generally being healthy. By striving to improve their health along this axis, individuals can shift toward the right and enhance their overall well-being. Additionally, it is crucial to consider the significance of generalized resistance resources. In order for an individual to transition from a state of illness to one of health, they must possess certain resources that can help them withstand stress, such as physical health, mental acuity, social support, and inner orientation and spirituality. Additionally, they must have a sense of coherence, which involves understanding, managing, and controlling their resources, as well as having a clear motive and reason for doing so. Antonovsky uses the analogy of a river to explain human life, likening individuals to those who have fallen into a deep river. To survive in a fast-flowing river, one must swim to the bank using their own power. Those who wish to avoid drifting should have generalized resistance resources and a sense of coherence to exert control over the available resources.

Salutogenesis presents the balance and resistance model, which is supported by other studies. For instance, Headey and Wearing's stock and flow model suggests that individual personalities and life events influence well-being (Headey & Wearing, 1991). Basic stocks of well-being are formed by individual socio-economic status, personality, and social network. The well-being stock fluctuates temporarily due to positive or negative life events, such as an increase in income or unemployment, but it is restored by factors such as status, personality, and network. In other words, as life's concrete challenges are successfully met, the well-being stock increases over the long term (flow). Cummins (2010) emphasizes homeostasis. Homeostasis refers to a mechanism that restores internal balance, even when psychological balance is disturbed. Subjective well-being is a psychological construct that can be maintained even when experiencing temporary stress. It allows for the restoration of balance and the ability to maintain daily life with satisfaction, happiness, and psychological flourishing. When homeostasis is disrupted, a negative challenge can become overwhelming and lead to depression. Subjective well-being can be maintained when facing a manageable challenge. However, if a strong challenge exceeds the critical point, subjective well-being rapidly declines. In summary, stable well-being is determined by the balance between psychological, social, and physical challenges that threaten individuals and the psychological, social, and physical resources that individuals can mobilize in response (Dodge et al., 2012).

3 Cultural Value Orientations and Institutional Quality

Cultural values shape people's attitudes and organizational rules. The functioning of the social system has a fundamental impact on individual well-being. Religion is known to have a profound impact on spirituality and the formation of inner values. Empirical evidence suggests that Southeast Asian Buddhist countries have higher life satisfaction than East Asian Confucian countries, even when controlling for GDP per capita. Nordic countries with Lutheran churches exhibit higher levels of happiness than Mediterranean Catholic countries.

Asian countries have distinct cultural orientations that differ from those of Western societies. Cultural value orientations are Weberian ideal types, and different approaches may reveal various value dimensions. This chapter focuses on two dimensions of cultural orientation and one dimension of institutional quality.

The first dimension refers to the individual's position within their social group. Recent research in sociology, comparative philosophy, and cultural psychology has revealed significant differences between collectivist (or personalist) and individualist cultures in terms of the social norms that regulate people's thoughts and actions (Chang, 1991; Hall & Ames, 1987; Hofstede et al., 2010). In individualist cultures, independence, autonomy, and self-determination are highly valued, while personal affect, loyalty, and harmony are prioritized in personalist ethics (Chang, 1991). The individualist tradition has nurtured a radical concept of individual freedom, which has served as the foundation for democracy and the market economy. However, it has also been a source of violence, alienation, and isolation. In collectivist cultures, the notion of the human being as a relational being is central. The individual is not independent but rather interdependent, embedded in the family, community, nation, and universe (Saraceno, 2016).

Hofstede distinguishes between individualism and collectivism. Individualism refers to the degree to which people feel independent, as opposed to interdependent as members of a larger whole. This means that individual choices and decisions are expected. Collectivism, on the other hand, does not necessarily imply closeness, but rather that one's place in life is socially determined. Similarly, Schwartz focuses on the relationship or boundaries between the individual and the group. The author explores the extent to which individuals are autonomous versus embedded in their groups. The cultural dimension is labeled as autonomy versus embeddedness. In autonomy cultures, individuals are viewed as autonomous, bounded entities. They are encouraged to cultivate and express their own preferences, feelings, ideas, and abilities, and to find meaning in their own uniqueness.[2] In embedded cultures, individuals are viewed as entities that are integrated into the collective. The significance of life is primarily derived from social relationships, identifying with the group, participating in its shared way of life, and striving toward its common objectives. Embedded cultures prioritize maintaining the status quo and discourage actions that may disrupt group solidarity or the traditional order. Important values in collectivist cultures include social order, respect for tradition, safety, obedience, and wisdom. Chang referred to this as personalist ethics, which is similar to the contrast between the economist's vision of the egocentric agent and the sociologist's vision of the social being, for whom obligation and compliance are important. Schwartz (2006) explains that in an embedded culture, individuals prioritize their extended family or in-group, while in an autonomous culture, they prioritize the nuclear family or themselves. Hofstede's concept of collectivism emphasizes the importance of the social network, while individualism prioritizes the individual's identity. In collectivism, education focuses on group harmony, whereas in individualism, education emphasizes personal honesty. Communication also differs between these two environments. In collectivist cultures, individuals convey meaning contextually, whereas in individualistic cultures, they tend to be less dependent on context in their communication. In collectivist cultures, those who violate the rules may suffer shame and loss of face, but they are not considered guilty in the same sense as in individualistic cultures. These differences are reflected in different management styles. In collectivist societies, employers and employees are often viewed as a family, while in individualist societies, employment is seen as an impersonal contractual relationship.

[2] There are two types of autonomy: intellectual autonomy and affective autonomy. Intellectual autonomy encourages individuals to pursue their own ideas and intellectual directions independently, valuing broadmindedness, curiosity, and creativity. Affective autonomy, on the other hand, encourages individuals to pursue positive emotional experiences, valuing pleasure, excitement, and variety in life.

Hofstede's second dimension relates to power distance, which refers to the extent to which less powerful members of organizations and institutions, such as families, accept and expect unequal distribution of power. Schwartz introduces the concept of a hierarchical culture, where people behave responsibly to preserve the social fabric. Individuals must be encouraged to consider the welfare of others, coordinate with them, and manage their inevitable interdependencies. The hierarchical culture accepts an unequal distribution of power, roles, and resources as legitimate. Individuals are socialized to take the hierarchical distribution of roles for granted and to comply with the obligations and rules associated with their roles. In such cultures, where power distance is large, agents interact through more hierarchical forms of coordination, which typically distinguish principal from agent or leader from follower. In a hierarchical society, there is a significant power distance index, which implies an authoritarian relationship between those in power and those without. An example of hierarchical domination is a gerontocracy, where age is valued as an informal standard and exerts a powerful influence. Additionally, a well-developed system of honorifics in everyday language and the development of courtesy are other indications of a hierarchical society (Choi, 1976). Individuals in lower ranks may face challenges expressing their opinions. Hierarchy is often perceived as a reflection of one's inherent abilities.

The polar solution labeled cultural egalitarianism seeks to get people to recognize each other as moral equals who share basic interests as human beings. They are expected to act for the benefit of others as a matter of choice. Important values in such cultures include equality, social justice, responsibility, helping others, and honesty. In the egalitarian culture, where power distance is short, equally endowed agents interact on an equal basis. Horizontal coordination is most important in this type. Those who grow up in a culture that allows for a short power distance expect power relations to be more consultative or democratic (Hofstede et al., 2010).

Other dimensions may also exist. Hofstede introduces the dimension of masculinity to measure the extent to which the use of violence is socially endorsed.[3] Schwartz introduces the contrast between harmony and mastery.[4] We will not discuss these dimensions in detail since they are not the focus of this chapter.

In summary, the author identifies several bipolar dimensions of culture that offer alternative solutions to the problems faced by all societies. These dimensions include embeddedness versus autonomy, hierarchy versus egalitarianism, and domination versus harmony. Societal emphasis on one cultural type on a dimension is typically

---

[3] In a society that values masculinity, men are expected to exhibit toughness and prioritize winning. In contrast, a society that values femininity tends to promote emotional closeness between genders and may not place as much emphasis on competition. Additionally, there may be greater sympathy for those who are perceived as underdogs.

[4] The response to this issue, known as harmony, emphasizes fitting into the world as it is, seeking to understand and appreciate rather than change, direct, or exploit. Important values in harmony cultures include a peaceful world, unity with nature, and environmental protection. Mastery is the opposite cultural response to this issue. It encourages active self-assertion to master, direct, and change the natural and social environment to achieve group or personal goals. Values such as ambition, success, daring, and competence are considered important in mastery cultures.

accompanied by a de-emphasis on the polar type with which it tends to conflict. As we will see below, American, and Canadian cultures tend to prioritize mastery and effective autonomy over harmony, while Chinese, Korean, and Thai cultures prioritize hierarchy over egalitarianism and intellectual autonomy. Many Southeast Asian countries, such as Malaysia, Singapore, and Indonesia, lean toward embeddedness rather than autonomy.

Hofstede identifies alternative cultural templates by intersecting individualism and power distance. According to his research, most Asian countries, including Indonesia, the Philippines, Thailand, Korea, and Singapore, exhibit high power distance and low individualism. In contrast, most continental European countries exhibit low power distance and high individualism. Mediterranean countries, on the other hand, exhibit high power distance and high individualism.

Analytically, there are four distinct cultural templates when crossing individualism and hierarchical culture. However, there is a strong empirical correlation between the two axes. Therefore, we can identify two ideal types of cultural templates: the clan-type society and the individual-type society.

The clan-type system is commonly found in hierarchical cultures where individuals are deeply rooted in their family, primary group, and village, and have strong obligations to one another. This system is characterized by closely linked social lives through robust social networks. Numerous examples in Asia demonstrate the significance of social networks in the patterning, accumulation, role, and value of social capital, emphasizing the primacy of social context. Kinship networks are prominent throughout the life course in China. Guanxi continues to be an important factor in the labor market and academic success of Chinese individuals, despite the transition from socialism to capitalism (Table 3).

In Chinese neighborhoods, neighbors cooperate while social control from above reinforces social hierarchy (Chua & Wellman, 2015a). Chua and Wellman reviewed studies on social networks and social capital in East and Southeast Asia and identified similarities and differences in how each country's social context affects the nature of its social networks. Chua and Wellman (2015b) define a version of networked individualism specific to Asian culture, characterized by close kinship and friendship, hierarchies, a strong work ethic, frequent travel, and the use of digital media.

Based on large data samples from worldwide surveys, a growing body of research has found a positive correlation between social context and subjective assessments of well-being, happiness, and health. Social capital, measured by the strength of family, neighborhood, religious, and community ties, supports both physical health and subjective well-being. Helliwell and Putnam confirm that social capital is significantly related to subjective well-being through various independent channels and in different forms. Marriage and family, ties to friends and neighbors, workplace relationships, civic engagement (both individual and collective), trustworthiness, and trust all appear to be independently and robustly related to happiness and life satisfaction, both directly and through their impact on health (Helliwell and Putnam, 2004). Traditionally, strong social networks have been a source of social support and longevity. They have also acted as an informal source of risk insurance for the poor and vulnerable in the event of natural disasters. Research has shown that the level of

Table 3 Ideal-typical comparison of clan, transitional, and individualist societies

Dimension	Clan-based society	Transitional (developmental) society	Individualist society
Power distance	Unequal, hierarchical	Decentralized	Equal, egalitarian
Actor trait	Embedded and obligational	De-personified	Autonomous
Radius of trust	Small	Medium	Large
Symptom of corruption	Oligarchy and official moguls	Elite cartel	Influence market (lobby)
Publicness	Low	Medium	High
Important goods	Material goods	Positional goods	Public goods
Well-being	High	Low	High
Religion	Traditional religion	Declining	Civic religion
Utopia	Rule of the right, philosopher king	Dynamic equilibrium	Tocquevillian democracy
Dystopia	Patrimonial oligarchy	Disarticulated hierarchy	Hobbesian struggle
Welfare regime	Informal security	Productivist regime	Welfare state regime (liberal, conservative, social democratic)

generalized trust, as measured by the question 'are most people trustworthy,' varies significantly across countries. Specifically, it is narrower in Confucian countries and wider in wealthy Protestant countries (Delhey et al., 2001; Rothstein, 2014; Rothstein & Stolle, 2008). Societies with a clan-like tradition tend to be islands of trust. However, when combined with legitimate leadership, they can become efficient and powerful. In Confucian culture, Mencius idealizes this as the "ideal Confucian Rule", like Plato's concept of the "philosopher-king". The leader's authority is derived from their charisma, respectable personal traits, and abilities.

Religion has a significant impact on spiritual well-being. Countries in Southeast Asia with Buddhist or Muslim populations tend to have higher levels of satisfaction compared to East Asian countries with a long tradition of Confucianism.

The quality of institutions plays a crucial role in shaping social welfare. It is widely acknowledged that social capital has a significant impact on well-being at the societal level. Studies conducted on national and international samples indicate that measures of social capital, particularly specific and general trust, have a considerable influence on well-being beyond economic factors. The quality of government has a significant impact on well-being, as evidenced by the research conducted by Helliwell (2006). To expand the concept of social capital from the strength of social networks to the quality of public rules at the societal level, it is necessary to focus on transparency. Transparency of rules is closely related to trust in the impartiality of public authorities and government. Rules are transparent when a set of universal rules is both publicly documented and respected by social actors. Violators can then be punished, in principle and without exception. The opacity of rules implies that there is no universal set of rules that govern social relations. Instead, these rules are continuously negotiated.

Physical and mental well-being, when measured at the individual level, is closely related to relational and collective well-being, which is measured at the macro level (White, 2017). It is important to note that personal well-being expresses the health of an individual's body and mind, while social quality refers to the desirable structure and process in society. In essence, high social quality is embodied in the public sphere. Junichi Saito identifies three elements that make up publicness (Saito, 2009). It comprises official activities, enforcement, power, and duty that the state implements through law or policy, as well as norms, concerns, common interests, or property that are relevant to all people. Additionally, it includes openness of space or information that does not deny access to anyone. Publicness is the foundation of a healthy society. Political scientists have traditionally analyzed the effect of politics on subjective well-being at the collective level. Studies have found that more liberal countries report greater subjective well-being (Okulicz-Kozaryn et al., 2014). Keyes proposes five dimensions of social well-being: social integration, social contribution, social coherence, social actualization, and social acceptance. After analyzing the social-structural sources of social well-being dimensions, Keyes (1998) reported a correlation between global well-being, physical health, and optimism.

Modernization in clan culture is characterized by rapid economic growth and political democratization. This leads to a growing concern for publicity and transparency, as competition for material goods is replaced by competition for positional goods. To avoid growing grievances in the development system, there must be an adequate level of transparency and sense of justice to match the growing inequalities. In the clan culture, informal security provided by family, village, and social networks manages old and new social risks. Family support remains the primary source of social protection due to the continued strength of family ties. However, rapid modernization brings new challenges.

4 The Rise of the Network Society and the Future of Social Welfare in Asia

Recent surveys of subjective well-being (SWB) in seven Asian countries reveal a stark contrast between Southeast Asian (SEA) and Northeast Asian (NEA) countries. SEA countries, such as Thailand, Vietnam, Indonesia, and the Philippines, are less developed and have a stronger clan-based system, while NEA countries, including Japan, Korea, and Taiwan, have a more transitional or developmental system. SEA countries exhibit higher levels of well-being at the personal, relational, and societal levels compared to NEA countries. Notably, despite lower levels of transparency, SEA countries report higher levels of societal well-being. It is worth mentioning that

SEA countries have a narrower radius of trust, but they still exhibit higher levels of happiness and more positive views on the progress of their society.

The results presented are based solely on the respondents' perceived well-being. This poses an interesting paradox for development, as NEA countries, despite decades of rapid development and democratization, exhibit lower levels of social well-being and happiness compared to SEA countries. The explanation for this phenomenon lies in the widening gap between modernization and the decline of traditional institutions that have historically served as a source of support and cohesion for people. Rapid modernization has improved the quality of life and expanded people's life chances. It has also transformed the social structure and fabric of social organization. The cultural heritage of NEA countries was closer to that of the clan system, combining personalistic ethics and large power distances. Rapid modernization in the NEA has brought about fundamental changes in three cultural dimensions.

The first dimension, which follows the direction of power distance, involves decentralization by distributing political power to the local level and reducing the power gap between the powerful and the powerless. NEA countries have slowly moved in this direction after democratization, but economic inequality has increased. The second dimension requires changes in the characteristics of actors. The NEA culture is still strongly embedded and obligatory. However, there is a trend toward individual culture. Institutional trust, measured as transparency, appears to be the most critical factor. Korea, Japan, Taiwan, Singapore, and Hong Kong share many similarities, particularly in terms of embeddedness and power distance. However, these city-states have transformed their societies by increasing transparency to the highest degree, resulting in high levels of competitiveness in the global market.

It is believed that NEA countries are in a transitional zone where the previous moral ethos, such as respect for a charismatic leader, has disappeared due to democratization. However, without a significant increase in transparency, these countries suffer from a lack of societal moral resources. The main component of such institutional capital comes from the accumulation of repeated execution of rational and legal authority based on fairness. However, despite the lack of transparency, relational social capital, such as *guanxi* and *yongo*, still plays a crucial role in resource allocation.

In Korea, a focused group interview identified critical factors as a fundamental cause of low social well-being (Cho et al., 2018). The first factor is gender role stereotyping, which has been strongly influenced by traditional culture. The disintegration of the traditional family has left serious problems for young women in particular. The labor market is seeing an increase in female participation. However, the public sector provides little care, making it challenging for women to balance work and family responsibilities. Another issue is relative deprivation, which is a serious concern. Korea has the highest penetration of the Internet and smartphones, and well-developed social media serves as a reference for conspicuous consumption. Koreans have transitioned from a clan-based society, but the existence of a dominant standard for consumption has significant implications for competition for positional goods, including education, employment, housing, and leisure activities. Another issue is the perception of unfairness that prevails in all areas, such as politics, the economy, the media, and the education system. The lack of fairness can cause frustration and anger. People are questioning the rules of the game, which can harm social well-being. A study on social well-being in Korea reveals that physical health is interconnected with mental, relational, and societal health. Excessive stress can lead to physical symptoms and disease. The experience of man-made disasters can cause depression, anxiety, and mental devastation. Disappointment with the government, a feeling of moral vacuum, and helplessness can contribute to low social well-being.

According to Wellman (2001), the advent of the Internet and the smartphone is causing a fundamental shift in cultural values, transforming traditional group-based societies into networked societies. High internet penetration rates have been observed in North America, Europe, and parts of the Asia–Pacific region. Access to the internet is considered vital. In 2016, the United Nations passed a non-binding resolution stating that disruption of internet access is a human rights violation. Governments and private companies are working to expand internet access globally, but many people in emerging markets and developing countries remain unconnected. According to the Pew Research Center, 75% of people in 39 countries either use the internet occasionally or own a smartphone. In advanced economies, over 90% of the population uses the Internet. South Korea leads with a 96% usage rate. Countries with higher gross domestic product per capita (purchasing power parity) tend to have higher rates of internet use, while poorer countries tend to have lower rates (Pew Research Center, 2018).

The study of social well-being faces a challenge in the networked society. People have altered their way of interacting with each other by incorporating the Internet and mobile phones into their lives. They are now more networked as individuals rather than being embedded in groups. In this world of networked individuals, the person has become more central than the family, work unit, neighborhood, and social group (Rainie & Wellman, 2012). Networked individualism is a shift away from classical social arrangements based on hierarchical bureaucracies or tightly knit social groups, such as households and work groups. Instead, networked individuals use the tools provided by the development of information and communication technology to seek different things as members of different groups. The networks that form these groups may be dispersed globally, resulting in a highly individualized and well-connected person.

References

Antonovsky, A. (1979). *Health, stress, and coping*. Jossey-Bass.

Antonovsky, A. (1987). *Unravelling the mystery of health: How people manage stress and stay well*. Jossey-Bass.

Antonovsky, A. (1993). *Some salutogenic word of wisdom to the conferees*. The Nordic School of Public Health.

Chang, Y. (1991). The personal ethic and the market in Korea. *Comparative Studies in Society and History, 33*, 106–129.

Cho, B.-H., Yee, J., Koo, H., You, M. S., & Park, S. (2018). *Beyond suffering Korea: Integration of the value and practice of social well-being*. 21 Century Books (in Korean).
Choi, J. (1976). *Hangukineui sahoejok seongkyeok (Social character of Koreans)*. Kaemunsa (in Korean).
Chua, V., & Wellman, B. (2015a). Social networks in East and Southeast Asia I: National characteristics, institutions, network capital, and Guanxi. *American Behavioral Scientist, 59*(8), 903–913.
Chua, V., & Wellman, B. (2015b). Social networks in East and Southeast Asia I: Labor migration, opportunity, social media, and well-being. *American Behavioral Scientist, 59*(9), 1055–1065.
Cummins, R. (2010). Subjective wellbeing, homeostatically protected mood and depression: A synthesis. *Journal of Happiness Studies, 11*, 1–17.
Delhey, J., Böhnke, P., & Zapf, W. (2001). The Euromodule: A new instrument for comparative welfare research. WZB Working Paper, No FS III 01-401.
Dodge, R., Daly, A. P., Huyton, J., & Sanders, L. D. (2012). The challenge of defining wellbeing. *International Journal of Wellbeing, 2*(3).
Easterlin. (1974). Does economic growth improve the human lot? In P. David & M. W. Reder (Eds.), *Nations and households in economic growth: Essays in honor of Moses Abramovitz*. Academic Press.
Hall, D. L., & Ames, R. T. (1987). *Thinking through Confucius*. State University of New York Press.
Headey, B., & Wearing, A. (1991). Subjective well-being: A stocks and flows framework. In F. E. Strack, M. E. Argyle, & N. E. Schwarz (Eds.), *Subjective well-being: An interdisciplinary perspective* (pp. 49–73). Pergamon Press.
Helliwell, J. F. (2006). Well-being, social capital and public policy: What's new? *The Economic Journal, 116*, C34–C44.
Helliwell, J. F., & Putnam, R. D. (2004). The social context of well-being. *Philosophical Transactions: Biological Sciences, 359*(1449). *The science of well-being: Integrating neurobiology, psychology and social science*, September 29, 2004 (pp. 1435–1446).
Hirsch, F. (1976). *Social limits to growth*. Harvard University Press.
Hofstede, G., Hofstede, G. J., & Minkov, M. (2010). *Cultures and organizations: Software of the mind* (3rd ed.). McGraw-Hill.
Inglehart, R., & Klingemann, H.-D. (2000). Genes, culture, democracy and happiness. In E. Diener & E. M. Suh (Eds.), *Subjective well-being across cultures*. MIT Press.
Inkeles, A., & Smith, D. H. (1974). *Becoming modern: Individual change in six developing countries*. Harvard University Press.
Jeon, S.-I. (2008). Social conflict and integration in the angry society. *Philosophy and Reality, 76* (in Korean).
Kemppainen, T. (2012). Well-being in socio-political context: European welfare regimes in comparison. In *Studies in social security and health 123* (93 pp.). The Social Insurance Institution of Finland.
Keyes, C. L. M. (1998). Social well-being. *Social Psychology Quarterly, 61*(2), 121–140.
Kim, K.-D. (2002). *Theory of social development in Korea*. Jipmundang (in Korean).
Kim, K.-D. (2017). *Alternative discourses on modernization and development: East Asian perspectives*. Palgrave Macmillan.
North, D. (1990). *Institutions, institutional change and economic performance*. Cambridge University Press.
Okulicz-Kozaryn, A., Oscar Holmes, I. V., & Avery, D. R. (2014). The subjective well-being political paradox: Happy welfare states and unhappy liberals. *Journal of Applied Psychology, 99*(6), 1300–1308.
Pew Research Center (Poushter, J., Bishop, C., & Chwe, H.). (2018). *Social media use continues to rise in developing countries but plateaus across developed ones: Digital divides remain, both within and across countries*. Pew Research Center.
Rainie, L., & Wellman, B. (2012). *Networked: The new social operating system*. MIT Press.
Ritzer, G. (1975). Sociology: A multiple paradigm science. *The American Sociologist*, 156–167.

Ritzer, G. (1981). *Toward an integrated sociological paradigm: The search for an exemplar and an image of the subject matter*. Longman.

Rothstein, B. (2014). *Human well-being and the lost relevance of political science*. European University Institute.

Rothstein, B., & Stolle, D. (2008). The state and social capital: An institutional theory of generalized trust. *Comparative Politics, 40*, 441–459.

Saito, J. (2009). *Democratic publicness* (translated from Japanese to Korean). EUM.

Saraceno, C. (2016). Varieties of familialism: Comparing four southern European and East Asian welfare regimes. *Journal of European Social Policy, 26*(4), 314–326.

Schwartz, S. H. (2006). A theory of cultural value orientations: Explication and applications. *Comparative Sociology, 5*(2–3).

Wallerstein, I. (1974) *Modern World-System I: Capitalist Agriculture and the Origins of European World-Economy in the 16th Century* (Studies in Social Discontinuity), New York: Academic Press.

Wellman, B. (2001). The rise of networked individualism. In L. Keeble (Ed.), *Community networks online*. Taylor & Francis.

White, S. C. (2017). Relational wellbeing: Re-centring the politics of happiness, policy and the self. *Policy & Politics, 45*(2), 121–136.

Wigglesworth, C. (2014). *Deep intelligence: The critical intelligences for leadership success in the 21st century*.

Jaeyeol Yee is a professor of sociology at Seoul National University and an international project member of the Center for Social Well-being Studies, Institute for the Development of Social Intelligence, Senshu University. He has contributed to the harmonization of social well-being surveys in Asia as director of the Korea Social Science Data Archives. His research interests include social quality, social well-being, social capital, disaster and safety issues, and sociological theory construction.

Social Well-Being in Asian Contexts

Hiroo Harada and Masayuki Kanai

Abstract This chapter delves into the concept of social well-being in Asia by examining it from historical, theoretical, and empirical perspectives. It traces the evolution of well-being from Aristotle's notion of "eudaimonia" to the present, emphasizing the necessity of adopting a comprehensive approach to human flourishing that extends beyond mere economic growth. The authors critique the reliance on GDP as the sole indicator of progress, drawing attention to arguments made by economists such as Pigou, who advocate for welfare economics as a means of assessing societal conditions. This chapter also discusses the impact of European colonization and modern global economic shifts on Asia's social fabric, noting the region's unique community-centric values influenced by the climate and natural features of tropical and subtropical monsoons. Additionally, this chapter introduces the work of the International Consortium for Social Well-Being Studies, which conducted the Social Well-Being Survey in Asia (SoWSA) across seven societies. The SoWSA findings challenge the correlation between economic prosperity and subjective well-being and reveal disparities between East and Southeast Asian societies. This research emphasizes the complexity of social well-being and advocates a multidimensional approach that incorporates cultural, social, and economic factors.

Keywords Eudaimonia · Economic growth versus happiness · Asia's economic and cultural contexts · International Consortium for Social Well-Being Studies · Social Well-Being Survey in Asia (SoWSA)

H. Harada · M. Kanai (✉)
School of Human Sciences, Senshu University, Kawasaki, Japan
e-mail: mkanai@senshu-u.jp

H. Harada
e-mail: h2@isc.senshu-u.ac.jp

H. Harada
Senshu University, Kawasaki, Japan

J. Yee et al. (eds.), *Social Well-Being, Development, and Multiple Modernities in Asia*,
https://doi.org/10.1007/978-981-97-3866-3_2

1 Social Well-Being in Asia in the Historical and Theoretical Contexts

1.1 Social Well-Being from a Historical Perspective

The philosopher Aristotle (1911) posited in 350 B.C. that "flourishing" (*eudaimonia*), which encompasses truth, goodness, and beauty, was most effectively attained through the exercise of reason. To sustainably improve the well-being of human beings, it is essential to focus on enhancing *eudaimonia* rather than merely seeking short-term happiness. In a society like ancient Athens, where democracy flourished, humans can thrive as social animals (*zoon politikon*).

The modern era, beginning with the Age of Discovery from the mid-fifteenth to mid-seventeenth centuries, the Industrial Revolution from the mid-eighteenth century to the nineteenth century, and the Napoleonic Wars in the early nineteenth century, led to the establishment of the nation-state system and economic prosperity in Europe. Since the latter part of the nineteenth century, social movements aimed at improving labor conditions have emerged in Europe as policy requests and gained social recognition. These movements gave rise to political parties advocating for socialism or labor unions, which were previously banned due to their opposition to the ruling regime. As a consequence, specific social policies, such as health and unemployment insurance, as well as the pension system, were introduced during this time period.

In the early twentieth century, two global conflicts—World War I and World War II—engulfed the world. These wars resulted in the widespread adoption of highly destructive weapons, causing extraordinary damage even in the victorious countries as well as the defeated ones. The political demands of the people led to the establishment of universal suffrage and increased social spending on medical services and facilities for the disabled. In contrast to World War I, which was confined to Europe, World War II saw battlefields expanding to include regions in Asia, the Middle East, and Africa.

Since the mid-twentieth century, the policies of most countries have been focused on economic growth under the Cold War Regime. According to Keynes (1936), economics has gained scientific grounds for analyzing macroeconomy and establishing theoretical foundations for making policies. The Gross Domestic Product (GDP), which aggregates the value added in a year within a country, has emerged as a crucial metric in macroeconomic analysis.[1] Under democratic pressure, social policies for people's needs have been adopted so that the average rate of social security expenditure to GDP in the world has dramatically increased.

[1] In economics, various scholars have engaged in a critique of GDP due to its ambiguity in accounting for household work, investment, and consumption of durable goods (e.g., Coyle, 2014; Drewnowski, 1974; Mishan, 1967; Nordhaus & Tobin, 1972).

The twenty-first century, however, has been characterized by a global state of VUCA (Volatility, Uncertainty, Complexity, and Ambiguity) due to several significant events such as the fall of the Berlin Wall in 1989, the financial crisis of 2007–08, the persistent issue of climate change, the turbulent COVID-19 pandemic of 2020–22, and the recent conflicts in Ukraine and Gaza since 2022. In light of these circumstances, it is crucial to develop alternative indices beyond GDP to effectively assess and maintain social well-being.

1.2 Social Well-Being from a Theoretical Perspective

Pigou (1920), who succeeded Marshall (1890) as the highest-ranking economist at Cambridge University, published a systematic book on welfare economics. Pigou's work laid the foundation for a rigorous and scientific analysis of social conditions by adopting the concept of welfare for value-neutral analysis. Since the mid-twentieth century, GDP has been widely used as a measure of economic and social progress, and most governments have made its growth a policy priority. However, it is uncertain whether GDP or economic prosperity is positively and closely related to individual well-being, which includes happiness and satisfaction (Karabell, 2014; Skidelsky & Skidelsky, 2012).

Hence, it is essential for the humanities and social sciences to elucidate the relationship between the mental and physical aspects of human beings, with the ancillary aim of eradicating obstacles that hinder advancement. These subjects, including psychology, sociology, economics, and political science, were prominent in the late twentieth century. In the twenty-first century, it is necessary to pursue innovation in the social sciences and use the concept of social well-being instead of GDP to address complex phenomena (Fleurbaey, 2009; Kahneman & Kruger, 2006).

Although the concept of well-being is subjective in nature, social factors have significantly influenced its formation. At the micro-level, family and relatives play a role in an individual's well-being, while at the meso-level, communities, friends, and jobs have an impact. At the macro-level, policies of municipal and central governments are relevant, and at the super macro-level, international and/or global institutions matter (Easterlin, 1974, 2021; Frey, 2008; Frey & Stutzer, 2002; Scitovsky, 1976). The interrelationships between these levels have been studied by various social sciences, such as economics and political science, since the twentieth century. However, in pursuit of scientific rigor and usefulness, these disciplines have tended to detach these interrelationships, resulting in extreme simplification. In contrast, the viewpoint of social well-being recognizes the overlapping situations between micro-, meso-, macro-, and super-level societies. Since the mid-twentieth century, it has been acknowledged that the natural environment of the globe has formed the foundation of human society, geographically and from generation to generation. Human beings have survived with the availabilities and constraints of their environment and can continue to do so in the future (Stiglitz et al., 2010).

1.3 Social Well-Being in the Asian Context

The history of the world has been significantly impacted by the extensive expansion and colonization carried out by European powers in Asia, Africa, the Middle East, and Latin America from the seventeenth to the mid-twentieth century (Helliwell et al., 2012; OECD, 2011). In Asia, social relationships at the community level have traditionally held importance due to the climate and natural features of tropical and subtropical monsoons. In contrast, Europe has historically seen global development driven by societal, institutional, and individual conduct (Myrdal, 1968). Japan, particularly in the late nineteenth century, was influenced by the West in terms of political economy, adopting democracy, and a market economy. However, Japan has maintained a distinct social perspective and approach within the broader Asian context.

During the latter half of the twentieth century, global economic development and significant advancements in transportation and information communication systems were prevalent throughout the world. Asia has risen to prominence in the world economy by surmounting international and ideological disagreements and incorporating itself into the global supply chain. In the twenty-first century, Asia has also become a key component of the global consumption chain. The economic rise of Asia can be attributed to the social values at the meso-level, which have been given greater importance (Deaton, 2013; Mahbubani, 2008; Pomeranz, 2000; Shambaugh, 2013). It is believed that animism and Confucianism, coexisting with religions, are deeply ingrained in the thinking of Asians and that bridging social capital (Putnam, 2000) has been strengthened through modernization and urbanization since the mid-twentieth century.

2 The International Consortium for Social Well-Being Studies

The influence of economic prosperity on individual happiness is substantial. In particular, how has economic growth positively impacted social well-being? Furthermore, how have the effects of economic growth at both macro- and super macro-levels affected the values of people in Asia, where the values at the meso-level, such as communities, have been emphasized?

To tackle these challenges, we commenced two research endeavors at the Institute for the Development of Social Intelligence at Senshu University: "Exploring Social Capital toward Sustainable Development in East Asia" (2009–2013) and "Forming a Social Well-being Research Consortium in Asia" (2014–2018). Both projects were overseen by Hiroo Harada and were financially supported by the MEXT-Supported Programs for the Strategic Research Foundation at Private Universities in Japan (Harada, 2016a, 2016b, 2019).

Table 1 Principal institutes of the International Consortium for Social Well-Being Studies

Country	Principal institute
Indonesia	Universitas Indonesia
Japan	Senshu University, Research Organization of Information and Systems
Korea	Seoul National University
Mongolia	Independent Research Institute of Mongolia
The Philippines	Ateneo de Manila University
Thailand	Chulalongkorn University
Taiwan	Academia Sinica
Vietnam	Vietnam Academy of Social Sciences

In the 2009–2013 project, which examined social capital, we underscored the importance of meso-level contexts in molding individuals' behaviors and thought processes in social settings. In contrast, the 2014–2018 project, which focused on social well-being, concentrated on formulating policies to enhance social conditions. We collaborated with eminent professors and researchers from esteemed universities and institutions across East and Southeast Asia, including Indonesia, Japan, Korea, Mongolia, the Philippines, Thailand, Taiwan, and Vietnam. These experts endorsed our methodology and objectives, leading to the establishment of the International Consortium for Social Well-Being Studies in 2014 (Table 1).

Since its inception, the Consortium has undertaken numerous research initiatives. In order to promote the dissemination of research findings, it has organized international conferences on an annual basis (Table 2). Additionally, the Consortium has published its yearly journal, *Social Well-Being Review*, commencing in 2015.[2]

3 Social Well-Being Survey in Asia (SoWSA)

The primary research endeavor undertaken by the Consortium was the "Social Well-Being Survey in Asia, 2015–2017 (SoWSA)," which was carried out in seven East and Southeast Asian societies (International Consortium for Social Well-Being Studies, 2020). While the 2009–2013 project on social capital had conducted several questionnaire surveys in Japan, Vietnam, Cambodia, and Laos, it had limitations, including small sample sizes, restricted geographic coverage, and immature questionnaire development. The SoWSA was established to address these shortcomings and to conduct a more well-organized comparative survey.

[2] The journal previously had the title of *The Senshu Social Well-Being Review* until its publication reached number eight in 2021. It is an open-access publication and can be accessed at https://senshu-u.repo.nii.ac.jp/search?search_type=2&q=919. Prior to this, the 2009–2013 project disseminated its yearly findings through a journal entitled *The Senshu Social Capital Review* (https://senshu-u.repo.nii.ac.jp/search?search_type=2&q=963).

Table 2 International conferences of the Consortium

No.	Year	Title	Venue
1	2016	Social well-being and sustainable development goals in Asia	Bangkok, Thailand
2	2017	Social well-being in the context of regional integration: searching for a joint ASEAN model	Hanoi, Vietnam
3	2018	Social well-being, social policy, and social transformation	Magelang, Indonesia
4	2018	Social well-being in the Asian context: from a comparative perspective	Seoul, Korea
5	2018	Balancing the outcomes of globalization: roles of social well-being	Tokyo, Japan
6	2019	Comparative well-being in East and Southeast Asian societies	Taipei, Taiwan
7	2023	Resilience and well-being in East and Southeast Asia	Tokyo, Japan
8	2024	Social well-being and resilience in developing societies of Asia	Tokyo, Japan

3.1 Sample Designs and Survey Modes

An overview of the survey, including sample design and implementation methods in each society, is given in Table 3. The survey mode was a web-based survey in East Asian societies (Japan, Korea, and Taiwan) and a face-to-face interview in Southeast Asian countries (Indonesia, the Philippines, Thailand, and Vietnam). The inconsistency in the survey mode was attributable to the annual budget limitations, while simultaneously considering the research expenses, socioeconomic conditions, and conventional practices in academic social research for each respective society. The sampling method employed was quota sampling, with slight variations in the two-stage or single-stage design and proportional or disproportionate representation (KOSSDA, 2020). The target population comprised males and females aged 20–69 across all societies.[3] The target area extended nationwide in all societies except Indonesia, where financial constraints hindered the conduct of a nationwide survey. The final sample size amounted to approximately 12,000 cases in Japan, where a substantial budget was allocated for a pilot survey; approximately 2000 and 2300 cases in Korea and Taiwan, respectively, where a web-based survey was implemented; and approximately 1000–1200 cases in the four Southeast Asian societies, where face-to-face interviews were conducted.

[3] The original datasets from some Southeast Asian societies included individuals outside of the 20–69 age range, due to the conventional methods of sampling and interviewing employed in each society. In the publication of the dataset as SoWSA v2.0 for general use, these individuals were removed for the purpose of comparison. Further information regarding the initial samples can be found in KOSSDA (2020).

Table 3 Sample designs and survey modes of SoWSA

Society	Timing	Area	Sampling	Mode	Sample size
Japan	February 2015	Nationwide	Proportionate quota sampling by sex, age, population of municipality, and region	Web survey	11,786
Korea	July 2015	Nationwide	Proportionate quota sampling by sex, age, and region	Web survey, partly telephone survey	2,000
Taiwan	July 2017	Nationwide (excluding off-shore islands)	Proportionate quota sampling by sex, age, population of municipality, and region	Web survey	2,303
Indonesia	July–August 2017	The islands of Java (6 provinces) and Bali (1 province), urban and sub urban areas only	Two-stage quota sampling and purposive sampling with snowball method for recruiting the non-Moslem	Face-to-face interview	1,248
The Philippines	June–December 2016	Nationwide	Two-stage quota sampling	Face-to-face interview	1,065
Thailand	October–December 2016	Nationwide	Proportionate quota sampling stratified by sex, population of municipality, and region	Face-to-face interview	995
Vietnam	July–December 2015	Nationwide	Two-stage quota sampling	Face-to-face interview	1,094

Source Assembled by the authors based on information from Appendix Table I and the main text in KOSSDA (2020)

3.2 *Questionnaire Development*

The survey instrument combines a standard module that asks the same questions in all societies and society-specific modules that are added independently at the discretion of the research team in each society. The standard module comprises four major groups of questions: (1) social well-being, (2) social capital, (3) risk and social safety net, and (4) face items.

The first group, "social well-being," corresponds to the dependent variables when analyzing the determinants of social well-being. To assess subjective well-being, we incorporated three instruments that have been employed in prior surveys: subjective happiness ("How happy are you currently?"), overall life satisfaction ("How satisfied are you currently with current life overall?"), and the Cantril ladder question[4] (Cantril, 1965; Helliwell et al., 2015) on an 11-point scale ranging from 0 to 10. No existing cross-national surveys covering East and Southeast Asian societies, such as the World Values Survey (e.g., Inglehart et al., 2018), the International Social Survey Program (e.g., ISSP Research Group, 2015), and the East Asian Social Survey (e.g., Li et al., 2021), asked these three questions simultaneously on the same scale. This represents a significant contribution of the SoWSA. In addition, the survey evaluated perceived inequality and discrimination, awareness of disparities, and other factors that indicate societal evaluation.

The second group of questions assesses "social capital," which represents the meso-level elements of social well-being. These questions were primarily sourced from our earlier surveys, which were conducted as part of the 2009–2013 social capital initiative. They encompass various aspects of trust, such as trust in family, relatives, neighbors, friends, and "most people," which is also referred to as generalized trust. Furthermore, the inquiries aimed to gather information on the degree of engagement with relatives, friends, and neighbors, as well as participation in community and organizational activities, including festivals.

The third cluster of questions pertains to the topic of "risk and social safety net" and encompasses meso- and macro-level factors that contribute to social well-being. Several of these questions were derived from previous surveys on social capital. These questions focused on individuals' experiences with a range of personal and collective risks, such as unemployment, poverty, natural disasters, and war. Additionally, they assess institutional trust in various organizations.

The final set of survey questions related to the respondents' demographic characteristics, socioeconomic status, and lifestyle. This includes inquiries about how they allocate their time. These questions reflect the micro-level determinants that contribute to social well-being.

3.3 Basic Observations

This section presents an overview of key descriptive statistics from the SoWSA dataset. In subsequent chapters, particularly Part III, readers can expect to find more comprehensive analyses and results from bivariate and multivariate statistical techniques.

[4] "Please imagine a ladder with steps numbered from 0 at the bottom to 10 at the top. Suppose we say that the top of the ladder represents the best possible life for you and the bottom of the ladder represents the worst possible life for you. On which step of the ladder would you say you personally feel you stand at this time, assuming that the higher the step the better you feel about your life, and the lower the step the worse you feel about it? Which step comes closest to the way you feel?"

In terms of subjective well-being, we will present descriptive statistics for two measures: subjective happiness and the Cantril ladder. The former represents an affective aspect of subjective well-being, while the latter reflects a cognitive and reflective aspect. As previously mentioned, both measures utilize an 11-point scale spanning from 0 (unhappy, the worst life possible) to 10 (happy, the best life possible). The data depicted in Figs. 1 and 2 indicate the mean and standard deviation of the two measures across the seven societies. The results reveal a significant disparity between the East and Southeast Asian societies. The East Asian societies showcase a low mean and high standard deviation for subjective well-being, while the Southeast Asian societies exhibit a reverse trend with a high mean and low standard deviation. Assuming a positive correlation exists between economic prosperity and subjective well-being, the finding that people in affluent East Asia are less happy and have more unequal happiness levels than those living in less developed Southeast Asian societies is counterintuitive. As discussed in the previous Chapter "Development, Culture, and Diverse Mechanisms of Social Well-Being in Asia," this apparent paradox serves as the starting point for the intellectual exploration presented in this book. The first chapter in Part III begins this exploration using multivariate analysis.

It is important to exercise caution when comparing univariate statistics, such as the mean and standard deviation, between societies with disparate cultural and psychological tendencies. Figures 3 and 4 offer a detailed look at the frequency distributions of these measures in seven different societies. Upon examination, it becomes clear that each society exhibits a unique pattern in the distribution of the data. For instance, the data from the Philippines suggest a preference for the middle point of the 11-point scale, which is option "5." To eliminate the influence of such cultural biases, it is recommended to compare the correlation structures of multiple variables across societies. This research approach is further discussed in the final chapter of this book.

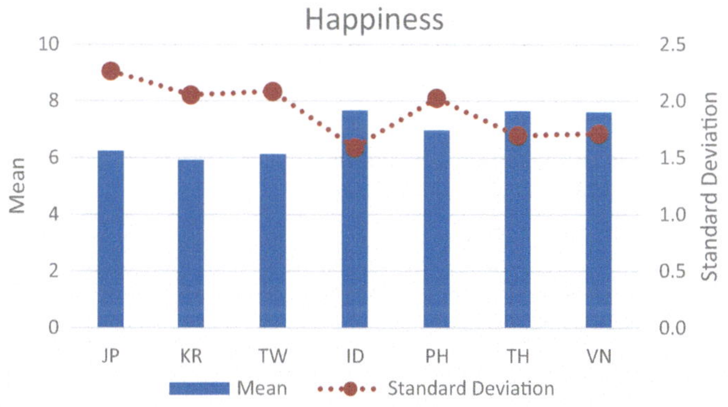

Fig. 1 Means and standard deviations of subjective happiness. Assembled by the authors based on SoWSA v2.0 (International Consortium for Social Well-Being Studies, 2020)

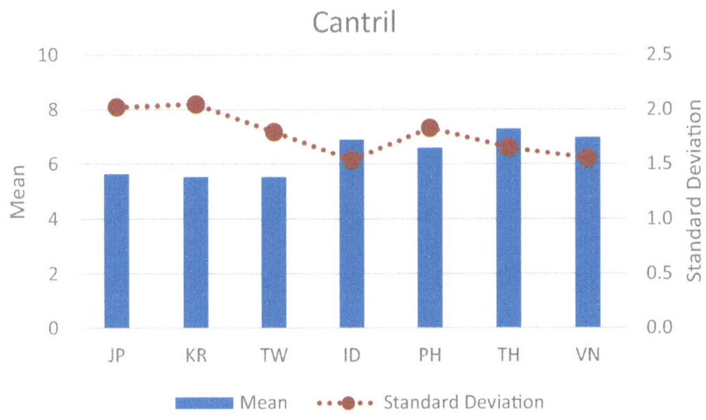

Fig. 2 Means and standard deviations of the Cantril ladder. Assembled by the authors based on SoWSA v2.0 (International Consortium for Social Well-Being Studies, 2020)

Undertaking a cross-national comparative analysis requires accounting for the demographic and socioeconomic structures of each society. Table 4 provides essential statistics, including the distributions of age, marital status, employment status, and education. A comparison of East and Southeast Asian societies reveals distinct contrasts. In East Asian societies, individuals are older, less likely to be married, more likely to be employed, and more likely to have received an education compared to Southeast Asian societies. These dissimilarities in the social context impact the interplay between the various elements and factors of social well-being at the micro-, meso-, and macro-levels.

Lastly, we extend our sincere gratitude to all the colleagues who were involved in the entire process of the SoWSA survey across the seven societies, including the development and localization of the questionnaire, the design of the sampling, the fieldwork, and the data cleaning. We also acknowledge the significant efforts of the colleagues from the Korea Social Science Data Archive (KOSSDA) and the Center for Social Data Structuring at the Joint Support-Center for Data Science Research at the Research Organization of Information and System, who played a crucial role in the harmonization of the data for its publication at KOSSDA. The details of this process are elaborated in the subsequent chapter.

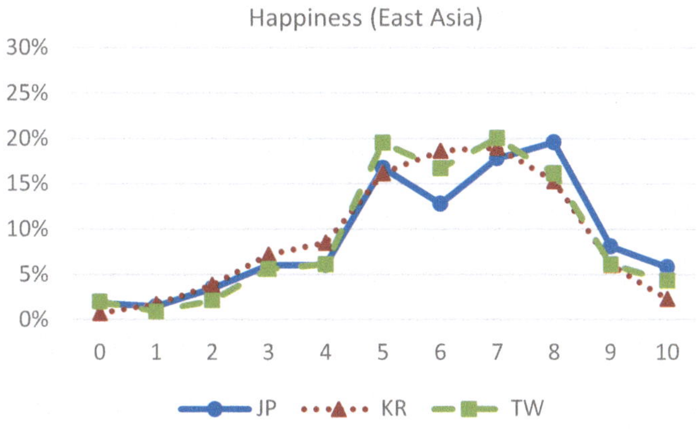

Panel A

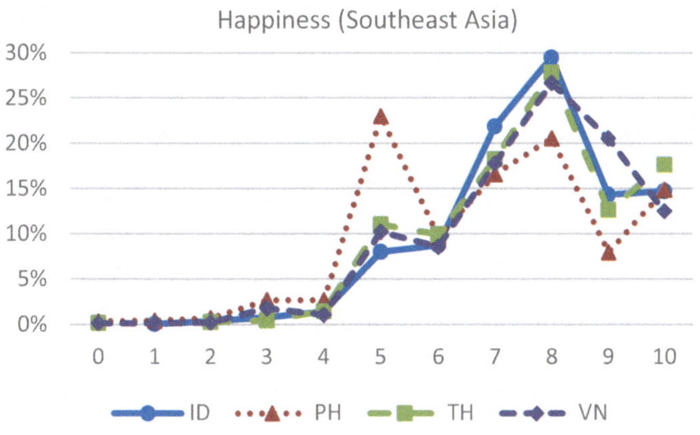

Panel B

Fig. 3 Distribution of subjective happiness in East Asia (Panel A) and Southeast Asia (Panel B). Assembled by the authors based on SoWSA v2.0 (International Consortium for Social Well-Being Studies, 2020)

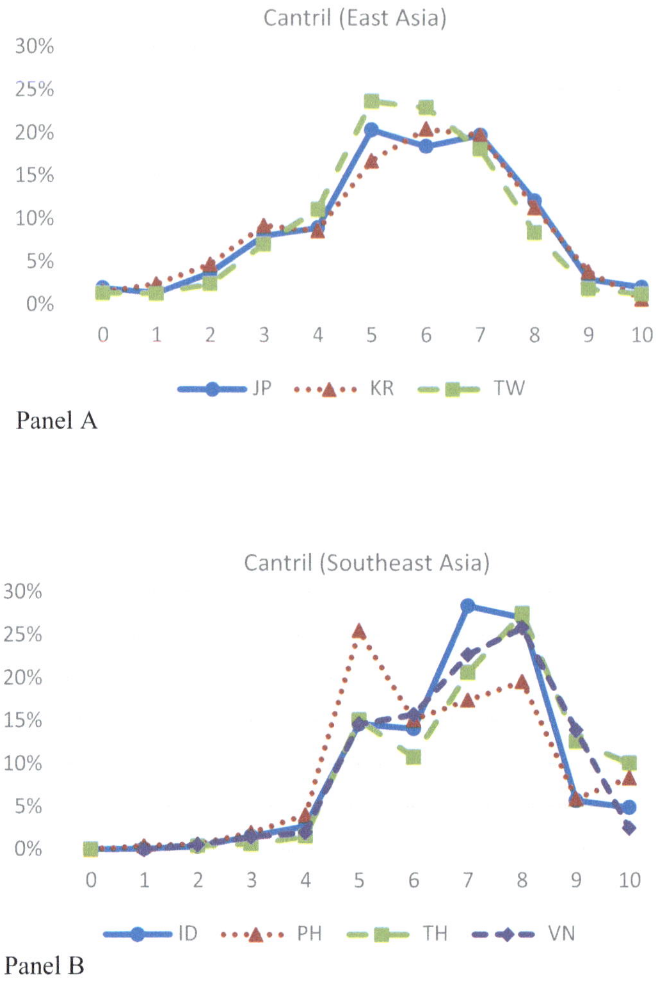

Fig. 4 Distribution of the Cantril ladder in East Asia (Panel A) and Southeast Asia (Panel B). Assembled by the authors based on SoWSA v2.0 (International Consortium for Social Well-Being Studies, 2020)

Table 4 Demographic and socioeconomic characteristics of the seven societies

	JP (%)	KR (%)	TW (%)	ID (%)	PH (%)	TH (%)	VN (%)
Age							
20s	19	18	21	29	21	17	30
30s	23	21	28	28	23	16	26
40s	18	25	25	21	22	22	22
50s	19	23	19	14	21	27	15
60s	21	13	7	8	13	18	8
Marriage							
Married	62	63	50	71	73	63	71
Never married	32	31	45	22	16	24	22
Divorced or widowed	6	6	5	7	10	13	7
Employment							
Standard	41	48	68	13	14	19	14
Non-standard	20	11	6	21	18	16	27
Self-employment	9	17	11	30	34	49	50
Unemployed or inactive	30	24	15	37	34	17	10
Education							
Lower secondary	1	1	1	35	30	52	44
Upper secondary	24	19	14	45	44	18	29
Short-cycle tertiary	22	14	20	6	14	5	4
Tertiary	45	55	46	13	11	21	21
Master or doctor	8	11	18	2	0	3	1
Non-tertiary	25	20	16	79	74	70	73
Tertiary or higher	75	80	84	21	26	30	27

Source Assembled by the authors based on SoWSA v2.0 (International Consortium for Social Well-Being Studies, 2020)

Acknowledgements This work was supported by the MEXT-Supported Program for the Strategic Research Foundation at Private Universities of Japan, 2014–18 (S1491003), JSPS KAKENHI Grant Number 19H01570, and ROIS-DS-JOINT 2017–23 (002RP2017, 003RP2018, 022RP2019, 028RP2020, 014RP2021, 014RP2022, and 059RP2023).

References

Aristotle. (1911). *The Nicomachean ethics of Aristotle* (D. P. Chase, Trans.). Dent.

Cantril, H. (1965). *The pattern of human concerns*. Rutgers University Press.

Coyle, D. (2014). *GDP: A brief but affectionate history*. Princeton University Press.

Deaton, A. (2013). *The great escape: Health, wealth, and the origins of inequality*. Princeton University Press.

Drewnowski, J. (1974). *On measuring and planning the quality of life*. Mouton.
Easterlin, R. A. (1974). Does economic growth improve the human lot? Some empirical evidence. In P. David & M. Reder (Eds.), *Nations and households in economic growth: Essays in honour of Moses Abramowitz* (pp. 89–125). Academic Press.
Easterlin, R. A. (2021). *An economist's lessons on happiness: Farewell dismal science!* Springer.
Fleurbaey, M. (2009). Beyond GDP: The quest for a measure of social welfare. *Journal of Economic Literature, 47*(4), 1029–1075.
Frey, B. S. (2008). *Happiness: A revolution in economics*. The MIT Press.
Frey, B. S., & Stutzer, A. (2002). *Happiness and economics: How the economy and institutions affect human well-being*. Princeton University Press.
Harada, H. (2016a). The significance and availability of happiness study. *The Senshu Social Well-Being Review, 2*, 9–39.
Harada, H. (2016b). Happiness in Japan: From the viewpoint of age, sex and relative wealthiness. *The Senshu Social Well-Being Review, 3*, 1–17.
Harada, H. (2019). Proposal for social well-being studies in Asia: A challenge beyond GDP. *The Senshu Social Well-Being Review, 6*, 3–11.
Helliwell, J. F., Layard, R., & Sachs, J. (Eds.). (2012). *World happiness report*. Earth Institute, Columbia University.
Helliwell, J. F., Layard, R., & Sachs, J. (Eds.). (2015). *World happiness report 2015*. Sustainable Development Solutions Network.
Inglehart, R., Haerpfer, C., Moreno, A., Welzel, C., Kizilova, K., Diez-Medrano, J., Lagos, M., Norris, P., Ponarin, E., & Puranen, B. (Eds.). (2018). *World values survey: Round six—country-pooled datafile*. JD Systems Institute & WVSA Secretariat. https://doi.org/10.14281/18241.8
International Consortium for Social Well-Being Studies. (2020, June 25). *Social well-being survey in Asia, 2015–2017*. (Indonesia) Universitas Indonesia, (Japan) Senshu University, (South Korea) Seoul National University, (The Philippines) Ateneo de Manila University, (Thailand) Chulalongkorn University, (Taiwan) Academia Sinica, (Vietnam) Vietnam Academy of Social Sciences [Producers]. Korea Social Science Data Archive (KOSSDA) [Distributors]. https://doi.org/10.22687/KOSSDA-A1-CUM-0022-V2.0
ISSP Research Group. (2015). *International social survey programme: Health and health care—ISSP 2011*. GESIS Data Archive, Cologne. ZA5800 Data File Version 3.0.0. https://doi.org/10.4232/1.12252
Kahneman, D., & Kruger, A. B. (2006). Developments in the measurements of subjective well-being. *Journal of Economic Perspective, 20*(1), 3–24.
Karabell, Z. (2014). *The leading indicators: A short history of the numbers that rule our world*. Simon & Schuster.
Keynes, J. M. (1936). *The general theory of employment, interest and money*. Macmillan.
KOSSDA. (Ed.). (2020). *Social well-being survey in Asia 2015–2017 survey report* (KOSSDA Survey Report A2001 Version 2.0). KOSSDA.
Li, L., Kim, S.-W., Iwai, N., & Fu, Y.-C. (2021). *East Asian Social Survey (EASS), cross-national survey data sets: Network social capital in East Asia, 2012*. Inter-University Consortium for Political and Social Research [Distributor]. https://doi.org/10.3886/ICPSR36277.v2
Mahbubani, K. (2008). *The new Asian hemisphere: The irresistible shift of global power to the east*. Public Affairs.
Marshal, A. (1890–1961). *Principles of economics* (9th ed.). Macmillan.
Mishan, E. J. (1967). *The costs of economic growth*. Staples Press.
Myrdal, K. G. (1968). *Asian drama: An inquiry into the poverty on nations*. Allen Lane.
Nordhaus, W. D., & Tobin, J. (1972). Is growth obsolete? *Economic Research: Retrospect and Prospect, 5*, 1–80.
OECD. (2011). *How's life? Measuring well-being*. OECD Publishing.
Pigou, A. C. (1920–1952). *The economics of welfare* (4th ed.). Macmillan.
Pomeranz, K. (2000). *The great divergence: China, Europe, and the making of the modern world economy*. Princeton University Press.

Putnam, R. D. (2000). *Bowling alone: The collapse and revival of American community*. Simon & Schuster.
Scitovsky, T. (1976). *The joyless economy: An inquiry into human satisfaction and consumer dissatisfaction*. Oxford University Press.
Shambaugh, D. (2013). *China goes global: The partial power*. Oxford University Press.
Skidelsky, R., & Skidelsky, E. (2012). *How much is enough? Money and the good life*. Other Press.
Stiglitz, J. E., Sen, A., & Fitoussi, J.-P. (2010). *Mis-measuring our lives: Why GDP doesn't add up?* The New Press.

Hiroo Harada is a Professor Emeritus of Economics at Senshu University. His research interests are in the fields of public finance, taxation, regional economy, public choice, and social capital/ well-being.

Masayuki Kanai is a Professor of Sociology at Senshu University. His research interests include subjective well-being, social capital, and social inequality.

Data Harmonization of Social Well-Being Survey in Asia

Hearan Koo, Hye-ok Heo, Yi-Fu Chen, and Tadahiko Maeda

Abstract In this chapter, we describe the process of integrating the SoWSA datasets of seven countries into a harmonized dataset in detail, mainly focusing on sociodemographic variables such as education, work status and occupation, and household income. We also briefly discuss the equivalence of the substantial variables that are considered the main concerns of comparative surveys. Drawing from our experience with harmonizing SoWSA data, we point out that a more coordinated and coherent data collection and integration strategy would be needed to ensure the quality of harmonized datasets. Given the rising demand for comparative research data, we concluded this chapter by highlighting the need for the development of more sophisticated and robust data integration methodologies in the future.

Keywords Social Well-Being Survey in Asia · SoWSA · Data harmonization · Cross-national survey · Data quality · Comparative analysis · Translation · Back-translation · Survey documentation · Conceptual equivalence · Measurement equivalence · Asian societies

---

The original version of the chapter has been revised: The affiliation of the second author has been removed. A correction to this chapter can be found at
https://doi.org/10.1007/978-981-97-3866-3_19

H. Koo · H. Heo (✉)
Korea Social Science Data Archive, Seoul National University, Seoul, Republic of Korea
e-mail: hyeokh@snu.ac.kr

Y.-F. Chen
Department of Sociology, National Taipei University, New Taipei City, Taiwan

T. Maeda
Center for Social Data Structuring, Joint Support-Center for Data Science Research, Research Organization of Information and Systems, Tokyo, Japan

J. Yee et al. (eds.), *Social Well-Being, Development, and Multiple Modernities in Asia*,
https://doi.org/10.1007/978-981-97-3866-3_3

1 Introduction

Over the past few decades, substantial advances have been made in comparative survey research. A significant amount of comparative survey data has been produced by numerous international survey programs in social science research, and they are available and accessible to the general research community. To enhance comparability and usability, separate individual country datasets are integrated and provided in a highly usable format. Concomitantly, notable innovations have been made in data harmonization methods (Dubrow & Tomescu-Dubrow, 2016; Granda et al., 2010; Hoffmeyer-Zlotnik & Warner, 2014).

Harmonization of survey data refers to a series of tasks that combine data from different surveys into a single integrated dataset. The primary aim is to improve comparability across time and place (Granda et al., 2010). Data harmonization is considered to add value to existing data, in the sense that it contributes to increasing usability and encouraging efficient secondary analysis of existing data. In practice, harmonization of variables in cross-national, multilingual, and multicultural surveys demands considerable resources and effort. Above all, experienced researchers or survey practitioners familiar with both the characteristics of the surveys and the diverse socioeconomic and cultural environments across a variety of societies and cultures that target surveys are implemented. Hence, collaboration between experts from different countries and cultures is inevitable.

The Social Well-being Survey in Asia (SoWSA) is not an exception. The SoWSA was conducted in seven Asian countries under the leadership of Japanese researchers. The Japanese team initiated and provided funding for data collection in the seven countries. The International Consortium for Social Well-Being Research (ICSWB) was organized and became a research network for collaborative studies. The researchers participating in the ICSWB agreed to share the data they collected and released it to the research community.

To publish the SoWSA data, a three-year project, funded by the Joint Support-Center for Data Science Research, Research Organization of Information and Systems (ROIS-DS), Japan, was created to harmonize and publish integrated data from the SoWSA. While experts from three East Asian countries have primary responsibilities for data harmonization, the researchers participating in the SoWSA project, who have been working closely with each other throughout the survey design, data collection, and data processing, provided the necessary information that was critical for integrating the data at every phase of data harmonization and final verification. For efficient communication and important decision making, a series of international workshops and meetings were held to bring researchers from the participating countries together. Rules and procedures for data coding, editing, and standardization were discussed and established at the meetings.

In this chapter, we describe the process of integrating the SoWSA datasets of seven countries into a harmonized dataset in detail, mainly focusing on sociodemographic variables. We also briefly discuss the equivalence of the substantial variables that are considered the main concerns of comparative surveys. We believe that this will contribute to the theoretical and methodological accumulation of data harmonization methods in the Asian region. The chapter begins with a brief overview of data harmonization approaches in general and illustrates the process of data harmonization of the SoWSA in particular. The following section explains the adjustments to the inconsistencies across national country surveys and ways of producing standardized background variables. Next, we briefly address the issue of conceptual and measurement equivalence of substantial variables and conclude with a few remarks for future data collection and harmonization based on our experience.

2 Harmonization Process of the SoWSA Data

2.1 Approaches to Data Harmonization

Data harmonization can be achieved using different strategies and procedures depending on the purpose and circumstances of data production. According to the "Guidelines for Best Practice in Cross-Cultural Surveys," there are two ways of harmonization: input harmonization and output harmonization (Survey Research Center, 2016). Input harmonization can be performed with data harmonization in mind from the design stage of the surveys. The input harmonization approach manages and imposes strict and shared rules and standards on which researchers of participating countries agree beforehand. For input harmonization, participating countries may consent to apply the same survey concepts and procedures and jointly get involved in developing a standard questionnaire and instruments. This approach aims to achieve a high degree of comparability.

Output harmonization, on the other hand, is used when there is a need to produce a harmonized dataset based on existing data that is not originally collected for comparative purposes. This approach examines whether variables are functionally equivalent and integrates them to maximize comparability. It is considered an alternative when there is a need for comparison, but no relevant data are available, or when the data collection process is difficult to coordinate at the initial stage.

Another approach, called ex-ante harmonization, is a mixture of these two approaches. This approach can be implemented if researchers of participating countries agree to measure a set of pre-defined target variables designed to be comparable; however, the detailed survey process and instruments are primarily determined at the level of individual countries. It is intended to reflect an individual country's contextual specificities of data collection practices and measurements.

Comparative analyses require data and information that are universally comprehensible but sensitive to particular social, economic, and cultural contexts. To satisfy this requirement, data harmonization of comparative surveys needs to consider both the commonalities of survey concepts and cultural and societal differences. However, it is not easy to come up with a common concept and measure shared with every country while considering differences across countries. The societal and cultural contexts of each country vary substantially, and even within a country, there exists a significant inconsistency in social institutions across time.

One way of resolving this difficulty is to rely on international standard classifications, such as the International Standard Classification of Occupations (ISCO) and the International Standard Classification of Education (ISCED) (Granda et al., 2010; Hoffmeyer-Zlotnik, 2016). They are viable options because they are based on unambiguous definitions for standardization, and researchers can easily access coding instructions to convert country-specific variables into comparable ones.

Whatever approach we take, the data harmonization of cross-national surveys is subject to systematic errors. They are caused by differences in national and cultural concepts underlying each variable or misconceptions and mistranslation of survey items (Hoffmeyer-Zlotnik & Warner, 2014). Because systematic errors cannot be completely controlled, it is important to document every decision made during the data harmonization process as well as the rules and criteria applied. Thorough documentation of surveys and data allows users to trace the sources of errors easily. It also helps users access detailed information about the data collection of each national survey and the characteristics of the original variables and their relationships to harmonized ones.

Regarding systematic errors, some researchers strongly urge that data harmonization should not be performed in the case of quota sampling or other types of non-probability sampling (e.g., Survey Research Center, 2016). This is because data collected from non-probability sampling has a high risk of bias and seriously destroys comparability. In principle, we believe that it is necessary to follow their advice. Nevertheless, we decided to provide a harmonized dataset of the SoWSA. There are two reasons for this decision. First, we found considerable data gaps between Western and Asian societies for social well-being studies. Recently, Asian societies have presented concerns regarding the social well-being of people and societies. This reflects their research and policy interest in whether the rapid economic progress they are experiencing can enrich people's lives and promote social well-being. To enhance our understanding and knowledge of social progress and well-being among Asian people, we need to have relevant data measuring social well-being in this region. Despite the growing demand for well-being data in the Asian region, existing well-being data have been predominantly produced in Western society. To fill this data gap, we believe that it would be helpful to publish a harmonized SoWSA dataset. Second, we found that survey administration and infrastructure are diverse across Asian countries. In some countries, quota sampling is dominant and may be the only feasible option for surveys. We believe that harmonized SoWSA data could be used with limited value in the absence of adequate data available for comparative studies of social well-being in the Asian region. We believe that extensive use of the integrated SoWSA will stimulate methodologically more rigorous data collection needs and lead to the generation of quality well-being data in the future.

2.2 Harmonization Process of the SoWSA

The type of data harmonization process of the SoWSA lies between ex-ante harmonization and ex-post output harmonization, in the sense that the data collection protocols are prepared at the beginning of fieldwork, but most of the harmonization protocols are set up after all surveys have been conducted. For comparative data collection, survey concepts and measurements were established before each country team joined the survey. The source questionnaire was drafted and provided by the Japanese team. The researchers of the participating countries shared this as a common instrument in their national surveys.

For substantial variables, national teams were requested to follow the "ask-the-same-questions" format. In principle, adaptation and modification are restricted to a minimum. On the other hand, for background variables, target variables were predetermined, and national teams could decide their own measurement formats under the condition of easy transfer into the target variables. The SoWSA applied ISCO-08, ISCED 2011, and decile response options for the target variables of occupation, education, and personal and household incomes, respectively. The key to the successful adaptation of international standards is how easily and accurately a national classification can be converted into an international classification system. However, in practice, conversion was not easily achieved, partly because of insufficient understanding and inappropriateness of the classification criteria. Consequently, modified or reduced coding schemes for standard variables were created.

National teams added other items of well-being measures that were considered relevant to individual countries to their fieldwork questionnaires. For example, the Philippines added relative deprivation items to their field questionnaire. Thailand and Taiwan attached health-related questions, such as anxiety and trauma (Thailand), CES-D, and subjective health evaluation (Taiwan). By adding relevant well-being items and instruments, each national team attempted to make up for the problem of their own country, initiating the development of question items and instruments. Despite the merits of such a flexible design of the field questionnaire, this modification led to significant deviations in the survey items and eventually limited data integration.

Translation problems were one of the most challenging tasks that we had to face. In the case of a multilingual cross-national survey, quality translation is crucial for collecting equivalent data and determining whether research results are sufficiently comparable. Usually, the translation of survey items does not involve word-by-word conversion. Instead, question wordings and formats were selected to capture the underlying concept of questions and hold identical meanings across countries. Harkness et al. suggested that quality survey translation needs to "keep the content of the questions semantically similar; within the bounds of the target language, keep the question format similar; retain measurement properties including the range of response options offered; and maintain the same stimulus (Harkness et al., 2010: 117)." To satisfy these requirements, they recommended evaluating translation as an integral part of the common questionnaire development process (Survey Research

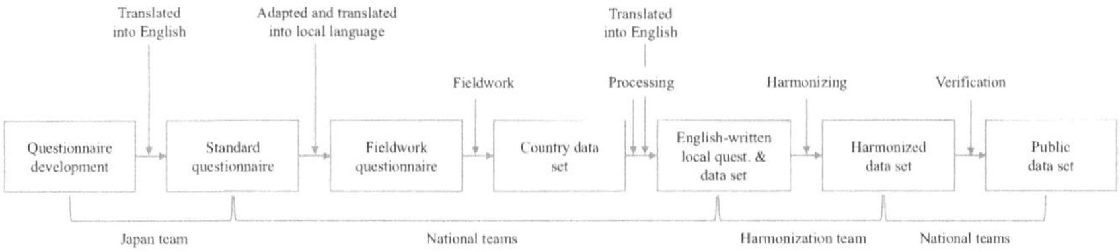

Fig. 1 Process of translation of survey instruments and SoWSA data

Center, 2016). In the case of the SoWSA, the equivalence of questions was examined after the data production of each participating country was completed, so that these requirements were not fully met.

As in other comparative surveys, the SoWSA underwent multiple steps of translation. Figure 1 presents the complicated process of translation of the questionnaire and the datasets of the SoWSA.

The source questionnaire for the SoWSA was first written in Japanese and then translated into English for sharing. Each national team translated the English written questionnaire to its national language and used it as a field questionnaire. The source questionnaire was translated into local languages under the responsibility of the national teams. The pre-defined variables were measured using country-specific questions and response categories and then later coded by national experts into standard variables. After all data production had been completed, the national teams translated the dataset into English and submitted it to the Japanese team using local field questionnaires.

To examine any deviations or misconceptualization in the national surveys, the national teams were requested to back-translate their national language-written field questionnaires into English. The back-translated questionnaires were then compared with the source questionnaire and checked to determine whether the questionnaire items used in each national questionnaire were identical in terms of substantial meaning and measurement scale. Any deviations from the source questionnaire, such as modified question wordings, adding or collapsing response categories, and changes in the order of set questions, were identified across countries. Data harmonization was performed with the translated datasets and back-translated questionnaires. After the data harmonization was completed, each national team examined any errors or misinformation in the harmonized dataset and documents and verified them.

This indirect and complicated process makes it difficult to minimize systematic errors (Harkness, 2003). Indirect examination of the adequacy of translation cannot correct errors resulting from errors in the original translation. Each stage of the multiple translation and back-translation processes is also subjected to error generation and accumulation. Therefore, there may exist a high risk of errors in harmonized SoWSA.

Harmonizing SoWSA is inherently limited in many respects. To produce as much comparable data as possible out of such constraints, we established the following basic principles: (1) to include variables from the source questionnaire only and to exclude all questions attached to the national questionnaire for their own additional survey purposes; (2) for background variables, to introduce variables with broader categories, taking the risk of the loss of information, if response categories are not identical or difficult to map; (3) to include variables with national measurement format as country-specific variables so that researchers can easily access and trace the original response options; and (4) to provide documentation describing data harmonization procedures, problems of integration, the degree of cross-national comparability of each variable, as well as information about national surveys and national statistical characteristics.

In the next section, we illustrate how we convert national variables in each country dataset into target variables in an integrated dataset, mainly focusing on background variables, such as education, work status and occupation, and household income.

2.3 Harmonizing Background Variables[1]

2.3.1 Educational Attainment

Educational attainment is an essential background variable that indicates the extent of human capital, competence, and qualification to access the labor market and the relative position of a hierarchical status structure. Education in the SoWSA was measured by asking the respondents their highest educational level. The target variable for measuring the level of education was a one-digit variable of ISCED 2011 standard. The ISCED one-digit classification consists of nine levels from 0 (early childhood education) to 8 (doctoral or equivalent level). The classification considers information about both general and vocational education qualifications.

Each country team measured the level of education in accordance with its education system and then assigned national response categories to equivalent ISCED codes. Table 1 gives how each national response option is mapped to ISCED codes.

As Table 1 gives, country-specific measures of education level do not match the full ISCED code scheme. Several response categories were omitted or collapsed in some countries. For instance, the primary education level is not differentiated from lower secondary education and below in Japan and Taiwan, while the doctoral or equivalent level is not differentiated from the master course and above in Vietnam. In addition, most of Southeast Asian countries (hereafter, SEA) capture people with "no

[1] Before harmonizing, we discussed how to set the age range of the integrated data set, since each country's survey has different population coverage from the lowest age of 17 to the highest age of 90. We decide to select respondents aged 20 ~ 69 for samples to be as comparable as possible. We should point out that the age range of East Asian countries was not significantly different, but the deviation was large in Southeast Asia. Therefore, the loss of sample in SEA is higher than that of EA (see Korea Social Science Data Archive, 2020, for detailed information about the age range of each country). The mapping of background variables across countries has been done with this selected data set.

Table 1 Education variable mapping to ISCED classification

Educ[a]	ISCED 2011	Japan	Korea	Taiwan	Indonesia	Philippines	Vietnam	Thailand
1	Other			8. 其他				
	No education				9. Tidak Sekolah	8 No education	0 No education	
	0 Early childhood education							0 Early childhood education
	1 Primary education		1. 초등학교 (국민학교)		0. SD/ Sederajat	0 Primary/ elementary	1 ~ 5 Tiểu học	1 Primary education
	2 Lower secondary education	1. 中学校 (旧制小学校, 旧制高等小学校)	2. 중학교	1. 國中以下	1. SMP/ Sederajat	1 Junior high school	6 ~ 9 Trung học cơ sở	2 Lower secondary education
2	3 Upper secondary education	2. 高等学校, 中等教育学校 (旧制中学校, 師範学校, 実業学校, 高等女学校)	3-1. 인문고등학교	2. 高中	2. SMA/ Sederajat	2 High school	10 ~ 12 Trung học phổ thông	3 Upper secondary education
			3-2. 실업계고등학교	3. 高職	3. Sekolah Keju-ruan/ SMK			
	4 Post-secondary non-tertiary education			4. 專科, 二技		3 Vocational school		4 Post-secondary non-tertiary education

(continued)

Table 1 (continued)

Educ[a]	ISCED 2011	Japan	Korea	Taiwan	Indonesia	Philippines	Vietnam	Thailand
3	5 Short-cycle tertiary education	3. 専門学校	4. 전문대학 (2·3 년제)		4. D3	4 Vocational high school	13 Trung cấp/Cao đẳng nghề	5 Short-cycle tertiary education
		4. 短期大学, 高等専門学校 (旧制高等学校)						
4	6 Bachelors or equivalent level	5. 四年制大学	5. 대학교 (4 년제)	5. 四年制大學/技術學院	5. D4/S1	5 Four-year university	14 Cao đẳng/Đại học	6 Bachelors or equivalent level
5	7 Masters or equivalent level	6. 大学院修士課程, 専門職大学院	6. 대학원 (석사과정)	6. 碩士	6. S2	6 Master's course, professional graduate school	15 Thạc sĩ/Tiến sĩ	7 Masters or equivalent level
	8 Doctoral or equivalent level	7. 大学院博士課程	7. 대학원 (박사과정)	7. 博士	7. S3	7 Doctorate course		8 Doctoral or equivalent level

[a] *1* lower secondary and below, *2* upper secondary, post-secondary non-tertiary, *3* short-cycle tertiary, *4* bachelors or equivalent, *5* masters or doctoral or equivalent

education," while East Asian countries (hereafter, EA) did not include this category in the response options.

The reduced differentiation of lower or upper secondary education may be related to the distribution of education among the people in each country. In fact, the proportion of primary education in the participating countries varies significantly. According to the UNESCO Institute for Statistics, for people aged 25 years and older, the share of primary education is 28.8% (as of 2015) for Indonesia, 24.6% for the Philippines (as of 2017), 20.6% (as of 2016) for Thailand, and 28.3% (as of 2009) for Vietnam. In contrast, it was 9.8% in Korea (as of 2015). Japan and Taiwan do not provide separate statistics of primary and lower secondary, and the proportion of combining the two categories is 16.7% (as of 2010) for Japan and 19.3% (as of 2016) for Taiwan.[2] These numbers are lower than the share of the primary education category only in SEA. This implies that it is more relevant for SEA to identify people with primary education separately from those with lower secondary education. However, EA does not seem to consider the primary education category as a significant indicator of educational qualifications.

Another interesting point worth noting is the difference in the "post-secondary non-tertiary education" category among participating countries. The definition of post-secondary non-tertiary education intends to capture those who have completed upper secondary education but have learned below the high level of complexity characteristic of tertiary education for both labor market entry and tertiary education. Table 1 gives that this category is not relevant or at least uncommon in countries, such as Japan, Korea, Indonesia, and Vietnam.

Due to the difficulty in mapping the levels of education categories to the full ISCED 2011 code scheme, we produced a 5-category educational attainment variable: 1 = lower secondary and below, 2 = upper secondary and post-secondary non-tertiary, 3 = short-cycle tertiary, 4 = bachelor's or equivalent, and 5 = master's or doctoral or equivalent. This reduced classification of ISCED may be a restraint to use when users attempt to compare variations in social well-being within lower or higher education groups.

2.3.2 Work Status and Occupation

The work status and occupation variables were designed to identify respondents' status regarding the labor market. They are key variables in determining the socioeconomic status of the respondent and analyzing social inequalities and labor market processes. The work status variable is also used to recognize the position of respondents in their life cycle, such as learning, working, and retirement stages (Hoffmeyer-Zlotnik & Warner, 2011: 11).

To identify the work status of the respondent, the SoWSA asks, "How do you work currently? If you have more than one job, please answer the most important one."

---

[2] Source: 2016 Yearbook of Manpower Survey Statistics. It is based on the population aged 20 ~ 69.

The source questionnaire provides six response options for those who are working and two for those who are not working. They are designed to distinguish between economically active and inactive, between the employee and the self-employed, and between full-time employment and part-time employment or casual employment.

In terms of question wording, the differences between individual countries are negligible. However, there is a notable difference in the response options of the SEAs (see Table 2) . We found that all SEAs added farmers or agriculture as an independent category. In general, farmers are classified as self-employed or employees, depending on whether they are working for profit or payment. However, researchers in SEA are reluctant to assign farmers to these categories. One of the reasons for this hesitation seems to be related to the share of farmers and agricultural workers in SEA. In SEA region, compared to EA, the share of employment in agriculture is greater than 25% of total employment, and agricultural employment is predominantly located in the informal sector. Their status may be inconsistent or complicated, making it difficult to clearly define. In particular, the boundary between self-employment and paid employment may not be straightforward because of the considerable diversity of informal employment situations in the agricultural sector.

To standardize work content, the SoWSA intends to provide an ISCO 4-digit coded variable. The format of the question was to ask the respondents what kinds of job they do in an open-ended question during the fieldwork, and later experts assigned the most appropriate code for the job description provided by the respondent. However, it is extremely challenging to code four-digit ISCO classifications. This requires the expertise and knowledge of the trained researchers. In addition, to classify distinctively, the respondent should describe his/her work in detail, and the description provided by the respondent should contain the necessary information for classification. However, the verbal description of a respondent is often insufficient and ambiguous when assigning an appropriate code. In some cases, it may not be easy to find an occupational title in a classification scheme. We faced the same problem and decided to create an occupation variable based on a one-digit code rather than a four-digit code.

The last but least thing we want to mention is related to the issue of expert coding versus the respondent's choice from the listed categories. During fieldwork, the Korean team used a different strategy to obtain occupational information. It used a closed question and provided a one-digit ISCO classification that was designed to be selected by the respondent, as well as the open-ended question. Whether the respondent's direct choice or the expert's indirect coding causes any systematic bias needs to be investigated further.

2.3.3 Household Income

Income is an important variable reflecting the standards of living or economic status of respondents. Hence, most surveys include questions on income. Nevertheless, income is one of the variables for which missing or non-response cases tend to be high. This is because it is difficult for the respondent to answer the income question. He/she

Table 2 Mapping of work status variables

Work status code[a]	Pre-determined response options	Japan	Korea	Taiwan	Indonesia	Philippines	Thailand	Vietnam
1	1 Chief executive, senior official, legislator						Manager	
	2 Regular employee/civil servant	Include (temporary leave due to illness or childcare)	Include (temporary leave due to illness or childcare)				Permanent worker	
2	3 Temporary/ part-time worker			Part time work	Include (ex: insurance agent)			
	4 Dispatched/ contracted employee			Dispatcher				
3	5 Self-employed, freelance, side work	Exclude side work		Exclude side work				
	6 Family worker							
					Farmer	Farmer-tenant Farmer-owner	Farmer with own land	Agriculture
3							Merchant	
5					Housewife			Home work
5					Student			

(continued)

Table 2 (continued)

Work status code[a]	Pre-determined response options	Japan	Korea	Taiwan	Indonesia	Philippines	Thailand	Vietnam
4	11 Not working but currently looking for jobs							
5	12 Not working and not looking for jobs		Include (housewife, student, retired etc.)					

[a] *1* regular employee, *2* non-regular employee, *3* self-employed, *4* unemployed, *5* economically not active

must enumerate all income sources to respond to it. In the case of household income, it is even more difficult to answer because respondents need to consider the income of all household members who contribute to household finance. Respondents often do not have sufficient information on the incomes of other household members. The income question is also a very sensitive one for certain groups of people. For example, high incomers or those who feel sensitive to privacy issues might be more reluctant to respond to the question. Consequently, a significant number of respondents often resist or refuse to provide information about their income. In the case of the SoWSA, the number of missing cases is not large, but varies across countries. While Korea and Taiwan have no "missing cases," and SEA has less than 0.5% non-response cases, Japan has 6.7% non-response cases.

The household income question in the source questionnaire asks for pre-tax and annual income. The question wording is, "Please indicate the past year's pre-tax income for your household (for family with shared finances). Include income from the rest of your family in your answer." As the question wording displays, the reference period for household income was a one-year period. However, it has not been uniformly adapted across countries. While Japan, Philippines, Thailand, and Vietnam used a one-year period as a reference, Korea, Taiwan, and Indonesia used one month period. Each reference period has its own advantages and disadvantages. For example, the shorter the reference period, the easier the respondent answers, because they are less likely to omit income sources that need to be included. However, if a country has a high proportion of the self-employed, a shorter period may result in a lower accuracy.

Household income can be asked to report the actual amount of income directly or select an income category from a list of response options. It has been observed that presenting response categories is better for obtaining responses to sensitive questions. However, in the case of income, it must accept a loss of information. The number of response options in a closed-ended question format is associated with the level of precision. The more the income category is presented, the higher the measurement accuracy. Two types of questions were used in the national surveys of the SoWSA. The Philippines, Thailand, and Vietnam asked about household income in exact amounts, while Japan, Korea, Taiwan, and Indonesia asked to select a category of income groups. We examined the distribution of income to identify any patterns resulting from such differences. Figure 2 presents a histogram of household incomes across countries. This shows that the response to the category-based question was more normally distributed. In contrast, the distributions of the responses from the exact number of income questions are highly skewed and heavily affected by outliers. How the differences in the reference period and response options affect the comparability of harmonized variables requires further investigation.

Because income information is based on national currencies, a direct comparison is not possible. One feasible option for standardizing is to employ an equal distribution of income across categories such as income deciles or quintiles. This allows us to produce a directly comparable variable; however, for classification, we need external information provided by official statistics or other reliable data sources to

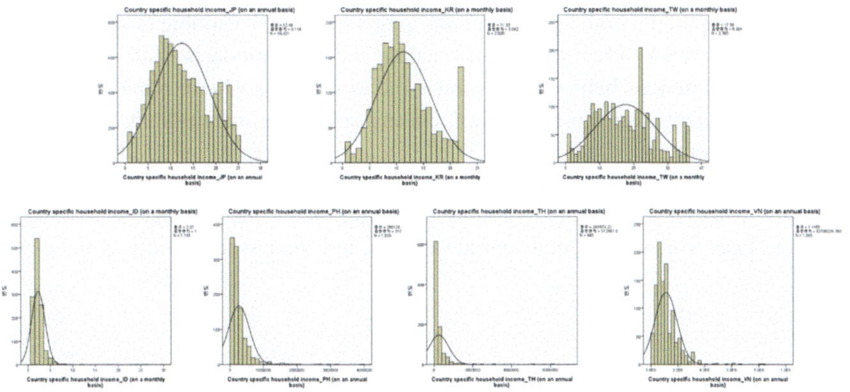

Fig. 2 Distribution of household income across countries

separate the boundaries between each category. The SoWSA was designed to identify respondents' position on the decile distribution of national household income statistics. National experts were asked to provide income decile codes based on respondents' answers to the household income question and external information. However, the target variable cannot be produced because necessary national statistics are not available in some countries, and it is difficult to convert the response into a decile income category.

2.4 Document Preparation and Dissemination

Researchers of the participating countries in the SoWSA and secondary users of the harmonized SoWSA data may utilize harmonized datasets with diverse interests and purposes, as well as with the original purpose of the SoWSA. Therefore, it is crucial to provide them with sufficient information about the data collection and harmonization process. The well-known International Social Survey Programme (ISSP) collects detailed technical and methodological information on how the survey was accomplished in each country and provides study monitoring reports containing detailed methodological and technical information on the surveys. We benchmarked its documentation processes. We collected information about surveys conducted in individual countries using the ISSP documentation format of study descriptions and characteristics of national populations and compiled them into the Survey Report. The survey report aimed to provide a comprehensive description of the survey and its variables. The report contains a brief overview of the SoWSA project and a description of individual SoWSA datasets, including bibliographic information, data collection methods, and data processing information. It also included the study description and population characteristics, background variable mapping tables, and sampling procedures.

We also prepared a coding guide containing variable-by-variable descriptions of harmonized SoWSA. The purpose of creating a coding guide is to describe similarities and differences between the source and target variables in terms of question universe statements, question wording, coding schemes, and missing data definitions. It also contains simple marks that indicate whether the individual variables are comparable across countries. Secondary users can refer to the coding guide to determine whether a concerned variable is asked in the same way across countries, how it deviates from the original source variable, and what to be cautious about using it.

3 Validating the Substantial Variables

While background variables are among the most frequently used variables in comparative research, they are generally not of primary interest or concern. The comparability of substantial variables is of great concern in these analyses. Therefore, the equivalence of the variables must be examined and validated. We briefly address this issue using a few examples.

3.1 Conceptual Equivalence

Conceptual equivalence is the first and the most important step in conducting cross-national surveys. Like most cross-national surveys, the SoWSA uses a common questionnaire in the data collection process. As illustrated above, the questionnaire provided by the Japanese team consisted of both English and Japanese. The local research teams translated the questionnaire into local languages. The idea of conceptual equivalence is that translation should capture the essence of a construct while ensuring the correct understanding of the construct among native speakers. Straus (1969) distinguished between the phenomenal identity and conceptual equivalence of a measurement. Phenomenal identity indicates the standardized quantification of data across nations. In a standard IQ test, researchers created standard questions, tasks, and scale items to assess intelligence. However, standardization does not necessarily ensure the validity of the assessment. For example, in a comprehensive test, the use of football (American football) as a keyword in a question may only make sense for people who are familiar with the sport. In this case, we need to use a conceptual equivalence approach, including culturally modified, ipsatized, and specific questions, tasks, and items in the translation process across research sites (Straus, 1969).

A local expert of the SoWSA ensured the conceptual equivalence. Primary investigators (PIs) from local teams carefully reviewed and translated the source questionnaire into local languages. The PIs considered cultural sensitivity when compiling local questionnaires. For example, to assess how active respondents were in neighborhood activities, the source questionnaire included neighborhood association activities. However, in Taiwan, neighborhood activities are often organized by village officers. In most areas, neighborhood associations do not exist or are not as active as those in other countries. The concept of neighborhood activities perceived by Taiwanese people is different from that of other countries. Therefore, the research team in Taiwan used activities organized by village officers.

In the harmonization process, conceptual equivalence requires not only identical definitions of a construct but also common understanding in local contexts (Tseng & Hsu, 1991). Even though the constructs are similar in terms of definition and meaning, instruments developed for the construct may not guarantee the measurement of the same construct in the same manner across countries. In addition, for scales, the process can ensure the inclusion of all domains under a construct (Olsen et al., 2013).

3.2 Measurement Equivalence

Even if the research team has prepared instruments for cross-national data collection, problems of measurement non-equivalence could still emerge due to various reasons. For example, items on a scale may exhibit different loading patterns across countries. It could also be an item of a scale with poor performance in a specific country. In either situation, we encounter the problem of measurement non-equivalence, indicating that the instruments (either the questions or items) could be problematic when conducting analyses of cross-national comparisons. This is problematic because non-equivalence confounds the findings of cross-national comparisons. The difference among nations could come from the "true" difference in subject matter, measurement non-equivalence, or both. Cross-national comparison (e.g., mean difference) without measurement equivalence simply compares oranges and apples (Dyer, 2015). To avoid this problem, researchers resort to a post hoc approach in which empirical data are carefully examined to secure measurement equivalence across nations.

From a generalized latent variable framework, Davidov et al. (2014) proposed a multigroup (countries as groups) confirmatory factor analysis to detect the levels of measurement equivalence. There are four hierarchies of measurement equivalence: configural, metric, scalar, and strict hierarchies. Higher levels of equivalence must impose restrictions on parameters across countries.[3] To detect whether levels of equivalence had been met, chi-square tests were used. To ensure comparability across countries, the data must meet at least (partial) metric equivalence. This approach can be used for continuous indicators; if categorical indicators are involved, multigroup item response theory (IRT) analysis can be used. In addition, researchers can use item-level analyses to detect problematic items. For example, we used a two-parameter IRT model to analyze the items of social unfairness in data from Japan, Korea, and

[3] For the definition of each level of equivalence, please see Davidov et al. (2014).

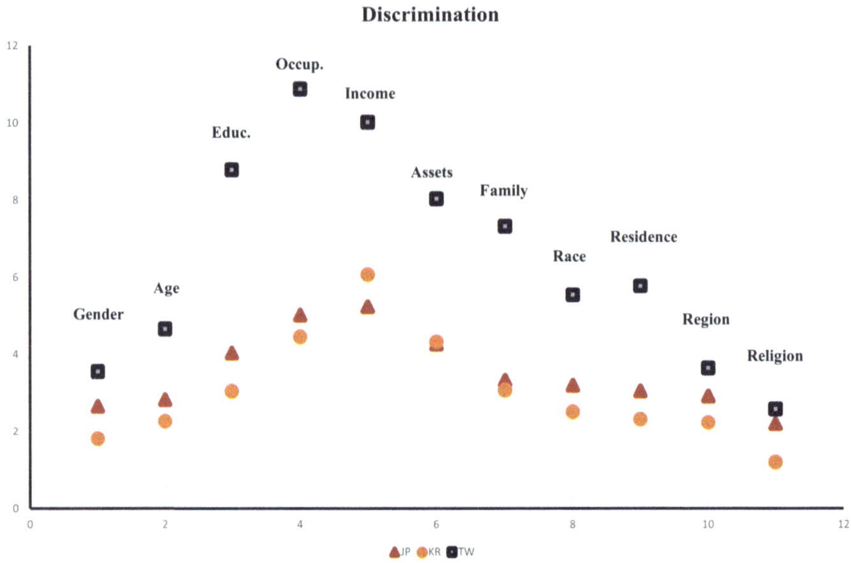

Fig. 3 Difficulty parameters of social unfairness in the three countries

Taiwan. Figures 3 and 4 show the difficulty and discrimination of each item across the three countries. A preliminary observation is that the item parameters of social unfairness in Japan and Korea are relatively similar for attribute-related items. After detecting differences in items, equating methods may be used to create a harmonized score for group comparisons. Further research can extend these analyses by including Southeast Asian countries. These findings can further inform the next run of data collection.

4 A Final Remark

The cross-national harmonization process presents a great challenge to the research team, as shown in the previous section. However, it also provides an exciting opportunity to learn from previous mistakes and design a better survey for the next run of the SoWSA. In this final section, we conclude with a few remarks about the lessons learned from our experience and recommendations.

As Wolf et al. (2016: 520) point out, harmonization is not just a "mechanical" work of pooling, mapping, and recoding. This requires considerable expert knowledge of the social, cultural, and political conditions of the countries concerned. It is also a complex and interrelated task that is linked to every process, from the design stage of the survey to the publishing stage of the final harmonized dataset. The selection of measurement, question wording, questionnaire design, sampling and fieldwork, data coding and editing, etc., may all contribute to the quality of harmonized data.

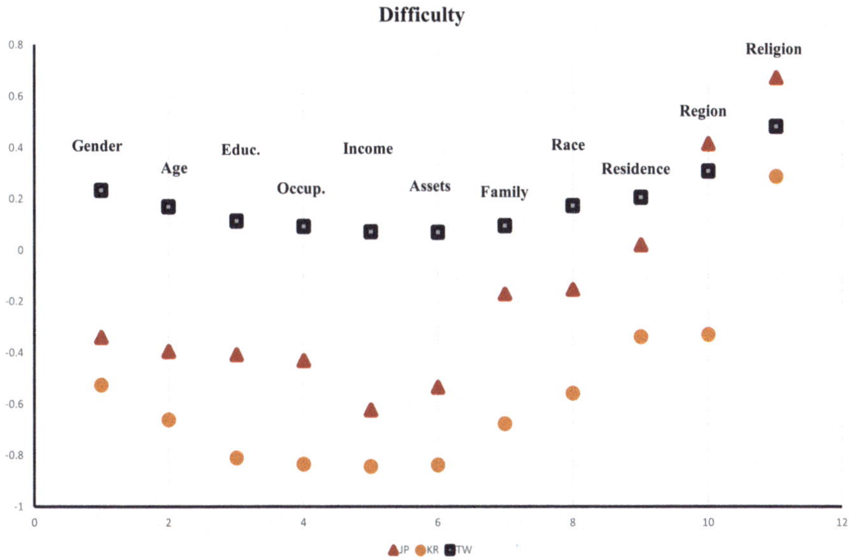

Fig. 4 Discrimination parameters of social unfairness in the three countries

Learning from the SoWSA harmonization experience, we believe that an a priori approach is required. If possible, research teams across countries should be involved in item development and discuss possible modifications to the questionnaires (questions, items, and response format) before data collection. As shown in the previous sections, the process is especially important for key demographic measures, such as educational attainment, occupational status, and religion/religiosity, to have a coordinated version of the instruments. In multinational surveys, tension inevitably exists between the need for measurement items that are relevant to a particular country and the need for consistency across countries. Tension is heightened when there is insufficient consensus on the best approach to measure demographic information and social well-being. Therefore, to ensure the quality of harmonized data, it would be better to adopt an ex-ante approach and a more coordinated data collection and harmonization strategy.

It should be noted that data harmonization means not only integration at the variable level, but also the assessment of comparability at the survey level. In this respect, the overall characteristics of the surveys, including sampling design and data collection methods, need to be examined and reported.

Regardless of how rigorous and comprehensive the procedure is, data harmonization cannot avoid adding its own errors. Therefore, harmonized data contain both the errors of the original source data and those produced in the harmonization process. In addition, there may be a loss of information resulting from the collapse of some of the response options or the categorization of continuous variables. Therefore, people who use harmonized datasets for their research questions should be aware of the limitations of the data and present and interpret their analysis results with great caution.

The harmonization of survey data requires the innovative development of methods for adjusting bias and errors arising from various phases of the data life cycle, the accumulation of knowledge about conceptual and methodological equivalence, and research on how different cultures and social contexts influence various survey errors. However, the theoretical and methodological basis for data harmonization has not been well established. Currently, where there is a high demand for comparative research data, extensive research, and discussion on more sophisticated data harmonization methods will be needed in the future.

References

Davidov, E., Meuleman, B., Cieciuch, J., Schmidt, P., & Billiet, J. (2014). Measurement equivalence in cross-national research. *Annual Review of Sociology, 40*, 55–75. https://doi.org/10.1146/annurev-soc-071913-043137

Dubrow, J. K., & Tomescu-Dubrow, I. (2016). The rise of cross-national survey data harmonization in the social sciences: Emergence of an interdisciplinary methodological field. *Quality & Quantity, 50*, 1449–1467. https://doi.org/10.1007/s11135-015-0215-z

Dyer, W. J. (2015). The vital role of measurement equivalence in family research. *Journal of Family Theory & Review, 7*(4), 415–431. https://doi.org/10.1111/jftr.12115

Granda, P., Wolf, C., & Hadorn, R. (2010). Harmonizing survey data. In J. A. Harkness, M. Braun, B. Edwards, T. P. Johnson, L. Lyberg, P. P. Mohler, B.-E. Pennell, & T. W. Smith (Eds.), *Survey methods in multinational, multiregional, and multicultural contexts*. https://doi.org/10.1002/9780470609927.ch17

Harkness, J. (2003). Questionnaire translation. In J. Harkness, F. van de Vijver, & P. Mohler (Eds.), *Crosscultural survey methods* (pp. 35–56). Wiley.

Harkness, J. A., Villar, A., & Edwards, B. (2010). Translation, adaptation, and design. In J. A. Harkness, M. Braun, B. Edwards, T. P. Johnson, L. Lyberg, P. P. Mohler, & T. W. Smith (Eds.), *Survey methods in multinational, multiregional, and multicultural contexts* (pp. 115–140). Wiley.

Hoffmeyer-Zlotnik, J. H. P. (2016). Standardisation and harmonisation of socio-demographic variables. In *GESIS survey guidelines*. GESIS—Leibniz Institute for the Social Sciences. https://doi.org/10.15465/gesis-sg_en_012

Hoffmeyer-Zlotnik, J. H. P., & Warner, U. (2011). *Measuring occupation and labour status in cross-national comparative surveys*. (GESIS-Schriftenreihe, 7). GESIS—Leibniz-Institut für Sozialwissenschaften. https://doi.org/10.21241/ssoar.32591

Hoffmeyer-Zlotnik, J. H. P., & Warner, U. (2014). *Harmonising demographic and socio-economic variables for cross-national comparative survey research*. Springer.

Korea Social Science Data Archive. (2020). *Social well-being survey in Asia, 2015–2017 survey report*. Retrieved from https://kossda.snu.ac.kr/bitstream/20.500.12236/23941/8/English_SurveyReport_CUM0022_V2.0.pdf

Olsen, M., Jensen, N. K., Tesfaye, M., & Holm, L. (2013). Conceptual equivalence of WHOQOL-HIV among people living with HIV in Ethiopia. *Quality of Life Research, 22*(2), 361–367. https://doi.org/10.1007/s11136-012-0141-7

Straus, M. A. (1969). Phenomenal identity and conceptual equivalence of measurement in cross-national comparative research. *Journal of Marriage and the Family, 31*(2), 233–239. https://doi.org/10.2307/349938

Survey Research Center. (2016). *Guidelines for best practice in cross-cultural surveys*. Survey Research Center, Institute for Social Research, University of Michigan. Retrieved November 30, 2023, from http://www.ccsg.isr.umich.edu/

Tseng, W.-S., & Hsu, J. (1991). *Culture and family: Problems and therapy*. The Haworth Press.

Wolf, C., Schneider, S., Behr, D., & Joye, D. (2016). Harmonizing survey questions between cultures and over time. In C. Wolf, D. Joye, T. W. Smith, & Y. Fu (Eds.), *The SAGE handbook of survey methodology* (pp. 502–524). Sage. https://doi.org/10.4135/9781473957893

Hearan Koo is a senior researcher at the Korea Social Science Data Archive (KOSSDA), Seoul National University. Her research interests are social well-being, mental health, and comparative sociological methods.

Hye-ok Heo is a researcher at the Korea Social Science Data Archive (KOSSDA), Seoul National University. Her research interests include the FAIR data sharing and best practices for teaching and learning quantitative data management.

Yi-Fu Chen is an associate professor with the Department of Sociology at National Taipei University. His main research areas include sociology of crime and deviance, sociology of the family, and life course research. His research includes the efficacy of parenting programs, gene-by-environment interaction effects on young adults' internalizing and externalizing problems, and adolescent violence. He is also interested in topics, such as adolescent sexting and the impact of SNS on adolescent physical and mental health. His recent research projects include topics on youth employment, financial socialization among young adults, and digital lives of Taiwanese adolescents.

Tadahiko Maeda is an associate professor of Center for Social Data Structuring, Joint Support-Center for Data Science Research, Research Organization of Information and Systems (ROIS-DS). His research interest includes social survey methodology and quantitative study of Japanese National Character.

Development and Social Well-Being

Introduction to Part Two

Jaeyeol Yee

Well-being is usually measured at an individual level. However, it is important to recognize that social well-being is not merely the sum of individual well-being. Instead, it is a dynamic process that emerges from the way people interact with the world around them. It is crucial to avoid viewing individuals as separate entities, disconnected from their social circumstances. Pursuing a good life should be done in socially acceptable ways, with consideration for others in society. This is why we organized Part 2 as a collection of country reports.

Social well-being emphasizes the importance of interpersonal and societal experiences and behaviors. By adding the term 'social' to well-being, we focus on the relational nature of individuals' everyday life and their interactions with institutional and aspects of society. Therefore, social aspects of well-being require revealing the quality of social relations and society.

The quality of society is also important for the quality of individual life. A well-functioning society provides a favorable environment for people's quality of life and encourages individual actions and interactions with others. Institutions and social norms in a well-functioning society enhance predictability in people's interactions with the world and contribute to the sustainability of society. Research has shown that an individual's well-being is greatly influenced by the institutional context of their society, including factors such as government quality, social protection expenditure, and resource distribution.

Part 2 consists of country-specific well-being issues in five Asian societies: Mongolia, the Philippines, Japan, Korea, and Taiwan. The chapters demonstrate the interrelationship between the social, economic, and political backgrounds of the countries with well-being issues. As a result, when the issue of social well-being is discussed, important issues are invoked as triggers for framing the issues.

J. Yee (✉)
Department of Sociology, Seoul National University, Seoul, Republic of Korea
e-mail: jyyee@snu.ac.kr

J. Yee et al. (eds.), *Social Well-Being, Development, and Multiple Modernities in Asia*,
https://doi.org/10.1007/978-981-97-3866-3_4

Analyzing social well-being in diverse Asian countries with different historical paths is challenging. However, many authentic issues can be classified into two levels. The first level is related to physical, climate, and natural background. For instance, understanding social well-being in the Philippines requires acknowledging the impact of frequent natural disasters on vulnerable communities. Mongolia's life satisfaction is closely linked to its rapidly expanding mining industry. This is due to the growing importance of underground resources in a nomadic nation with a small population and vast territory consisting of grasslands and deserts.

Another issue is closely related to the level of institutional development and the quality of social life. In comparison to Mongolia or Southeast Asian countries like Vietnam, the Philippines, Indonesia, and Thailand, East Asian countries such as Japan, Korea, and Taiwan have achieved higher income levels and more commercialized social lives. However, to fully understand the well-being of the Japanese, it is necessary to consider the aftermath of the thirty-year recession that followed the 1990s, as well as the persisting effects of a dominant one-party system that is less responsive to the needs of the people. Similarly, while Korea and Taiwan have achieved rapid economic growth and democratization in recent decades, they are currently facing the paradox of affluence and democracy.

Chapter "Social Well-Being in the Extractive Economy in Mongolia: The Case of Mining Sector Trust and Social License" analyzes the impact of the expanding mining industry on the social well-being of Mongolia. Economic growth in Mongolia has a significant effect on community cohesion, which in turn affects individual well-being. While the mining industry is a major contributor to the country's economic growth, companies must maintain socially acceptable levels of trust and legitimacy to avoid harming social well-being. This chapter examines the social impact of the mining industry in the South Gobi region through the lens of social licensing. The authors strive to provide an objective evaluation of the industry's effects on the local community. The study shows that residents' well-being remains high, and there is no significant difference in trust compared to other groups. The findings suggest that mining companies must accommodate communities without disintegrating or negatively impacting them, requiring many aspects of social licensing.

Chapter "Social Capital and Well-Being: Interrogating Vulnerabilities and Adaptive Capacities and Resilience in Disaster-Prone Communities in the Philippines" discusses the Philippines, where vulnerabilities and well-being are closely linked to adaptive capacity and resilience in the face of disasters caused by heavy rain, typhoons, and earthquakes. The Philippines is widely recognized as one of the most disaster-prone countries globally. Therefore, the resilience of communities in the face of disasters is crucial in determining societal well-being. The authors suggest that trust and social capital are important during and after a disaster. Studies have shown that social capital, including bonding, bridging, and linking capital, helps communities build resilience. Trust in institutions is especially important, and the structure of social capital plays a crucial role in enhancing community resilience. The paper also emphasizes the significance of gender and regional differences.

Chapter "Social and Subjective Well-Being in Post-growth Japan: Adapting to New Inequalities" discusses Japan, where social and subjective well-being has declined since the 1990s. During the period of high growth, Japan was a relatively homogeneous and optimistic middle-class society. However, after experiencing a severe 30-year recession, it has transformed into a 'gap society', resulting in disparities in the labor market, marriage, and retirement. Moreover, social connections that were once robust are now weakening. The number of individuals who lack social support and are isolated is increasing, leading to a decline in hope for a better society. It is worth noting that despite this trend, the younger generation maintains a positive attitude.

Chapter "Beyond the Paradox of Affluence: The Korean Experience" discusses Korea, where despite rapid growth and democratization, Koreans are experiencing a paradox of affluence. This is evidenced by rising suicide rates, declining fertility rates, and decreasing happiness. The case of Korea exemplifies the paradox of declining social well-being despite remarkable economic growth and successful democratization. The chapter emphasizes the importance of social quality, particularly civil society capacity, in determining happiness. It is also demonstrated that competition based on status-seeking or sign-winning can have detrimental effects on happiness. The author emphasizes the importance of strengthening the basic pillars of society, such as fairness and transparency.

Chapter "When Economic Growth Is Gone: The Global Generation and Disparities in Happiness in Taiwan" discusses Taiwan, where the younger generation reports exceptionally high and well-maintained levels of happiness compared to other Asian and European countries. Taiwanese people, including the younger generation and the whole population, show higher life satisfaction compared to their East Asian neighbors. The study controlled for the effects of age, period, and cohort using the APC model. Contrary to the predictions of the global generation thesis, the younger generation holds an optimistic view of their current and future situations. The author explains that in Taiwan, the bond within families remains strong due to parents' financial support for their children's college education and allowing them to live with them until they find employment and settle down. This reduces conflicts between work and family. Cooperation and social capital facilitate the younger generation's optimism toward the future.

Jaeyeol Yee is a professor of sociology at Seoul National University and an international project member of the Center for Social Well-being Studies, Institute for the Development of Social Intelligence, Senshu University. He has contributed to the harmonization of social well-being surveys in Asia as director of the Korea Social Science Data Archives. His research interests include social quality, social well-being, social capital, disaster and safety issues, and sociological theory construction.

Social Well-Being in the Extractive Economy in Mongolia: The Case of Mining Sector Trust and Social License

Tselmegsaikhan Lkhagva, Bold Tsevegdorj, Batsugar Tsedendamba, Dashzeveg Lkhagvanorov, and Byambasuren Yadmaa

Abstract Debates about the relationship between economic growth and individual well-being, and between economic growth and community cohesion, are widespread. Resource-rich developing countries, especially those with extractive economies, grapple with challenging decisions, navigating the balance between economic growth and social well-being. This paper presents a case study that examines the state of trust among mining-affected communities and the relationship among different social groups, institutions, and mining companies in the Mongolia's extractive economy. Mongolia's recent mining expansion has brought boom and bust effects to the country's economic, social, and political life. The case study uses survey data collected from residents of the resource-rich South Gobi region, and we compare the results to those of the Mongolia's nationwide Social Well-being Survey. To measure trust in mining companies, we used Boutilier and Thomson's four dimensions of social license to operate in mining credibility, including economic legitimacy, sociopolitical legitimacy, interactional trust, and institutional trust. To measure societal trust and subjective well-being, we used methodologies aligned with the World Values Survey (WVS), the Organization for Economic Cooperation and Development (OECD), and the Asian Social Well-being Consortium. The results of the study show that the people in the South Gobi report higher levels of subjective well-being

T. Lkhagva (✉) · B. Tsedendamba · D. Lkhagvanorov
Independent Research Institute of Mongolia, Ulaanbaatar, Mongolia
e-mail: tselmegsaikhan@irim.mn

B. Tsedendamba
e-mail: batsugar@irim.mn

D. Lkhagvanorov
e-mail: dashzeveg@irim.mn

B. Yadmaa
National Academy of Governance, Ulaanbaatar, Mongolia
e-mail: ya.byambasuren@irim.mn

B. Tsevegdorj
National University of Mongolia, Ulaanbaatar, Mongolia
e-mail: bold@irim.mn

J. Yee et al. (eds.), *Social Well-Being, Development, and Multiple Modernities in Asia*,
https://doi.org/10.1007/978-981-97-3866-3_5

than the national average, while trust in social groups does not differ from the national trend. In terms of different dimensions of social license to operate and trust, citizens' economic acceptance of mining companies was relatively high, but sociopolitical acceptance and institutional trust were low. Thus, the paper attempts to explore the implications of communities' trust in the mining industry for their subjective well-being and social cohesion.

Keywords Subjective well-being · Trust · Mining · Social license to operate · Mongolia

1 Introduction

1.1 Social Well-Being and Trust

Which holds greater primacy—economic growth or social well-being? People are constantly searching for new concepts of social development that encompass more than economic growth, and one of them is social well-being. Scholars, such as Nussbaum and Sen, have noted that it is one-sided to measure the level of social development by economic indicators such as GDP per capita (Nussbaum & Sen, 1993). In countries around the world, the issues of social well-being issues have been studied in various ways. However, quantitative research on the impact of economic and social relations on the well-being of Mongolians is relatively rare.

It is interesting to see whether Easterlin's paradox that economic growth does not improve the well-being of ordinary citizens (Easterlin, 1974) or Veenhoven's thesis that economic growth improves the well-being of ordinary citizens (Veenhoven & Vergunst, 2014) can explain the current socioeconomic situation in Mongolia.

Over the past 30 years, migration from rural to urban areas has dominated in Mongolia, but recently, migration has increased to the new destination, the South Gobi Province.

What is driving this new trend? Is it the economic growth or improved social well-being? The South Gobi Province is a burgeoning mining center known for its growing importance in the extraction of valuable minerals, which has a significant impact on both the regional and national economies, making it a good place to assess social issues affected by mining. As noted by researcher Gundsambuu, "Mongolian society in the twentieth century is a remarkable laboratory for cognitive science" (Gundsambuu, 2002). We assumed that this was a perfect opportunity to test the conclusions of Eastirlin and Veenhoven by examining the well-being of the mining-affected area by comparing it to the overall well-being of Mongolia.

While the traditional approach to the study of well-being has primarily emphasized economic factors, recent trends, as exemplified by Portela et al. (2013), indicate a notable shift toward a heightened focus on social elements, particularly the significance of trust (Helliwell & Wang, 2010), bringing novel research perspectives to the field. Trust enhances subjective well-being and strengthens social cohesion.

We categorize trust into general trust and trust in social groups. Assessing citizens' trust in entrepreneurs helps gauge social cohesion and comprehend how business influence affects community well-being. Companies can operate peacefully as long as they do not harm community well-being. That is why it is crucial for companies, especially in the mining industry, to secure the recognition and support of the local community. Operating within the legal bounds is not enough; it is essential for companies to earn the gratitude and trust of local communities, emphasizing a critical aspect of corporate social responsibility. In this study, we measured social well-being, including *life satisfaction, cooperation, and trust,* using Cantril's ladder scale. The survey questionnaire, aligned with the OECD's Better Life Index manual, consisted of 11 chapters and 185 questions.

1.2 Social License to Operate

Social license is a sign of an organization's activities by its stakeholders, especially by the affected local community (Boutilier & Thomson, 2011). Today, in the age of ESG, the world's leading corporations are seriously trying to meet not only the legal and regulatory requirements, but also the expectations of the stakeholders, particularly local communities. Failure to meet these expectations not only risks business reputation, but also reduces business opportunities. In addition, it may lead to public resistance, strikes, and vandalism, or it may result in legal measures and financial risks, as a result of these actions. A lot of studies on public trust in mining areas in Australia, Chile, and China (Moffat & Zhang, 2014) show that trust is the basis on which the social license of mining business is attained from the local communities and stakeholders.

1.3 Analytical Approach for Categorizing the Social License to Operate (SLO)

Researcher Jeol Gehman explained that there are three different concepts to describe the social license to operate: the pyramid model (Boutilier & Thomson, 2011), the three strands model (Gunningham et al., 2004), and the triangle model (Wüstenhagen et al., 2007). **The pyramid model** describes the acceptance of the mining business hierarchically as a pyramid. In this model, acceptance through administrative tools is located at the bottom of the pyramid, acceptance through the result of active organizational collaboration is located in the middle section, and acceptance through the trust, communication, and shared value of all parties is located at the top. The

three-strand model considers that the operative social license is obtained as a result of three interdependent factors: legal license by ensuring legal requirements, social license by ensuring local requirements and the demands of other stakeholders, such as environmental activists, and economic license by ensuring the interests of investors and business owners. **The triangle model** considers three dimensions: the social, political, and legal acceptance; community acceptance; and market acceptance.

Furthermore, the recent study by Moffat and Zhang suggested that three types of integrity are required to acquire the social license to operate in mining and recommended that the most important factor is trust. Their analyses revealed that building trust with local communities is vital for mining firms to acquire and maintain a social license to operate. Negative impacts on social infrastructure, perceived contact quality, and procedural fairness significantly influenced community acceptance. This underscores the crucial role of equitable treatment, effective engagement, and impact mitigation for mining companies in securing and retaining a social license to operate (Moffat & Zhang, 2014).

In our study, we used Boutilier and Thomson's (2011) pyramid model, which is likely to focus on the framing of corporate social responsibility, and may be advantageous for assessing social license in Mongolian mining sector. In 2011, they tested a set of 15 items, that, according to their analysis, loaded on four latent factors, dubbed economic legitimacy, sociopolitical legitimacy, interactional trust, and institutionalized trust. On the other hand, this model has the advantage for comparison, as the model was tested in nine different languages in 11 countries (Boutilier, 2017).

The pyramid model illustrates the fluctuation in social license to operate (SLO) levels based on varying scores of the four factors (Fig. 1). In the bottom panel, with only economic legitimacy, SLO is confined to a high-risk region, and stakeholders mostly grant minimal acceptance. The middle panel, lacking sociopolitical legitimacy and institutionalized trust, results in fluctuating SLO, mostly at an acceptance level. The top panel, with economic and sociopolitical legitimacy and interactional trust, significantly increases the likelihood of SLO acceptance, with stakeholders often oscillating between acceptance and approval levels.

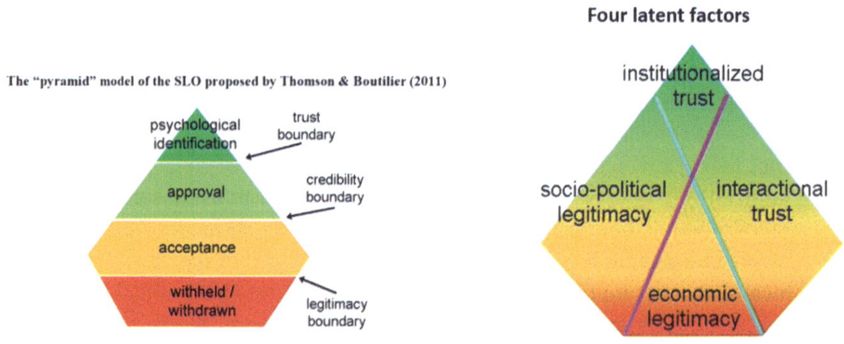

Fig. 1 Pyramid model of the social license to operate and four latent factors

2 Country Context

Mongolia is a landlocked country in Asia and is sandwiched between Russia to the north and China to the south. It is surrounded by the Altai Mountains in the west, the Khangai Khentii Mountains in the north, the Khyangan Mountains in the east, and the Great Gobi Desert in the south. The country has various types of land, including the Gobi, steppe, forest-steppe, and Siberian forest, so climate changes significantly affect the livelihood of the population. The administrative unit consists of 330 *soums* and 21 provinces along with the capital city of Ulaanbaatar. With a total population of 3.3 million, over 1.5 million (NSO, 2019), or 47%, live in the capital city Ulaanbaatar, while others live in the countryside. Certain researchers consider that Mongolia is a unique country with a distinctive lifestyle that combines both nomadic and sedentary lifestyles.

Mongolia's societal evolution, shaped by three historical revolutions, has moved from independence in 1911 to socialism in 1921 and, eventually, to a democratic system in 1990. This transformation involved a significant shift from a centrally planned to a free market economy, marked by the closure of state-owned industrial factories, resulting in economic challenges (Gundsambuu, 2002). Amidst this, the mining sector emerged as a pivotal economic force, accounting for a substantial portion of GDP, industrial production, exports, and foreign investment (NSO, 2019).

While the mining-driven economic development has had some positive effects on Mongolian society, it has also created a number of challenges. Issues such as social inequality, poverty, and the disproportionate increase in average salaries within and outside the mining sector have emerged. Moreover, the expansion of mining activities and population migration has led to problems such as negative public attitudes toward the sector, conflicts over coal transportation, and environmental degradation (NSO, 2018). A study on "Mining and Water Management in the South Gobi" revealed citizen distrust in the responsible use of water resources by mining companies (IRIM, 2013). Conflicts among herders over transport routes and environmental concerns have triggered opposition from citizens, NGOs, and interest groups (IRIM, 2012).

This underscores the need to measure the country's development, particularly citizens' well-being, not only through economic growth indicators, but also by evaluating individual opportunities for social well-being. Ronnås (2011) suggests that the emphasis should be on creating opportunities for each person rather than just measuring economic growth and GDP per capita.

Table 1 Results of the studies on the well-being of Mongolians

Name of the study	Date	Relevant indicator	Scale	Results	International average
Mongolia Happiness Index (NSO)	2016	Happy planet index	–	14.3	26.4
		Well being	0–10	4.9	5.4
Happiness, Hope, Economic Optimism (Gallup International)	2015	Happiness index	Percentage	71%	56%
		Hope index	Percentage	12%	38%
		Economic optimism index	Percentage	– 32%	23%
The Social Well-being Survey of Mongolia (IRIM)	2018	Happiness	0–10	8	5.3[1]; 4.9[2]
		Life satisfaction	0–10	7.8	6.8[3]; 6.5[4]
		Trust	0–10	4.7	5.4

3 Main Findings

3.1 General Trends in the Social Well-Being of Mongolians

Research and data on social cohesion and trust, pivotal indicators of societal and individual well-being derived from social development, are limited in Mongolia. In recent years, however, there has been a surge of innovative studies exploring the happiness and well-being of Mongolians. Table 1 presents the key findings from the primary research on the well-being of Mongolians.

A 2016 study by the National Statistical Office of Mongolia revealed that the happiness index in Mongolia is 1.8 times lower than the global average, ranking 136th out of 140 countries. In particular, it is 3.1 times lower than Costa Rica, the top-ranked country. In terms of well-being indicators, Mongolia ranks 90th, 2.9 points behind Switzerland and 2 points ahead of Togo.

According to the "Happiness, Hope, Economic Optimism" study conducted in 68 countries by Gallup International, Mongolians' trust and economic trust indexes were lower than the global average. However, the happiness index was found to be 15% higher than the global average.

Additionally, results from IRIM's "Social Well-being Survey of Mongolia" indicate that Mongolians have a relatively high levels of self-esteem and consider themselves to be happy—about 3 points higher than the global average. This level in line with Nordic countries, which are known for their high levels of happiness. The survey also revealed significant differences in happiness responses based on demographic characteristics. For instance, people living in rural areas, those who were married, and those who were employed tended to report higher levels of happiness than their

[1] World Happiness Report, 2018.

[2] Gallup World Poll, 2018.

[3] World Values Survey, 2014.

[4] OECD (Better Life Index), 2017.

counterparts living in urban areas, those who were unmarried, and those who were the unemployed.

3.2 *Life Satisfaction*

Mongolians are highly satisfied with their lives (7.8), with happiness indicators surpassing the international average (6.8). By comparison, Scandinavian countries have an average life satisfaction rate of 7.5, while Syrians, Burundians, and Central Africans have the lowest life satisfaction at 3.0. Notably, factors such as education, employment, and income levels did not affect life satisfaction among Mongolians. However, responses varied based on health status, social support, freedom to make decisions, and whether individuals lived in rural or urban areas.

3.3 *Cooperation*

To assess the propensity to cooperate with various groups, representatives of various segments of society were queried about their willingness to cooperate with nine different groups. Results are shown in Fig. 2.

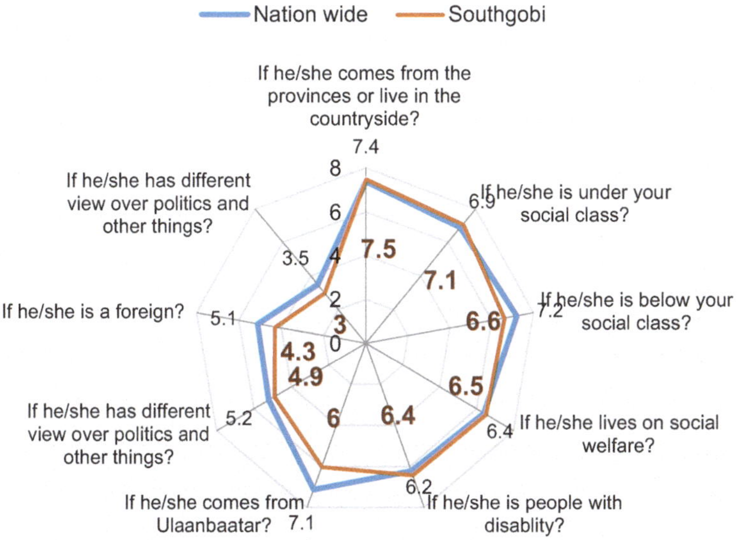

Fig. 2 Willingness to cooperate with others (10 very interested in cooperating; 0-not interested in cooperating)

These results show that citizens have limited interest in cooperating with LGBT people and foreigners. The low willingness to cooperate with the LGBT community can be explained by the lack of understanding and information among the public. Notably, the South Gobi Province has a large number of foreign-invested mining companies, but trust in foreigners is lower than the national average of 0.8. This indicates that foreign workers are struggling to gain the trust of local citizens.

Table 2 shows the results of whether the respondents were willing to help different groups in the community and, conversely, whether these groups were willing to reciprocate.

Interesting results were found in the mutual willingness to help, as most of the people rated themselves as willing to help others rather than relying on other groups to help them. People are willing to help their surrounding community or the close people in the social circle, anticipating reciprocal help from them. This suggests that a greater social distance weakens willingness to help. Notably, people show less willingness to help people of different nationalities, different religious beliefs, and LGBT people. These findings are consistent with the assertion that "*the social cohesion of Mongolians is traditional and is family-centered*".

Table 2 Willingness to help others

	Classifications	I am willing to help people if they are... (%)	I think people are willing to help me if they are... (%)	Difference (%)
1	Family members	99.6	99.1	0.5
2	Relatives	99.1	97.2	0.9
3	Co-workers/ colleagues	98.9	96.3	2.6
4	Friends	98.3	95.9	2.4
5	People with disability	96.9	73.2	23.7
6	My neighbors	93.0	86.3	6.7
7	People from different provinces	90.2	73.4	16.8
8	Strangers	70.2	38.8	31.4
9	People of different nationalities	68.2	48.4	19.8
10	People with different religious beliefs	64.3	52.9	11.4
11	LGBT people	45.5	34.0	11.5

3.4 *Trust*

Although Mongolians generally have cautious tendencies in their interactions with others, as reflected in relatively low scores on trusting fellow individuals, Larsen's analysis of the 2014 World Value Survey data indicates that only five out of 52 countries responded positively to the statement "can trust most people." Mongolians exhibit a tendency toward traditional and mechanical solidarity, demonstrating trust and a willingness to cooperate with groups that share similar characteristics. This can be attributed to Mongolia's preservation of traditional social attributes. Mutual trust forms the foundation of social cohesion, with higher levels of cohesion contingent upon mutual credibility, cooperation, trust, and mutual assistance among diverse social groups. The study posits that "the social cohesion of Mongolians is traditional and family-centered".

3.4.1 General Trust

We aimed to explore whether the enhancement of the economic conditions of the residents in the mining province, brings a change in the general trust. Our hypothesis suggested that the general trust of citizens in South Gobi Province differs from the national level. The results reveal that the overall level of general trust among local respondents is low. When asked about trusting other people and the need for caution in communication, the average score was 4.6 (compared to the national average of 4.7).

On the question of whether most people would use them or be fair, respondents gave an average score of 6.2, relatively high compared to the national average of 4.7. Despite the changes brought about by the mining boom, the traditional social relations have remained unchanged, with nomadic people helping each other to survive in the face of harsh climatic conditions and a sparse population.

3.4.2 Trust in Social Groups

Figure 3 shows the average level of trust people have for different groups of people.

The survey indicates significant differences in trust levels among different groups. Trust is higher for close relationships, but it decreases as social distance increases. The level of trust among South Gobi residents toward other groups is 1.0 point higher than that of the general Mongolian population. Despite this higher level of trust, the general pattern of trust remains the same, as a family-centered type. Contrary to the hypothesis, the general trust of citizens in the mining area is consistent with the general trust pattern in Mongolia, which has not unchanged over a decade of mining activity. However, the trust toward foreigners of South Gobi residents is lower than that of the national sample, indicating that general trust may change in the future.

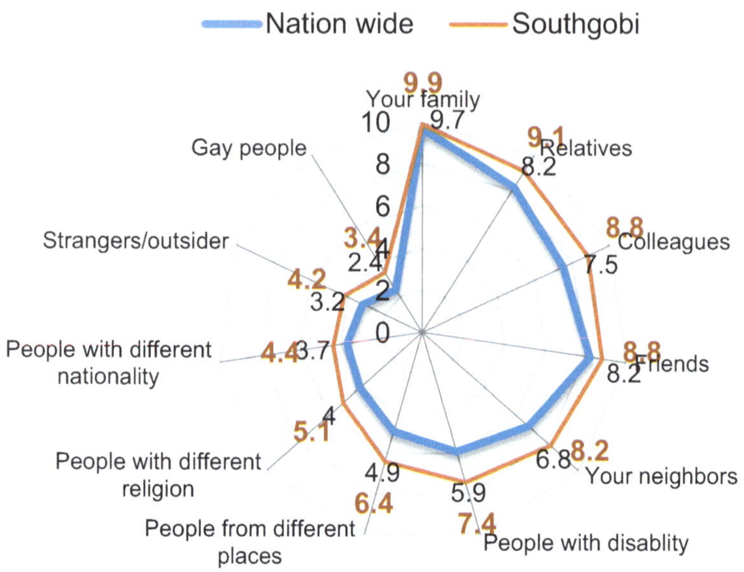

Fig. 3 Trust in others, by average

3.5 *Factor Analysis on the Model of Social License*

A key component of this study was an assessment of the social license to operate of mining companies. This assessment was conducted using four factors—economic legitimacy, interactional trust, sociopolitical legitimacy, and institutional trust—comprising a total of 15 indicators. To ensure the accuracy of the classification of these 15 indicators into the four factors, a reliability analysis was performed.

Four factors were equally weighed as ¼. In addition, each indicator belonging to each factor was equally weighed. For instance, the indicators belonging to the economical legitimacy of mining company were weighed 1/12 (1/4 * 3). ($\sum_{i=1}^{d} w_i = 1$) (Table 3).

The assessment of economic legitimacy of mining company was 7.29 as the correlation of its component was KMO $= 0.69$, $\chi^2(10) = 581.52, p < 0.001$ as Bartlett's test of sphericity, and the main factor explains 77% of the total variation. 581.52, $p < 0.001$ as Bartlett's test of sphericity, and the main factor in this chapter explains 77% of the total variation. As for interactional trust, the result was 4.8, KMO $= 0.74$ for the components, Bartlett's test of sphericity result was $\chi^2(10) = 376.31, p < 0.001$, and the main factor explains 80% of the total variation. The assessment result of the sociopolitical legitimacy of mining company was 5.5, KMO $= 0.81$ for the components of this factor, Bartlett's test of sphericity result was $\chi^2(10) = 471.25, p < 0.001$, and the main factor explains 80% of the total variation.

The result of the assessment of institutional trust was 3.73, as the correlation of its component was KMO $= 0.84$, Bartlett's test of sphericity result was $\chi^2(10) =$

Table 3 Assessment results on factors and indicators

	Question	Average	Weigh
1. *Economic legitimacy of mining company—7.29*			1/4
M1	We can gain from a relationship with the mining company	7.29	1/12
M2	We need to have the cooperation of the mining company to reach our most important goals	7.52	1/12
M5	The presence of the mining company is a benefit to us	7.35	1/12
2. *Interactional trust of mining company—4.8*			1/4
M3	The mining company does what is says it will do in its relations with our organization	5.13	1/12
M4	We are very satisfied with our relation with the mining company	4.96	1/12
M6	The mining company listens to us	4.45	1/12
3. *Sociopolitical legitimacy of mining company—5.5*			1/4
M7	In the long term, the mining company makes a contribution to the well-being of the whole region	6.72	1/16
M8	The mining company treats everyone fairly	4.03	1/16
M9	The mining company respects our way of doing things	4.91	1/16
M10	Our organization and the mining company have a similar vision for the future of this region	5.67	1/16
4. *Institutionalized trust of mining company—3.73*			1/4
M11	The mining company gives more support to those who it negatively affects	5.05	1/20
M12	The mining company shares decision-making with us	3.98	1/20
M13	The mining company takes account of our interests	2.96	1/20
M14	The mining company is concerned about our interests	2.96	1/20
M15	The mining company openly shares information that is relevant to us	3.29	1/20
The average value of trust given to the mining organization		4.40	

Table 4 Alpha coefficients of Cronbach

Factor	#of variables in the given factor	Alpha coefficients of Cronbach
Economic legitimacy of mining company	3	0.85
Interactional trust of mining company	3	0.86
Sociopolitical legitimacy of mining company	4	0.85
Institutional trust	5	0.91
Total factors	15	0.94

1140.31, $p < 0.001$, and the factor explains 77% of the total variation. Compared with the other factors, the rate of economical legitimacy is much higher. Table 4 shows the results of reliability analysis on the abovementioned four factors by Alpha coefficients of Cronbach.

For all factors, the alpha coefficient is greater than 0.85, indicating that all four factors are reliable. In addition, the alpha coefficient is 0.94 for all components, indicating that the factors are entirely reliable.

3.6 Evaluation on Social License

When conducting the assessment, the 11 scales (starting from 0 to 10) used to measure subjective well-being were conferted to Boutlilier's scaling (starting from 1 to 5) using detailed statistical calculations, and the following corresponding values were obtained (Table 5).

As a result of the study, the legitimacy boundary is indicated by a value above 2.5, the credibility boundary is determined by a value above 5.5, while the trust boundary is reached at a relatively high value of 8.5. The comparison of this study with the study on trust in the South Gobi Province shows that in order to overcome the trust boundary of the citizens, the operating mining companies must be rated in the ranks of family (9.9), relative (9.1), co-workers (8.8), and friends (8.8). If the mining companies operating in the South Gobi Province are rated at the neighborhood level, the operations will be fully approved. If the rating is below 2.5, the initiative to stop mining operations in South Gobi Province will be instigated by local communities. In detailed estimates, the economic legitimacy (7.29) of mining companies in South Gobi reaches a fully operational level, and as shown in the Tomson and Boutilier model, basic social licensing is consistent with "economic legitimacy". However, their institutional trust (3.73) is somewhat recognized.

The overall assessment of social license is 4.4, which indicates that the mining companies in the South Gobi have reached a "fully recognized" level by crossing the legitimacy boundaries and are closer to the credibility boundary. To reach this level,

Table 5 Equivalence of the scaling

Related mean of Tomson and Boutilier's evaluation gap	Related level	Related mean of IRIM's evaluation gap
1–2.40	Withheld/withdrawn	0–2.5
Legitimacy boundary		
2.4–3.08	Low acceptance/tolerance	2.5–4.2
3.08–3.56	High acceptance/tolerance	4.2–5.5
Credibility boundary		
3.56–3.93	Low approval	5.5–6.6
3.93–4.3	High approval	6.6–8.5
Trust boundary		
4.3–5	Full trust	8.5–10

Source Results of research conducted by IRIM and "A Measure of the Social License to Operate for Infrastructure and Extractive Projects" by Boutilier (2017)

the economic acceptability has increased significantly, but the institutional trust has decreased. The fact that mining companies do not take local interests into account has influenced the assessment.

Responses to the general trust question "*Generally, do you think people are kind and helpful to each other, or just mind their own business?*" were compared with responses to 15 questions about social license. Citizens answered "mining companies will contribute to the local well-being in the long term", with a negative statistical significance (− 0.31) indicating that people assume mining to have a negative impact on their well-being in the long run. When compared to the life satisfaction question of "*out of 10 ladders, on which step of the ladder would you say you personally feel you stand at this time?*", all responses were statistically insignificant. Although the economic legitimacy factor of the social license to operate reflects the full level of acceptance, the negative and statistically insignificant results indicate that the citizens do not provide answers that confirm that the mining-related economic development improves well-being. This supports the argument that economic development in the South Gobi does not significantly contribute to the enhanced well-being of its citizens, which is consistent with Easterlin's paradox that economic growth does not necessarily translate into improved well-being for the general population. At the same time, the findings of the study do not agree woyj Veenhoven's thesis that there is a positive correlation between economic growth and the well-being of ordinary citizens.

4 Conclusion

In Mongolia, there is a critical need for research that focuses on subjective well-being, a key measure of social well-being, along with factors such as social cohesion and trust that regulate social development. The study reveals that Mongolians generally hold a high self-esteem about their happiness and exhibit higher life satisfaction compared to similarly developed countries.

In terms of trust, individuals are willing to help close friends and their immediate community, but this willingness diminishes as the social circle extends. Trust toward strangers, including those of different nationalities, religions, and sexual orientations, is relatively low, supporting the hypothesis that Mongolian social cohesion is traditional and family-centered.

However, there is no significant shift in the nature of trust in the mining development area of South Gobi Province. While the level of trust among South Gobi residents is 1.0 point higher than the national average, the general pattern of trust is very similar to the national sample, refuting the hypothesis of a distinct general trust in mining development areas.

If one equates Boutilier's social license evaluation on a scale of 0–10, the legitimacy threshold is set above 2.5, the credibility threshold above 5.5, and the trust threshold at a relatively high value of 8.5. A score below 2.5 could lead local communities to advocate for a halt to mining operations in the South Gobi. However, mining companies with a social license score of 4.4, which is close crossing the credibility boundary, fare reasonably well.

The study finds that general issues of trust and life satisfaction are not strongly linked to social license considerations. This suggests a common perception among citizens that mining-related economic development does not improve their well-being. This indicates that people expect mining growth to have a negative impact on their well-being and doubt about the idea that mining-driven economic development improves well-being. Despite objective measures of social well-being, such as rising GDP per capita, chronic poverty, and increased inequality, which support Easterlin's paradox, citizens maintain skeptical about the positive effects of mining-related economic development on their overall well-being.

Acknowledgements The contributions and thoughtful analysis in the development of this chapter are sincerely appreciated. Gratitude is extended to Byambasuren Yadmaa, Byambasuren Dorjnyambuu, and Dolgion Aldar for their invaluable efforts. The quality and depth of the work has been significantly enhanced by their expertise and dedication.

Bibliography

Boutilier, R. (2017). *A measure of the social license to operate for infrastructure and extractive projects*. Available at SSRN 3204005.

Boutilier, R., & Thomson, I. (2011). Modelling and measuring the social license to operate: fruits of a dialogue between theory and practice. *Social Licence, 1*, 1–10.
Easterlin, R. A. (1974). *Does economic growth improve the human lot? some empirical evidence.* in *nations and households in economic growth* (pp. 89–125). Academic Press.
Gundsambuu, Kh. (2002). *Mongolian social stratification: Development and trends.* Academy of Science.
Gunningham, N., Kagan, R. A., & Thornton, D. (2004). Social license and environmental protection: why businesses go beyond compliance. *Law & Social Inquiry, 29*(2), 307–341.
Helliwell, J. F., & Wang, S. (2010). *Trust and well-being.* (No. w15911). National Bureau of Economic Research. Working paper series.
IRIM. (2012). *Truck drivers survey.* Commissioned by ADB.
IRIM. (2013). *Public perception survey of mining and groundwater management in the South Gobi.*
Moffat, K., & Zhang, A. (2014). The paths to social licence to operate: An integrative model explaining community acceptance of mining. *Resources Policy, 39*, 61–70.
National Statistical Office of Mongolia. (2018). *Economic growth, poverty and unemployment relations survey.*
National Statistical Office of Mongolia. (2019). *Annual inflation rate.*
Nussbaum, M., & Sen, A. (Eds.). (1993). *The quality of life.* Clarendon Press.
Portela, M., Neira, I., & Salinas-Jiménez, M. D. M. (2013). Social capital and subjective wellbeing in Europe: A new approach on social capital. *Social Indicators Research, 114*, 493–511.
Ronnås, P. (2011). *Challenges for achieving job-rich and inclusive growth in Mongolia* (No. 994658443402676). International Labour Organization.
Veenhoven, R., & Vergunst, F. (2014). The Easterlin illusion: Economic growth does go with greater happiness. *International Journal of Happiness and Development, 1*(4), 311–343.
Wüstenhagen, R., Wolsink, M., & Bürer, M. J. (2007). Social acceptance of renewable energy innovation: An introduction to the concept. *Energy Policy, 35*(5), 2683–2691.

Tselmegsaikhan Lkhagva holds Master of Sociology and Development Studies, and she is Executive Director of the Independent Research Institute of Mongolia (IRIM). She studies social impact and gender dimensions in the extractive sector, and urban and rural changes.

Bold Tsevegdorj holds a master's degree in Sociology, is a founder and board member of the Independent Research Institute of Mongolia (IRIM). His research areas include social changes, social wellbeing and democracy.

Batsugar Tsedendamba is a Master of Sociology, and he works at the Independent Research Institute of Mongolia (IRIM) as a consultant. His study areas are governance, democracy and civic space.

Dashzeveg Lkhagvanorov is a Master of Sociology, works as a senior researcher at the Independent Research Institute of Mongolia (IRIM). His areas of specialization include social surveys, social impact assessments, monitoring and evaluation, workshop facilitation, and project management.

Byambasuren Yadmaa is a Board Member of IRIM and serves as the faculty at the National Academy of Governance, Mongolia. With a PhD in Public Administration, he brings over 30 years of experience in public administration, public policy and social development.

Social Capital and Well-Being: Interrogating Vulnerabilities and Adaptive Capacities and Resilience in Disaster-Prone Communities in the Philippines

Emma Porio and Justin See

Abstract A burgeoning literature has found that social capital and trust networks play a central role in disaster recovery and developing community resilience. However, little is known about the structure of social capital, trust networks, and other infrastructural ties among disaster-prone communities in the Philippines. To address this gap, this study interrogates the role that social capital play among vulnerable groups in the Philippines and unpacks its implications in advancing resilience building initiatives. Drawing on a national survey of 1200 respondents, this study has three key findings. First, there is a significant difference on trust levels according to gender: males tend to have stronger institutional ties than females. Second, there exists a regional imbalance in terms of the distribution of social capital and social well-being. The farther the respondents are from Metro Manila, the higher their trust networks and social well-being outcomes are. Third, formally organized groups like neighborhood associations, civic organizations, national/local government units, and their agencies have a critical role to play in working with communities to build resilience to natural disasters. The study ultimately finds that social well-being is highly correlated with social capital: those who are included in social networks tend to exhibit better health and well-being outcomes across the country.

E. Porio (✉)
Department of Sociology and Anthropology, Ateneo de Manila University, Quezon City, Philippines
e-mail: eporio@ateneo.edu

Manila Observatory, Quezon City, Philippines

J. See
Anthropology and Development Studies, The University of Melbourne, Parkville, Victoria, Australia
e-mail: justin.see@unimelb.edu.au

J. Yee et al. (eds.), *Social Well-Being, Development, and Multiple Modernities in Asia*,
https://doi.org/10.1007/978-981-97-3866-3_6

1 Introduction

The Philippines is highly at risk to climate disasters. The 2018 World Risk Report ranks the Philippines as the third most vulnerable country in the world to natural disasters (Heintz et al., 2018). Thus, it is very important to understand the contextual drivers of disaster preparedness, response, recovery, and resilience of disaster-prone communities. Previous studies (e.g., Aldrich, 2018; Porio, 2015) found that social capital and trust networks play a central role in disaster recovery and developing community resilience. For example, Dapilah et al. (2020) demonstrate how membership in organized groups enhanced the adaptive capacity of a rural community in Ghana by facilitating livelihood diversification and the introduction of new farming techniques. Likewise, Moore and Westley (2011) contend that social networks enable the sharing of knowledge and information, which can help build adaptive capacity.

Meanwhile, climate and disaster impacts to marginal and vulnerable communities (Porio, 2016; Porio & See, 2023; Baptiste et al., 2011), especially women, children, and elderly, who usually bear the brunt of the impacts of floods, typhoons, and drought have not received much attention. In the aftermath of the 2009 Tropical Storm Ketsana in Metro Manila, Porio (2014) found that women-headed households incurred more losses and expenditures for basic necessities before, during, and after the storm. In the 2020 post-Ulysses (international name, Vampo) assessment, Karaos and Nicolas (2021) found that relocatees, originally from poor, marginal, and environmentally insecure riverine communities of the Pasig riverlines, were adversely affected by the strong winds and floods. In their relocation, communities of Kasiglahan, Montalban, described their experience as worse than in their original slum and squatter community. Relocated residents, inundated with floods with some of their houses washed out, told the authors, "it seemed like our lives jumped from the frying pan to the fire"! They survived during the first three days after the floods with the help of their families, relatives, and neighbors. After that, relief goods came in trickles from non-governmental organisations (NGOs) and the local government, because the latter was also a victim of the typhoon and flooding in the area.

In many post-disaster stories of survival and resilience, community residents always talk of social relations among families, relatives, and community networks providing support for recovery and rehabilitation. But while women leaders and social networks are central to the disaster response and recovery of communities, rarely are their roles and functions as embedded in these social, political, economic structures and processes discussed in disaster resilience efforts. This study interrogates the role of social capital among vulnerable groups, especially women and their families, neighbors and community members, and their efforts toward recovery and resilience. This chapter is structured as follows. First, we introduce the concepts of social capital, trust networks, social infrastructural ties, and community resilience. Second, we present the research questions that this paper seeks to address. Third, we present the key findings from our national survey on social capital and trust networks. Finally, we discuss what the findings mean and how it contributes to our knowledge in understanding social capital, trust networks, and how it contributes to building community resilience in the Philippines, especially among the vulnerable groups and communities who are highly exposed to climate and disaster risks such as typhoons, floods, and earthquakes. In some conflict-ridden areas in Mindanao, impacts from climate disasters are greatly heightened by displacement of people and their livelihoods.

This paper argues that in post-disaster communities, different components of social capital are mobilized according to their levels of social and locational vulnerabilities and capacities. More importantly, the mobilization of community and/or institutional resources by different genders and socioeconomic groups can be differentiated according to the dimension of social capital being mobilized in various types of political and cultural spaces for transforming capacities and building community resilience. These types of social capital mobilization reflect how people employ strategically the social infrastructure and civic ties in their community's significant spaces and places to construct and maintain their social ties and trust networks to support their quality of life (Aldrich, 2018; Porio, 2022). This is especially crucial in hazard-prone areas, where both bridging and linking capital are low, especially among low-income communities.

By analyzing how different components of social capital are mobilized by different status groups in different urban and rural regions of the Philippines, the paper hopes to contribute to understanding the structure of adaptive capacities and community resilience in post-disaster Philippines and Southeast Asia. It draws from the International Survey of Social Well Being Regional Consortium or SWB database organized by the Senshu University. The insights and analysis in this chapter weaves together the findings from the national survey in the Philippines in 2016[1] and the presentations of SWB consortium members and/or colleagues at the Social Well-Being Consortium Conferences in the region.[2]

2 Social Capital, Trust Networks, and Post-disaster Recovery and Community Resilience

Every year, the Philippines experiences an average of 20 typhoons and tropical storms, and the eventual flooding inundation to cities and communities threaten the lives, strength, and stability of the urban–rural poor in many highly exposed and vulnerable coastal and upland communities (Porio, 2011, 2014; Porio and See, 2023). Yet responses to the challenges of building community recovery and resilience nationwide vary greatly and cannot be explained by the magnitude of the catastrophic

---

[1] I am very grateful to the intellectual generosity of Professor Hiroo Harada, Professor Masayuki Kanai, Dr. Keitaro Yazaki, Professor Jaeyeol Yee, Dr. Surichai Wungaeo, Dr. Czarina Saloma, Dr. Jowel Canuday, Dr Enrique Leviste and Professor Ricardo Abad for their support of this study.

[2] SWB Regional Conferences in Senshu University (February 2015 and June 2016), Chulalongkorn University (March 2017), University of Indonesia (March 2018).

hazards that hit them nor the amount of aid received from their national governments and the international humanitarian community (Aldrich, 2018; Porio, 2014). In his classic work, Aldrich (2018) succinctly explained that the difference between social resilience and despair in disaster-prone communities is social capital and how these are ***differentially*** mobilized by different status groups and localities in finding solutions to their everyday problems and most especially during and post-disaster situations.

Aldrich (2018), in *Building Resilience,* highlights the critical role of social capital in the ability of a community to withstand disaster and rebuild both the infrastructure and the personal and institutional ties that are at the foundation of any community. Aldrich examines the post-disaster responses of four distinct communities—Tokyo following the 1923 earthquake, Kobe after the 1995 earthquake, Tamil Nadu after the 2004 Indian Ocean Tsunami, and New Orleans after 2005 hurricane Katrina—and finds that those with robust social networks were better able to coordinate community recovery activities. In the process, they were able to build their families' and communities' immediate, medium, and long-term recovery initiatives toward resilience (Porio, 2017a, 2017b, 2017c). Social capital and trust networks were crucial in quickly disseminating information and financial and physical assistance. Communities, then, with abundance of social capital were able to minimize the out-migration and displacement of people and valuable resources out of the area, which contributed to their long-term recovery, robustness of their social structure, and institutions. Aldrich (2018) concluded that the difference between resilience and disrepair lies in the depth of communities' social capital and summarized this in his concept of social infrastructural ties. In Aldrich (2021),[3] however, he advances the concept of social infrastructure, but this paper prefers the original concept.

Aside from the established link between social capital and community resilience, a number of studies in disaster-prone communities in Southeast Asia have linked social capital to a variety of health outcomes and measures of well-being. Yee et al. (2016) argue that social well-being does not only depend on economic and market forces but on non-economic ones like social capital. Wun'gaeo et al. (2017) found that social capital in Bangkok and its surrounds has a higher effect on social well-being than measures of economic development. Kawachi et al. (2004) discovered that there is an association between social capital indicators such as civic engagement and membership in organizations and lower mortality and better mental health.

Social capital. In understanding disasters and community resilience, earlier works (Aldrich, 2013, 2017; Bourdieu, 1985; Cai, 2017; Portes, 1998; Putnam, 2000a, 2000b; Porio, 2017a, 2017b, 2017c) have noted how there has been a neglect of attention toward social infrastructure. Much attention has been given toward physical infrastructures such as the establishment of buildings, bridges, roads, and walls/levees to protect people from risks brought about by natural hazards. Aldrich and Meyer (2015) explained that there should be a redirection of attention from the physical to

[3] In his webinar presentation, Social Resilience in a Disrupted World, March 25, 2021, Aldrich uses the word social infrastructure, but in this paper, I will stick to the word, social infrastructural ties.

the social infrastructure (e.g., social capital, trust networks, strength of institutional ties, etc.) as alternative factors in addressing or mitigating disasters.

Social capital, as a component of the social infrastructure, is referred to as "the networks that connect individuals to each other" (Aldrich, 2017). This connection exhibits a mutual benefit between and among the individuals and communities (Porio, 2016; Portes, 1998; Putnam, 2000a, 2000b). This relationship is conversational and impartial, which may be classified in either of the three types—bonding, bridging, and linking social capital. Putnam (2000a, 2000b: 22) makes a distinction between bonding and bridging social capital, arguing that bridging social capital is "outward looking and encompasses people across diverse social cleavages" while bonding social capital consists of "inward looking networks that tend to reinforce exclusive identities and homogeneous groups". Another kind of social capital—linking capital—was proposed by Woolcock (1998) as links formed by communities with economic, political, and social institutions. It refers to relationships established with people in authority, such as the government. According to Aldrich and Meyer (2015), both bonding and bridging social capital are classified as horizontal ties, while linking social capital is at the vertical tie (Aldrich and Meyer 2015). Abad (2005, 2017), Putnam (2000a, 2000b), and others, however, argue that bridging social capital reflects the associational or institutional ties that people have and could either have horizontal and/or vertical dimensions and effects in terms of status, power, and authority. Eventually, these factors would shape the structure of distribution of resources in pre- and post-disaster communities.

Implicit in these above-mentioned works is the idea that bonding social capital is good for "getting by" but bridging and linking social capital are essential for "getting ahead" (Leonard, 2004). Previous studies[4] (e.g., Abad 2006, 2017; Adger et al., 2007; Aldrich 2018), however, have argued that the distribution of social capital by socioeconomic status (i.e., income, education, and occupation) and gender in the Philippines is uneven, with low-income groups and women possessing less bridging and linking social capital. This uneven distribution of social capital affects the social and political capacities of different status groups (gender, ethnicity, and class) to mobilize resources beyond the domestic sphere of influence toward building climate and disaster resilience in their communities, institutions, and beyond. Yet the domestic care and well-being of household members hinged largely on the hands of women and low-salaried service workers, given the structure and design of the country's community health care and social services systems. This uneven distribution of social capital affects their capacities to mobilize community/institutional resources for recovery and building resilience, especially during and after flooding disasters. This paper seeks to contribute to these on-going debates by examining the structure of social capital in disaster-prone communities in the Philippines according to their social location (i.e., gender, socioeconomic strata, and related factors of inherent vulnerability) and geo-physical/locational vulnerability.

Embedded in these structural processes are issues of distributive and procedural justice. Distributive justice involves the "distribution of benefits, costs, risks, and

[4] I am grateful to Ms. Faye Gutierrez for her assistance in doing the review of literature.

harms among human beings" (Ali, 2006, p. 2) while procedural justice includes questions of who participates, on what terms, and how decisions are made (Martin et al., 2014). Both types of justice are not only associated with recovery assistance programs; they are also inextricably linked to social capital, trust, and social infrastructural ties in the community. In their survey of post-Haiyan communities in the municipalities of Eastern and Western Samar, See and Porio (2015) found that those who had strong political and institutional ties with the local health system and local governments declared they received timely help and assistance which eventually resulted in better health outcomes. Conversely, those who did not have routine contact with barangay health workers felt isolated, did not receive much help, and did not enjoy good health status before or after Haiyan (See & Porio, 2015). Upon closer scrutiny, See and Porio (2015) found that the ways that administrative and legislative procedures were crafted to favor those with better social capital compared to those who did not, and these were linked to better resource access and outcomes for these particular groups. And women, with their ease in constructing relationships with social workers, community health workers, and local education officials/teachers before, during, and after disaster situations, are able to source aid and help from social protection agencies and the like. But our study also found that those women with higher income, higher education, and leader capacities within marginal communities are more efficient in mobilizing these social-political–economic infrastructural ties (See & Porio, 2015).

Levels of trust in institutions. Trust in institutions has also been found by the World Values Survey (1981) to account for societal progress and stability. According to Lars Tragardh of the Ersta Skondal University College (Stockholm), Nordic societies have maintained their level of progress and development through "statist individualism" where the Nordics believe that the state's main job is to promote individual autonomy and social stability. Thus, any policy or law like the family laws in recent years provide for universal free education for students of all backgrounds to achieve their potential. Separate taxation of spouses puts wives on equal footing with their husbands while universal day care for children makes it possible for both parents to work full-time. Both maternity and paternity leaves are also available (The Economist Special Report 2013). The World Values Survey (2014) also showed that while in most Nordic countries, about 60 percent of their citizens have trust in state institutions and other social systems, in countries like Mexico, Turkey, and Philippines, only about 10 percent of the population have trust in state-related institutions (cited in Porio, 2015). Meanwhile, with governments increasingly overstretched by the increasing incidence and intensity of natural and human-induced disasters, a thorough understanding of what contributes to efficient disaster relief and reconstruction is more important than ever. Aldrich (2018) underscores a critical component of an effective disaster response, which leads us to a better understanding of how the foundation for community resilience can and should not be constructed (Porio 2014, 2017a, 2017b, 2017c).

Community resilience. According to Aldrich (2018), community recovery after climate disasters is more than just a bottle of water and batteries. By this, he means that post-disaster recovery is not just a matter of distributing rice, noodles, sardines, and old clothes/blankets. Instead, it demands a far more strategic framework of developing livelihood, and physical and social infrastructure resilience (Porio 2017a, 2017b, 2017c). Montana-Leblanc (2008), in discussing the disastrous post-Katrina recovery efforts, argues that the reason widows were excluded was not because of social capital but because of their exclusion from the community and their being marginalized from the councils responsible for the allocation and distribution of relief aid and goods to the neighborhoods and districts. Meanwhile in the Indian tsunami post-disaster recovery, Aldrich (2018) points to the exclusion of widows from post-tsunami aid. He argues that this exclusion was not the result of women being outside their societies but the effect of their being politically impotent in the councils that managed aid delivery. And oftentimes, this impotence is rooted in the patron–client relationships embedded in the systems of power and privilege in the community social structure. As will be shown later in this paper, social capital and other social infrastructural ties do not really explain the uneven distribution of post-disaster relief, rehabilitation and recovery assistance, and eventual disrepair or resilience but rather how the ***structure of social capital*** shaped the crafting and design of institutional procedures associated with allocation of resources in post-disaster communities (Porio 2017a, 2017b, 2017c).

Social ties play a vital role in providing services, assistance, and aid before, during, and after disasters. As Aldrich (2018) describes it, social capital and social ties are the "real drivers of resilience." This is manifested in the different types of social capital—bonding (horizontal), bridging (horizontal-vertical),[5] and linking (vertical). The neighbors, which had shared spaces with that of the other neighbors, are described as the "first responders" (Aldrich and Meyer 2015; Porio, 2018). The assistance offered by neighbors could be caused by their shared interests and/or associations. This could be the same as those ties with family, relatives, and friends, still found with horizontal ties. The vertical connections found in bridging and/or the linking ties are the best predictors or measurement of a community's resilience (Porio, 2015; Aldrich, 2018). If individuals and communities are capable enough of establishing a connection or network with people of authority, then the level of resiliency of that community is high. But Aldrich (2018) argues that bridging and bonding social capitals only reduces the feeling of despair or anxiety of the community. That such social capital "helps people 'get by' but does not boost them enough to 'get ahead' (Aldrich, 2011)." But as Abad (2006) and I argued earlier (Porio, 2018), bridging social capital represents associational ties with community-based organizations and/ or civil society organizations who have different capacities from the local residents and can provide links to external resources during relief and recovery efforts. In fact, in the Philippines, while most of the ***ayuda*** or assistance to urban poor communities or informal settlements were supplied by the CSOs and the private sector, these

[5] I added the vertical dimension of bridging social capital representing associational ties as they represent social ties to groups different from that of their relatives and neighbors, as analyzed by Abad (2006). Here, we would acknowledge our debt of gratitude to Dr. Ricardo Abad's intellectual generosity ever!

were delivered to the community with the help of the following departments and/or units of the Philippine Government: (1) Social Welfare and Development, (2) Interior and Local Government, and (3) Office of the Civil Defense (Porio, 2023). So, in this case, both bridging and linking capital intertwined to provide relief from the covid-19 pandemic and community lockdown to the informal settler communities.

Contrary to Putnam's (2000a, 2000b) argument, Aldrich (2011) associated much importance with the vertical ties, while Putnam (2000a, 2000b) assigned an opposite weight to that of the horizontal ties. Putnam (2000a, 2000b) notes the story of success and prosperity of Northern Italy, compared to those in the South which did not achieve the same. The northern part of Italy achieved its success status because of the existing relationship found between its community or citizens and government. North Italy directed their attention in developing and strengthening their horizontal and vertical relationships with associations and institutions. Although Aldrich (2011, 2018) insists that the real drivers are the internal stakeholders, it is yes and no, because it is the intersectionality of their desire and motivation to recover and improve, on one hand, and their trust in the workings of the institutional systems, on the other hand (Porio, 2018). This argument is supported by the behavioral patterns we see in the SWB Survey data in the Philippines. We will pursue this analysis through the embedded procedures of beneficiary selection in the distribution of goods and services in pre-/post-disaster areas of post-Haiyan (Eastern Visayas), post-Washi (Mindanao), and post-Ketsana (Metro Manila and Luzon) communities.

The above analysis will also be complemented here by Manyena's (UNISDR, 2014) definition of resilience as the capacity of groups and communities to "bounce forward better". In Manyena's model of resilience (see below) to bounce forward better after a disaster hits the community, "response is dominated by local people", and "disasters provide opportunity and not cause of risk and power relations are addressed and lead to social change" (UNISDR, 2014). Meanwhile, Combaz (2014) also argued that the following component elements shape community resilience: (1) contextual factors or drivers (e.g., socioeconomic and political conditions), (2) disturbance or shock (e.g., floods or earthquakes), (3) capacity of the system to respond or deal with the shock, and (4) reaction or response of the group or community. The above frameworks of disaster response and recovery will be utilized in assessing the role of social capital, trust networks, and other social infrastructural ties before, during, and after disasters in disaster-prone communities in the Philippines (Fig. 1).

More importantly, Manyena's framework will be supplemented with the following illustration of the relationships of social capital, social infrastructural ties, and community resilience. This will be further elaborated in the discussion section.

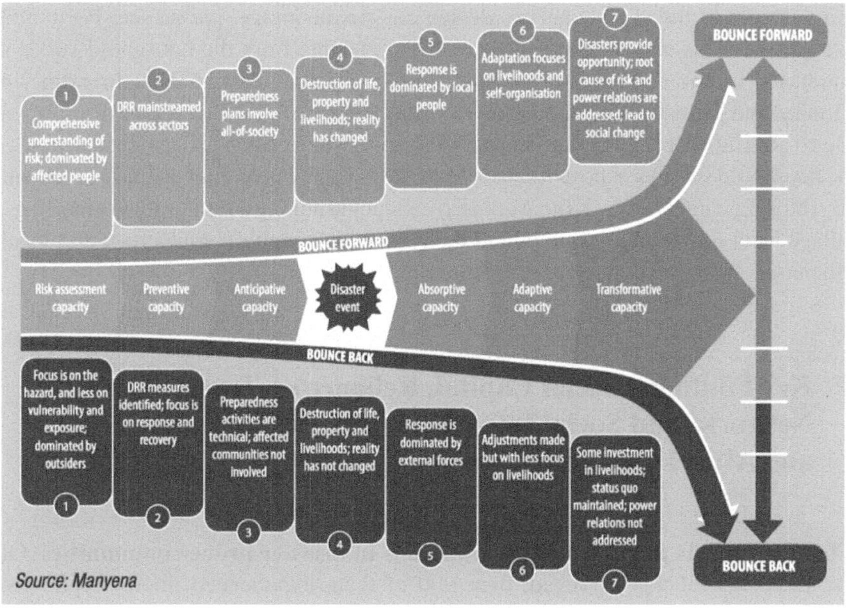

Fig. 1 Manyena's (2014) conceptualization of community resilience

3 Research Questions

Research questions, both empirical and analytical. The analytical trajectories here in this paper focus on the role of social capital, trust networks, and other social infrastructural ties in pre-/during and after flooding disasters. We separated this group (about 892 households of the total 1200 sample households in the SWB survey). We were concerned with the following questions: What is the structure of social capital, trust networks, and other social infrastructural ties among Filipinos, in general? By regions, by gender, and by socioeconomic status? What are the implications of these patterns of trust in organizing disaster response and resilience-driven institutions and groups? How should local populations and their community-based organizations focused on disaster response and resilience organize and reconfigure their strategies of engagements in these regions?

3.1 Methods, Data Sources, and Analysis

The main database utilized here is the 2016 Survey of Social Wellbeing, organized by the Senshu University Consortium of Social Well-Being. Conducted in the three island groups of the Philippines, the study surveyed 1200 households. For more details of the sample survey design and methodology, please see, Porio and See (2017). This was supplemented with the insights from the household surveys conducted by the authors, who are part of the Coastal Cities at Risk: Investing in Climate and Disaster Resilience, A Transdisciplinary Action Research Project, in Metro Manila (2014, 2018) and in post-Haiyan, Eastern Samar (2015). In addition to the household surveys in post-Ketsana Metro Manila and post-Haiyan Eastern Samar, key informant interviews (KIIs) were also conducted among community leaders (e.g., village head or barangay captain and the community health volunteer(s)) and local officials.

4 Key Findings: Social Capital, Reliance on Trust Networks and Social Infrastructural Ties During and After Disasters

Climate impacts to vulnerable populations in disaster-prone communities. Of the 1,200 households surveyed, over 900 of them experienced floods, typhoons, earthquakes, and droughts. This is not surprising as the Philippines is located in the so-called Ring of Fire, with many disaster hazards. The following sections will describe the gender and distribution of social capital and trust networks embedded in the local institutions and community social structure.

Gender, socioeconomic status, and reliance on trust networks. Although both genders have varying levels of trust, males compared to females seem to have higher trust and reliance on their families, relatives, friends, neighbors, employers, co-workers, armed forces, neighborhood associations, volunteers of civil society/civic groups, and institutions like church or religious groups. Are men naïve or just have a stronger trust base compared to women? Or are women more realistic or just do not have strong associational or institutional ties? We think the answer is in the middle. But this finding reinforces the previous findings of Abad (2005, 2017), Porio and See (2017, 2023), See and Porio (2015), and Porio 2017a, 2017b, 2017c that men appear to be more trusting to their social networks. Perhaps, this could be accounted by the fact that men have more "connectedness" to formal institutions in their communities like the barangay council and committees on disaster risk reduction and management (DRRM), environment, etc.

Interestingly between Metro Manila and the provinces in Mindanao, the latter seem to have more gender parity in terms of their levels of trust in their families, relatives, friends, neighbors, employers, faith-based organization (FBOs like church, temple, etc.), schools, hospitals, firefighting organizations except trust with co-workers, neighborhood associations, and local governments where females seem to have less trust in them during disasters (see Table 1). But in terms of civil status, Mindanao's married respondents, compared to singles and the widowed/separated, have higher trust levels with their families, relatives, friends, neighbors, employers, co-workers, except with the armed forces, neighborhood associations, civic organizations, temples/churches/mosques and FBOs, where the level of trust among married and separated/widowed households were almost equal and/or higher compared to those from Luzon and Metro Manila respondents. Although, overall, the singles seem to have less trust in temples/churches and FBOs, schools and hospitals, police, firefighting organizations, local governments, and political parties during disasters.

Formal employment is very much associated with high levels of trust in their families, neighborhood associations, and most of all in national/local government institutions (schools/hospitals, armed forces, police, and firefighting organizations) and faith-based organizations and associated places (temples, mosques, and churches/chapels). Being formally integrated into the labor market through regular employment seems to be the key in increasing their trust with public institutions who do not fail them during disasters. The above pattern of differential levels of trust by gender (i.e., women trusting less) with local institutions can be explained by the women's low levels of community engagements in sports, community development, elderly/child support, crime prevention, and disaster preparedness. This is especially true in Metro Manila and Luzon.

The region of Mindanao, however, displayed a different pattern, where women seem to have a higher level of community engagements compared to their counterparts in Metro Manila and Luzon. This is counter-intuitive as living in more urbanized areas is supposed to make women more engaged in broader community activities. Perhaps, this differential also explains why there is higher levels of trust in Mindanao with their formal institutions like the police, armed forces, civic organizations, schools/hospitals, and firefighting organizations during disasters. Perhaps the distance from the metropolis and that these local institutions were the only ones delivering them the services, made them trustworthy before the residents.

Social well-being and trust levels are highly correlated. Those having high SWB scores also have higher trust levels with their families, neighborhood associations, local institutions, and service agencies. This relationship was also affirmed in the authors' survey in post-Haiyan Eastern Samar, where those who have high trust levels with their local health system also enjoyed high health status (See & Porio, 2015).

Table 1 Level of trust and regions in the Philippines

	Metro Manila (%)	Luzon (%)	Visayas (%)	Mindanao (%)
Family and relatives	81	76	75	76
Friends and acquaintances	48	55	55	43
Co-workers	7	7	16	18
Local government	23	27	24	35
Neighbors	36	38	31	41
Strangers	4	6	3	6

Source Authors. Based on the survey question: "*Based on this list, who do you trust the most?*"

Regional imbalance in distribution of social well-being, social capital, and trust levels during disasters. The above studies have also shown that the distribution of social capital and trust networks vary by region. As observed previously by Porio and See (2017), the farther they were from Metro Manila, the higher they trust government institutions and faith-based organizations (FBOs). As reinforced by our expanded analysis of the SWB database here, those from outside of Metro Manila, especially Mindanao, have higher trust in associations (temple, church, and other faith-based organizations or FBOs) and government institutions (police, armed forces, schools/ hospitals, and firefighting organizations). Alternatively, there is less trust in these institutions among self-employed, farmers, and the unemployed, except in trust in FBOs which seem to enjoy high levels of trust (90% or more) in formally/informally employed, unemployed, and farmers/fisherfolks. Also, significant here is that women have higher levels of community engagements, which seem to explain why both men and women in Mindanao have higher trust levels with government and other formal institutions. Thus, bridging and linking capital among women seem to be higher in Mindanao compared to those in Luzon and Visayas (Table 2).

Integration to formal institutions through employment and faith-based community activities/organizations is linked to higher levels of trust in civic associations and government institutions. While Filipinos, in general, have high levels of trust with their immediate families, relative, and friends, integration into formal institutions through employment seems to foster higher trust (60–90%) in formally organized groups like neighborhood associations, civic organizations, national/local government units, and their agencies (police/armed forces, health/hospitals, schools, firefighting organizations, etc.).

This has implications to relief, rehabilitation, and recovery efforts and building toward community resilience by local governments, civil society, and humanitarian agencies and by the communities and households and families of respondents. First, community resilience can be achieved through the combined structures and processes

Table 2 Level of trust in specific government institutions and other organizations

	Metro Manila (%)	Luzon (%)	Visayas (%)	Mindanao (%)
Hospital	68.3	66.3	60	68.7
Police	46.6	48	51.7	53.7
Firefighting organization	69.3	69.3	70.7	49.7
Armed forced	48.4	49.3	57.3	60.6
Political parties	37.7	40.7	23	34.7
Volunteers and civic groups	62	58.3	47	64
Church and religious groups	77.3	71.7	57.3	83.3

Source Authors. Based on the survey question "*who do you trust to help you with your everyday problems?*"

of both formal and informal networks, supported by a collective effort by community groups as well as formal agencies and organizations. Second, formal institutions have an important role to play in engaging with communities to build collaboration and trust, which is critical to resilience building efforts. Third, formal institutions have a strong track record in mobilizing local communities in disaster recovery and are therefore well-placed to support resilience building work alongside local communities.

The above patterns of trust by gender, civil status, and education (social location) with formal institutions are reinforced highly in Mindanao. Perhaps, due to the more than 40 years of low-intensity conflict in this region, which also have the highest population of Muslims, both Christian-oriented groups (e.g., basic ecclesiastical communities, and humanitarian initiatives), Islamic organizations, and resistance groups from various ethnicities and political groupings, people have learned to trust more those associated with formal institutions. In fact, in areas like Zamboanga, Sulu, and Marawi, natural hazards like floods interact with human-induced disasters that intensify and escalate the disastrous effects of these events.

Trust and reliance in local institutions is very crucial in far flung areas where the only source of emergency and recovery services could only be the national/local government agencies/units (e.g., police, armed forces, schools, hospitals, and firefighting units) and faith-based organizations like the mosque, church, and other humanitarian groups.

Social infrastructural ties expanded through the community systems' procedures of resource distribution. The intersections of gender, ethnicity, and social capital/trust networks are the foundations of social infrastructural ties of people in disaster-prone communities. The above patterns of mobilization show that social infrastructural ties are articulated through the normative processes embedded in the social interactions. Based on the component patterns of social well-being, social capital and trust networks serve as the glue to the social infrastructure ties of the community. We will elaborate, in this section, what constitutes social infrastructural ties that Aldrich (2018) did not expound very much in his works. As articulated in earlier analysis of SWB data (Porio & See, 2017) and in the Appendix Figures of this paper, social well-being is highly correlated with social capital and trust networks that are mobilized during disasters. Social capital is just the tip of the iceberg of social infrastructural ties in the community's social structure.

Reconstituting social capital, trust, and social infrastructural ties for community resilience. The above analysis shows how social capital and trust networks are implicated with other dimensions of social infrastructural ties, which are integral in disaster recovery and building community resilience. The ability to recover from shocks like flooding disasters and "bounce forward better" comes from tight bonding connections with others—both vertical and horizontal ties—that link communities to civil society, faith-based organizations, and public institutions (schools, hospitals, police, and local government service agencies) that provide the best defense against disasters and serve as the foundational base for community resilience. Trust levels with associations, especially with those groups that are perceived to care for the

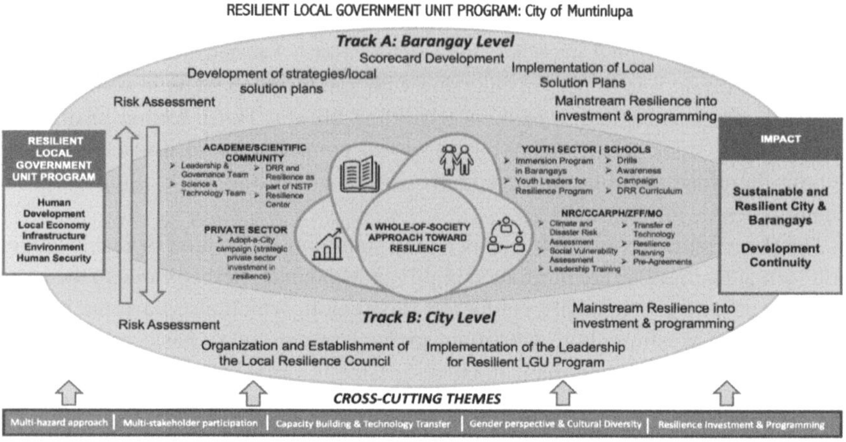

Fig. 2 Context of mobilizing bonding, bridging, and linking social capital in the Local Government Unit (LGU) Resilient Program in Muntinlupa City, Philippines. *Source* National Resilience Council (NRC) and Porio (2021)

people's welfare and can be relied upon to provide services during disasters (e.g., schools, hospitals, police, local government, and their service units), are central to developing community resilience.

Adger (2000) made a clear link between social and ecological resilience, particularly where social groups or communities are dependent on ecosystems and environmental resources for their livelihoods. Moreover, people can create novel approaches to change the dynamics of community resilience by the ways they mobilize their social capital and trust networks for better access of resources for recovery after disasters (See & Porio, 2015). They can also increase their social capital and trust networks by deepening their interactions among each other through activities and programs that engage them collectively with critical bridging and linking institutions toward adaptation and social transformation. See Fig. 2 for illustrative programmatic context of mobilization of social capital by local officials, academy, youth, private sector, and community groups. Notably, the representation of vulnerable women's groups like that of the Gender and Development Committee of the city is not very visible, although they are included in the Human Development Group in the Local Government Unit's (LGU) Resilient Local Government Program.

In the above illustration of the Muntinlupa City's Resilient Barangay Local Government Unit Program, the "Whole of Society Approach Towards Resilience" is implemented through collaborative networks in academe/scientific community, youth programs in schools, private sector, and the NRC-CCARPH-ZFF-MO Consortium.[6] This section will discuss how gender, especially women, are implicated in

[6] The consortium is composed of the National Resilience Council (NRC), Coastal Cities at Risk in the Philippines (CCARPH), the Zuellig Family Foundation (ZFF), and the Manila Observatory (MO), providing capacity building programs to the Local Government Unit (LGU) Resilient Program.

the mobilization of social capital in disaster-prone communities, especially during response and recovery periods. Although the status of women in the Philippines is quite high in the gender inequality index, this is not really reflective of women in low-income and marginal communities in urban and rural poor areas of the country. In the above program, while the barangay leadership are mostly held by male leaders, those managing the health, education, and other social services are mostly occupied by women. So, while male leaders seem to make decisions at the barangay/community councils, the women leaders in different committees (e.g., social protection, education, health, gender and development, etc.) implement the delivery of services to the urban poor communities. So, ultimately the mobilization of resources (e.g., relief goods and emergency health services) are facilitated by the women leaders and service providers with their barangay/village leaders, local chief executive, private sector/business groups, civil society organizations (CSOs), and community-based organizations. Thus, within this context of overlapping trust networks, the structure of social capital embedded in these networks shapes the crafting and design of institutional procedures associated with allocation of resources in post-disaster communities (Porio 2017a, 2017b, 2017c).

Social capital under the covid-19 lockdown. Social capital, especially bridging and linking social capital, has also been implicated under covid-19 pandemic and lockdown. In March 2021, under the height of second layer surge of covid-19 infections, one resident in Maginhawa St, Quezon City organized a community pantry in a cart in front of her house in Quezon City with the sign: *Magbigay ayon sa kakayahan, kumuha alin sa pangangailangan* (Give according to your capacity, get according to your need), posted an appeal in a cart in Quezon City, Metro Manila. The "first responders", i.e., those who donated vegetables, rice, and canned goods, were her neighbors and nearby friends and the second layer were her friends/colleagues from her university networks, who heard about her initiative and drove by to drop their contributions. The first to get food aid "ayuda" or help were her neighbors from the informal settlers nearby who knew the community pantry organizer. In a May 5, 2021, New York Times article, writer Amada Rosa, reported that Asians have become the most vaccinated group because of the latter's social capital and/or trust networks with their community-based organizations. She reported that "though it may be difficult to quantify the effect community-based organizations have made in the vaccination effort, these groups have been a lifeline for their most vulnerable community members" She further asserted that despite widening disparities within the community, income inequality has not become a barrier to their community wide vaccination. Commenting on this article, the Philippine Government's Interagency Task Force for Covid-19 Management consultant, Dr. John Wong commented that "it is the higher level of social capital among Asians which is also a protective factor against disasters."

While covid-19 pandemic and lockdown effects have also intensified the climate impacts (floods during typhoon season and extreme urban heat during summer) to already poor and impoverished urban–rural women and children, their hunger had been reduced with the emergence of food exchange networks driven by bonding and bridging social capital. Assistance (popularly known as ***ayuda (thus, the term, ayuda-centric)*** from the government (linking capital) cannot respond adequately to the rising food needs of the people, thus the emergence of community pantries all over the country the past two months because of dire need.

In conclusion, this study explored the structure of social capital, trust networks, and other social infrastructural ties among Filipinos in climate-related disasters contexts. It finds that in post-disaster communities, different components of social capital are mobilized according to their levels of social and locational vulnerabilities and capacities. In general, men as well as those who are formally employed tend to have the highest levels of trust and reliance on their families, relatives, friends, neighbors, and employers. In terms of location, the study finds that those from Mindanao tend to have the highest trust in associations (temple, church, and other faith-based organizations or FBOs) and government institutions (police, armed forces, schools/hospitals, and firefighting organizations). Additionally, the study finds that those who are well-integrated into formal institutions and organizations tend to have higher levels of trust in other people. The paper ends with a brief account of the status of social capital during the covid-19 pandemic and lockdowns in the Philippines. It finds that social capital, embodied through community pantries and the *ayuda* (assistance), played a critical role in responding to the food and health needs of different communities. The paper ultimately calls for more approaches that can strengthen social capital in climate-related and post-pandemic contexts, as communities with high levels of inclusion and positive engagement with formal leadership tend to be better placed in their recovery and resilience.

Appendix

See Table 3, 4, 5, 6 and 7.

Table 3 People who respondents trust the most, disaggregated by location

Level of trust/social capital and networks					
	Philippines (%)	Metro Manila (%)	Luzon (%)	Visayas (%)	Mindanao (%)
Most People	26	30	28	17	28
Family & Relatives	75	81	76	75	76
Friends & Acquaintances	45	48	55	55	43
Co-workers	12	7	7	16	18
Local Government, Police	27	23	27	24	35
Neighbors	37	36	38	31	41
Strangers	5	4	6	3	6

Table 4 People who respondents trust the most to help deal with their problems

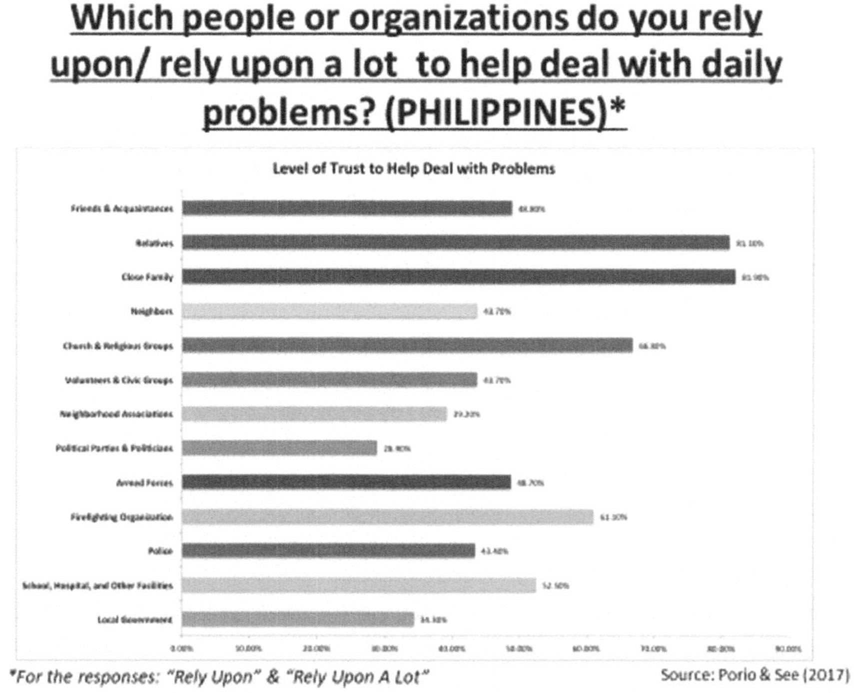

Table 5 Institutions that respondents trust the most to help deal with their daily problems

Summary: Level of Trust with Daily Problems					
Type of people	Philippines (%)	Metro Manila (%)	Luzon (%)	Visayas (%)	Mindanao (%)
Local government	34.3	29.4	39	29.3	39.4
School, hospital, and other facilities	52.5	49.7	52	50.3	58
Police	43.4	38.7	40.3	48.6	45.6
Firefighting organization	61.1	64.7	61	68	50.7
Armed forces	48.7	45.3	45	49.7	54.6
Political parties and politicians	28.9	27	32.3	21.3	34.7
Neighborhood associations	39.2	41.6	46.4	26	43
Volunteers and civic groups	43.7	47.7	49.3	32.6	45
Church and religious groups	66.8	68.6	66	55	77.7
Neighbors	43.7	42.3	52.4	33.7	46.4
Close family	81.9	80.3	79.3	84.3	83.3
Relatives	81.1	83	81.7	78.6	81
Friends and acquaintances	48.8	52.3	62	33.3	47.7

Table 6 People who respondents trust the most to help deal them during disasters (in Mindanao)

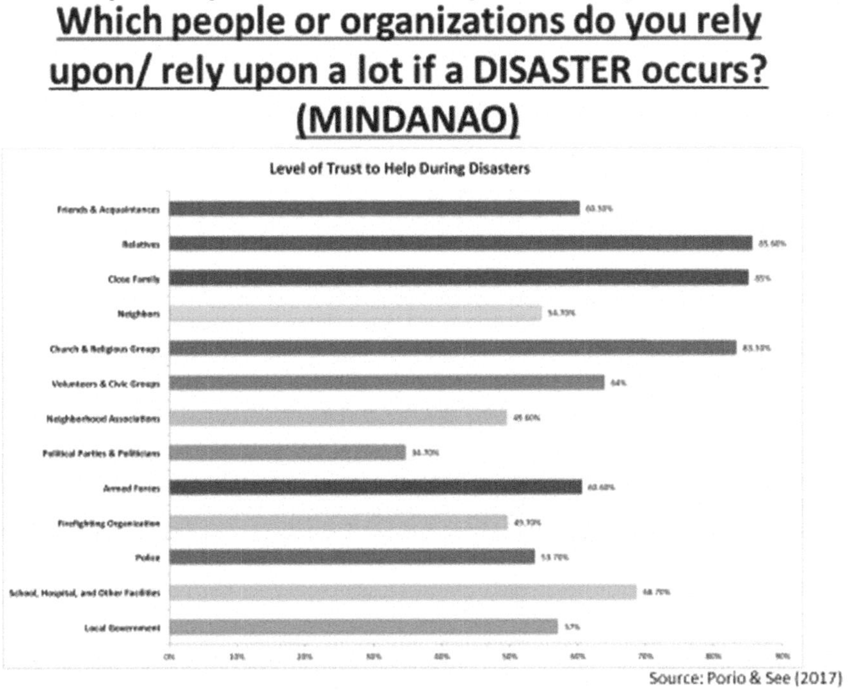

Table 7 People who respondents trust the most to help deal them during disasters (for the Philippines)

Summary: level of trust during disasters					
Type of people	Philippines	Metro Manila	Luzon	Visayas	Mindanao
Local government	53.4	52	59	45.6	57
School, hospital, and other facilities	65.9	68.3	66.3	60	68.7
Police	50	46.6	48	51.7	53.7
Firefighting organization	64.8	69.3	69.3	70.7	49.7
Armed forces	53.9	48.4	49.3	57.3	60.6
Political parties & politicians	33.9	37.7	40.7	23	34.7
Neighborhood associations	47.1	52.3	53.7	33	49.6
Volunteers and civic groups	57.9	62	58.3	47	64
Church and religious groups	72.5	77.3	71.7	57.3	83.3
Neighbors	48.8	51.4	54.7	34.7	54.7
Close family	84.7	85	82.7	86	85
relatives	83.9	87	83.3	79.7	85.6
Friends and acquaintances	53.8	54.3	64.4	36.3	60.3

References

Abad, R. G. (2005). Social capital in the Philippines: results from a national survey. *Philippine Sociological Review*.

Abad, R. G. (2006). Aspects of Social Capital in the Philippines: Findings from a National Survey. Social Weather Stations' Occasional Papers Series.

Abad, R. G. (2017). *"Citizenship participation in the Philippines" selected results from a 2014 National Survey*. Ateneo de Manila University.

Adger, W. N. (2000). Social and ecological resilience: Are they related? *Progress in Human Geography, 24*(3), 347–364. https://doi.org/10.1191/030913200701540465

Adger, W. N., Agrawal, S., Mirza, M., Conde, C., O'brien, K., Pulhin, J., Pulwarty, R., Smit, B., & Takahashi, K. (2007). Assessment of adaptation practices, options, constraints and capacity (Climate Change 2007: Impacts, Adaptation and Vulnerability. Contribution of Working Group II to the Fourth Assessment Report of the Intergovernmental Panel on Climate Change, Issue.

Ali, A. (2006). A conceptual framework for environmental justice based on shared but differentiated responsibilities. In T. Shallcross & J. Robinson (Eds.), *Global citizenship and environmental justice* (pp. 41–77). Brill.

Aldrich, D. P. (2011). The power of people: Social capital's role in recovery from the 1995 Kobe earthquake. *Natural Hazards, 56*(3), 595–611. https://doi.org/10.1007/s11069-010-9577-7

Aldrich, D. P. (2013). *Response to my critics*. Hazards and Crisis in Public Policy.

Aldrich, D. P. (2017). *The importance of social capital in building community resilience*. Policy Studies Organization.

Aldrich, D. P. (2018). The right way to build resilience to climate change. *Current History, 117*(795), 16–21. https://www.jstor.org/stable/48614311

Aldrich, D.P. (2021). *Social Capital and Community Social Structure*. Presented in the webinar, Singapore Together.

Aldrich, D. P., & Meyer, M. A. (2015). *Social capital and community resilience* (pp. 254–269). SAGE Publications.

Bourdieu, P. (1985). The social space and the genesis of groups. *Theory and Society, 14*(6), 723–744. http://www.jstor.org/stable/657373

Cai, Y. (2017). Bonding, bridging, and linking: photovoice for resilience through social capital. *Natural Hazards*, 1169–1195.

Combaz, E. (2014). *Disaster resilience: Topic guide*. https://gsdrc.org/wp-content/uploads/2014/02/GSDRC_DR_topic_guide.pdf

Dapilah, F., Nielsen, J., & Friis, C. (2020). The role of social networks in building adaptive capacity and resilience to climate change: a case study from northern Ghana. *Climate and Development, 12*(1), 42–56

Kawachi, I., Kim, D., Coutts, A., & Subramanian, S. V. (2004). Commentary: Reconciling the three accounts of social capital. *International Journal of Epidemiology, 33*(4), 682–690. https://doi.org/10.1093/ije/dyh177

Heintz, H.-J., Kirch, L., Küppers, B., Mann, H., Mischo, F., Mucke, P., Pazdzierny, T., Prütz, R., Radtke, K., Strube, F., & Weller, D. (2018). *World Risk Report 2018*. https://weltrisikobericht.de/wp-content/uploads/2019/03/190318_WRR_2018_EN_RZonline_1.pdf

Jean-Baptiste, N., Kuhlicke, C., Kunath, A., & Kabisch, S. (2011). *Review and evaluation of existing vulnerability indicators for assessing climate related vulnerability in Africa*.

Karaos, A. M. & Nicolas, G. (2021). *Towards a science-informed and people-centered resettlement program*. John J. Carroll Institute of Church and Social Issues Policy Paper.

Leonard, M. (2004). Bonding and bridging social capital: Reflections from Belfast. *Sociology, 38(5)*, 927–944. https://doi.org/10.1177/0038038504047176

Martin, A., Coolsaet, B., Corbera, E., Dawson, N. M., Fraser, J. A., Lehmann, I., & Manyena, S. B. (2014). Disaster resilience: A question of 'multiple faces' and 'multiple spaces'? *International Journal of Disaster Risk Reduction, 8*, 1–9. https://doi.org/10.1016/j.ijdrr.2013.12.010

Montana-Leblanc, P. (2008). *Not just the levees broke: My story during and after Hurricane Katrina.* Simon and Schuster.

Moore, M.-L., & Westley, F. (2011). Surmountable chasms: networks and social innovation for resilient systems. *Ecology and Society, 16*(1). Retrieved from http://dlc.dlib.indiana.edu/dlc/bitstream/handle/10535/7513/ES-2010-3812.pdf?sequence=1&isAllowed=y

Porio, E. (2011). Vulnerability, adaptation, and resilience to floods and climate change- related risks among Marginal, Riverine Communities in Metro Manila. *Asian Journal of Social Science, 39*(4), 425–445. https://doi.org/10.1163/156853111X597260

Porio, E. (2014). Climate change vulnerability and adaptation in Metro Manila challenging governance and human security of urban poor communities. *Asian Journal of Social Science, 42*(1–2), 75–102. https://doi.org/10.1163/15685314-04201006

Porio, E. (2016). Prosperity and inequality in Metro Manila: Reflections on climate disasters, social housing and governance. *Globalization and democracy in southeast Asia: challenges, responses, and alternative futures.* London: Palgrave Macmillan.

Porio, E. (2018). *Gender, climate adaptation and resilience in Metro Manila.* Paper presented in the ICLEI World Congress on Urban Areas, Montreal International Convention Center, July 17–22, Montreal: Canada.

Porio, E. (2022). Urban poor community strategies: Towards a resilient recovery from natural disasters and the covid-19 pandemic in the Philippines. In J. M. Fritz & J. Rheaume (Eds.), *Community intervention: Clinical sociology perspectives.* Springer Publication.

Porio, E. E. (2015). *Sustainable development goals and quality of life targets: Insights from Metro Manila in current sociology.* Sage Publications.

Porio, E. E. (2017a). Citizen participation, environmental security and risk governance: Integrating climate change adaptation and mitigation and disaster risk reduction and management (CCAM-DRRM) in Metro Cebu. Misereor Foundation (Aachen, Germany) and the PagTambayayong, Foundation for Mutual Aid, Inc.

Porio, E. E. (2017b). Risk and resilience: interrogating prosperity, inequality and climate- disaster impacts in Metro Manila. Philippine Institute of Development Studies.

Porio, E. E. (2017c). *Social well-being in the Philippines: Indicators and patterns in Senshu Journal of Social Well-Being.* Senshu University Press.

Porio, E., & See, J. (2017). Social well-being in the philippines: indicators and patterns. *Senshu Social Well-being Review, 4*, 95–116. https://core.ac.uk/download/pdf/156952967.pdf

Porio, E., & See, J 2023). Manila: Aspiring to be an inclusive, resilient, and sustainable city amidst climate and disaster risks. In *Routledge handbook of Asian cities* (pp. 392–404). Routledge.

Porio E. E. (2021). *Bridging Science-Policy-practice nexus through transdisciplinary research and resilience innovations: Science and technology for society.* Presented in the Capacity-Building for Science Teachers in the Pamantasan ng Lunsod ng Muntinlupa (University of the City of Muntinlupa), 7 May 2021.

Portes, A. (1998). Social capital: Its origins and applications in modern sociology. *Annual Reviews*, 1–24.

Putnam, R. (2000a). Social capital: Measurement and consequences. *Canadian Journal of Policy Research.*

Putnam, R. D. (2000b). *Bowling alone: The collapse and revival of American community.* Simon and Schuster.

See, J., & Porio, E. E. (2015). Assessing social vulnerability to flooding in Metro Manila using principal component analysis. *Philippine Sociological Review, 63*, 53–80.

The Economist Special Report. (2013). The secret of their success. *The Economist.*

The World Values Survey. (2014). World Values Survey.

UNISDR (United Nations International Strategy for Disaster Reduction). (2014). *Fifth Africa regional platform and third ministerial meeting for disaster risk reduction.* Abuja: UNISDR

Woolcock, M. (1998). Social Capital and economic development: Toward a theoretical synthesis and policy framework. *Theory and Society, 27*, 151–208.

Wun'gaeo, S., Jumnianpol, S., Nuangjamnong, N., Srisupan, P., & Chimmamee, M. (2017). Social well-being in Thailand 2016: Survey Report. *The Senshu Social Well-being Review, 4*, 75–93. http://www.cusri.chula.ac.th/en/archives/4266

Yee, J., Lim, H., Nam, E., Kim, D., & Kim, E. (2016). Survey design and descriptive outcomes of Korean Survey. *The Senshu Social Well-being Review, 3*. https://senshu-u.repo.nii.ac.jp/records/8034

Emma Porio is Professor of Sociology at the Ateneo de Manila University and Science Research Fellow at the Manila Observatory. Her research interests include marginality, social vulnerability, climate and disaster resilience.

Justin See is a lecturer in Development Studies at the University of Melbourne. His research investigates issues of power, injustice, and inequality within climate change adaptation projects.

Social and Subjective Well-Being in Post-growth Japan: Adapting to New Inequalities

Carola Hommerich

Abstract Japan has transformed in recent decades from a strongly growing, economically successful country regarded as a prime example of social equality and inclusion, to one with a stagnating economy, a shrinking population, and a considerable proportion of elderly citizens. New forms of inequality have emerged and deepened, and a new perception of Japan as a "gap society" (*kakusa shakai*) is commonly acknowledged. With the ongoing dualization of the labor market, the standard life course prevalent in the years of economic growth (e.g., marriage, lifetime employment, and gradual social upgrading via a seniority-based renumeration system) has become less attainable, although many still covet it as the template for a "good life." Meanwhile, formerly strong social bonds in the family, local community, and work have weakened, leaving an increasing share of the population without a social network to rely on in times of need. These two developments have resulted in increased feelings of vulnerability and anxiety across all social strata. However, there seems to be a shift among younger generations about what is imagined as a "good life," with lesser emphasis on materialistic values and a greater focus on enjoying the moment. This can be considered as an adaptation process to Japan's new social reality.

Keywords Happiness · Well-being · Social inequality · Japan

1 Introduction

As a highly developed and affluent nation, Japan is still widely perceived to be a success story of relatively equitable economic growth. Its speedy ascent to becoming the world's second largest economy in the late 1960s, and its ability to keep that position for years thereafter, earned Japan praise from the World Bank (1993) for spearheading the "East Asian Miracle" of swift growth paired with reduced inequality.

C. Hommerich (✉)
Sophia University, Tokyo, Japan
e-mail: hommerich@sophia.ac.jp

J. Yee et al. (eds.), *Social Well-Being, Development, and Multiple Modernities in Asia*,
https://doi.org/10.1007/978-981-97-3866-3_7

Rapid educational expansion (Ishida, 2007: 69) and the fundamental shift of the occupational composition from agriculture to blue-collar and white-collar jobs in the post-war years (Fig. 1) resulted not only in large-scale migration from rural to urban areas, but in tangible social upgrades and higher living standards for major parts of the population. By the mid-1970s, more than 90% of the population identified as middle class—a result that became the foundation for Japan's longstanding self-view as a homogenous middle-class society (Chiavacci, 2006; Hommerich & Kikkawa, 2019).

Today, the average quality of life in Japan in terms of income, health, and access to education remains relatively high. In 2022, Japan ranked 19th out of 189 countries and territories included in the Human Development Index (UNDP, 2022), sporting one of the highest life expectancies in the world, as well as high levels of educational attainment and per capita income. However, in more in-depth comparisons with countries at similar levels of economic development, Japan is not among the top runners. In the OECD's Better Life Index, which evaluates the 38 OECD member countries and key partners Brazil, Russia, and South Africa in 11 categories measuring material well-being and quality of life, Japan ranked 30 out of 41 in 2023 (OECD, 2023). Japan scores highly on personal security, education, and employment, and is above the OECD average regarding household wealth, housing, and environmental quality. However, subjective health and life satisfaction are below the OECD average. The comparatively low level of subjective well-being, despite the generally high standard of living, is mirrored in the UN's World Happiness Report 2023 (Helliwell et al., 2023): Japan ranks 47 out 137 nations in average self-reported happiness for 2020–2022 and is outranked by countries with lower levels of objective quality of life. The reasons for this are manifold. Work–life balance remains poor, with 17.9%

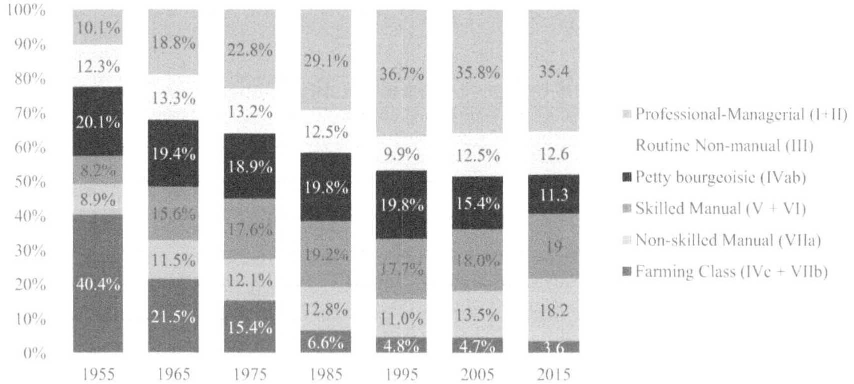

Fig. 1 Japan's social structure, 1955–2015. *Source* Data from the SSM survey series. The data for 1955–2005 are quoted from Ishida and Miwa (2009: 652), and data for 2015 are quoted from Hommerich and Kikkawa (2019: 15). *Note* The data quoted here comprise men aged 25–64 years. Women have been included in the surveys since 1985 but are excluded from this sample for reasons of comparability

of employees working more than 50 h per week (OECD average = 11%).[1] This especially affects men, forcing women to take on the lion's share of housework and childcare, which in turn makes it difficult for them to combine a full-time job with family life. As a result, Japan still lags far behind other highly developed nations in terms of gender equality. Although 75% of 15–64-year-olds are in paid employment (OECD average = 68%), 83% of men are in paid employment compared with 67% of women, and women are more likely to be engaged in precarious employment than men. Another well-being dimension in which Japan falls below the OECD average is civic engagement, with low voter turnout, indicating weak political interest and participation (Hommerich, 2015). This disinterest in political matters is not necessarily the result of a carefree life that does not necessitate political action, but rather seems to reflect low expectations held against political leaders and the lack of time to engage in anything beyond managing one's own personal life.

Overall, Japan presents itself as another example of the so-called Easterlin paradox (Musikanski et al., 2019: 28), having passed a point of development beyond which further economic growth and affluence no longer translate into an increase in subjective well-being. Instead, reports of increasing cases of social isolation or withdrawal, depression, and suicide paint a rather bleak picture of East Asia's former economic superstar.

The fact that well-being in Japan is not as high as expected has garnered attention. In 2010, the Japanese government, briefly led by the Democratic Party of Japan (DPJ) then, set up a "Commission on Measuring Well-being"[2] comprising Japanese experts in happiness research to develop a fine-tuned measurement tool to gain a deeper understanding of why Japanese subjective well-being was comparatively low (Commission on Measuring Well-being, 2011). However, with the return of the Liberal Democratic Party (LDP) to power in December 2012, well-being quickly vanished from the political agenda, giving way to a renewed focus on economic growth. The National Survey of Lifestyle Preferences, a longitudinal survey measuring well-being that had been carried out annually since 1995, was discontinued, and the Commission on Measuring Well-being was dissolved rather abruptly before it could implement its measurement tool at the national level.

This notwithstanding, interest in well-being—especially its low level—has not dwindled in Japan. It has remained a prominent topic in public discourse and academic research, tapping into various aspects of well-being (see Holthus & Manzenreiter, 2017; Tsai & Iwai, 2020). Among the multiple layers that shape social and subjective well-being, this chapter discusses mainly two topics that seem to be strongly connected to the low level of subjective well-being among the Japanese: (a) an increase in economic inequality triggered by the growing segmentation of the labor market, which has resulted in a shift of self-image from a homogeneous middle-class society to that of a gap society (*kakusa shakai*); and (b) a weakening of

---

[1] https://www.oecdbetterlifeindex.org/topics/work-life-balance/ (Accessed December 15, 2023).

[2] Minutes of the commission's meetings as well as information on the measurement tool developed by it are available here: https://www5.cao.go.jp/keizai2/koufukudo/koufukudo.html (Accessed December 15, 2023).

social bonds which has led to the creation of the term "society without bonds" (*muen shakai*). The chapter closes with a look at possible new definitions of "the good life," which seem to exist among younger generations who have grown up and adapted to the social reality of post-growth Japan.

2 Acknowledging Inequality

Interest in the topic of well-being was sparked when Japan had to relinquish the idea of eternal economic growth. With the bursting of the speculation bubbles in the real estate and stock markets (the so-called "bubble economy") in the early 1990s, Japan abruptly entered a phase of economic downturn and later stagnation after three decades of rapid economic growth. Academic analyses of social inequalities started to boom, with some scholars pointing to fundamental structural changes leading to new disparities (Kariya, 2001; Satō, 2000; Tachibanaki, 1998; Yamada, 2004), whereas others identified only limited changes and claimed that Japan had never been as egalitarian as often assumed (Hara & Seiyama, 2005; Ishida, 2001; Ōtake, 2005; Sato, 2007).

The recession was initially perceived as a transitory stage that would pass quickly, but after being hit hard by the Lehman shock two decades later, it became clear that economic growth would not return anytime soon. Slowly, the notion of Japan as an unequal society entered public discourse as well, with some semi-academic publications on the topic becoming national bestsellers (Miura, 2005). However, it took some time for topics of social inequality to make it onto the political agenda and, as is often the case in Japan, it involved an external wake-up call. It was only after the OECD (2008) attested to Japan's levels of income inequality and poverty being above the OECD average that the Japanese government acknowledged the growing social disparities and, for the first time, announced an official relative poverty rate in 2009, stating that 15.7% of the population fell below the poverty line.[3] China's overtaking of Japan as the world's second largest economy in 2010 further added to the realization that the years of constant expansion and social upgrading were over and called for a reassessment of Japan's self-image and position in the world.

The main drivers of the rising economic inequality have been fundamental changes in Japan's labor market (Sato & Imai, 2011). Although the occupational structure may have stabilized over the past three decades (see Fig. 1), there has been a drastic shift in the quality and safety of employment. Lifetime employment, seniority-based wages, and harmonious industrial relations—formerly the cornerstones of the Japanese employment system—have all weakened after the bubble economy ended in the early 1990s. Since then, gradual deregulation has led to a dualization of the labor market, with the share of non-regular employment doubling to more than one-third of the working population by the late 2000s and remaining at the same level

[3] The relative poverty rate is calculated as the share of people with incomes below 50% of the median disposable income.

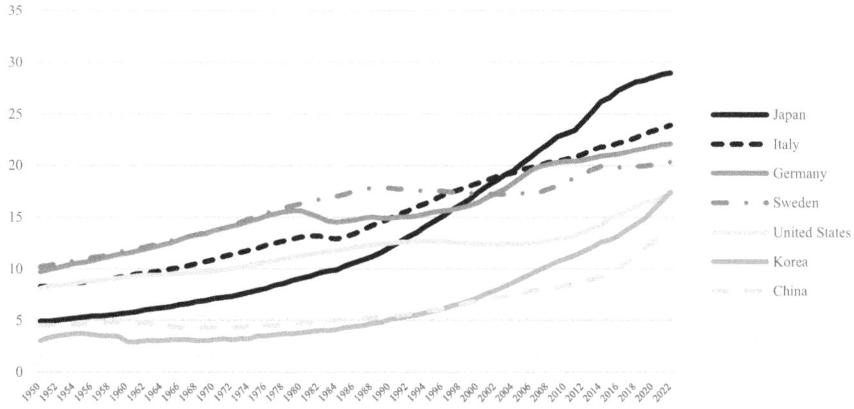

Fig. 2 Proportion of elderly population (aged 65 and older), 1950–2022. *Source* Assembled by the author based on data taken from OECD (2023), elderly population (indicator). DOI: https://doi.org/10.1787/8d805ea1-en (Accessed December 15, 2023)

since then (Heinrich, 2013; MIAC, 2017).[4] This trend is tangible also in economic terms, with the average monthly household income of workers declining steadily by more than 10% from about 595,000 yen in 1997 to 525,000 yen in 2003 and then stagnating (MIAC, 1984–2017).

During the same period, Japan underwent a fundamental demographic change, becoming a demographically stagnant and hyper-aging society (Coulmas et al., 2008). Within 15 years from the late 1980s to the early 2000s, Japan went from being the youngest advanced industrial society to the demographically oldest nation in the world (Fig. 2). With rapid demographic aging and a total fertility rate that remains far below replacement level, the number of people who are not part of the working-age population is growing. This means that the current workforce will have to shoulder an increasing financial burden associated with caring for the elderly.

It is now accepted that social inequality exists in Japan and that an increasing share of the population is struggling with precarious living conditions (Allison, 2013; Chiavacci & Hommerich, 2017; Ishida & Slater, 2010; Kawano et al., 2014; Shirahase, 2014). As large corporations cut back on the extensive welfare packages they used to provide, the Japanese government is confronted with the necessity of taking on the role of provider for the needy and has been compelled to expand its welfare state (Tachibanaki, 2005: 42). Slowly, some reforms are being enacted, but major deficiencies remain. The elderly worry about their pensions, while the young have little hope of achieving financial independence (Yamada, 2004). Mechanisms of social security and public assistance, which were shaped in an era of growth, have become dysfunctional and fail to provide for those in need (Hommerich, 2012).

[4] In 2017, 37.5% of the labour force worked in non-regular employment (MIAC, 2017).

3 Weakening of Social Bonds

However, adapting to widening socioeconomic cleavages and demographic aging has not been the only challenge Japan has faced in recent decades. In 2010, a much-discussed TV documentary by public broadcaster NHK further added fuel to the still relatively new debate on inequality and precariousness by calling attention to an increase in social isolation in Japan (NHK, 2010).[5] The topic was addressed by economist Toshiaki Tachibanaki in his popular book on "The true colors of a society without bonds" (2011), which was followed by numerous other publications discussing the weakening of social ties (Genda, 2013; Hommerich, 2015; Ishida, 2011; Kankonsôsaigojokyôkai, 2012; Miyamoto, 2012). The disintegration of social networks, however, was not merely a topic used by the media to play on common anxieties. Social bonds had been weakening for some time. A 2007 white paper, for instance, noted a loss of social capital in three areas of social interaction: the family, the local community, and the workplace (Cabinet Office, 2007).

With regard to the family, as in other post-industrial countries, changing living arrangements have weakened family ties: in 2010, one-third of all households comprised people living alone (NIPSSR, 2018). This proportion has continued to grow since then and is projected to reach 40% by 2040. The proportion of elderly living alone is particularly high. This is partly due to the breakup of the three-generation household: among households with members aged 65 and older, the share of married children living with their parents has dropped from 44.8% in 1986 to 9.4% in 2019 (MHLW, 2020). Since not living together results in reduced communication among family members, this has had a negative impact on the intensity of family relationships (Cabinet Office, 2007). Moreover, family formation is occurring later in the life course or, as evidenced by the increasing share of unmarried 50-year-olds, not at all (Cabinet Office, 2019b).[6] More people stay alone throughout their lives.

A similar development can be witnessed in ties within the local community. Since the 1970s, relationships with neighbors and the local community have been declining, and the share of Japanese people who are closely associated with their neighbors dropped from 53% in 1975 to 11% in 2007 (Cabinet Office, 2007). In the same year, 31% of the Japanese believed that ties in the local community had weakened over the past 10 years (Cabinet Office, 2007). Although this development is voluntary in part, especially among younger Japanese who find the obligatory small talk with their neighbors' bothersome (ibid.), it goes hand in hand with increased anxiety about the safety of the local neighborhood.

Major changes in the Japanese work environment have further contributed to the loss of once strong networks. In the wake of the economic recession, Japanese

[5] The documentary particularly caused a stir by drawing attention to the rising number of elderly people who die alone and are discovered only weeks or sometimes months later, because they lived alone with no or only distant social connections. This phenomenon has been called "lonely death" (*kodokushi*).

[6] In 2015, the share of unmarried 50-year-olds was 23.4% for men and 14.1% for women, up from 3.9% and 4.3%, respectively, in 1985.

companies have downsized their core workforce and are no longer able to offer all their employees the promise of lifelong employment and generous social security packages that were once the hallmark of the Japanese employment system. Instead, as outlined above, they are hiring non-regular workers, paying them lower wages, and providing negligible social security benefits. Working side by side, but under very different conditions, it is difficult for regular and non-regular employees to bond or develop a team spirit of working toward the same goal. Meanwhile, regular employees are also experiencing increasing pressure at their workplace and are worried about losing their jobs. As a result, workers feel that communication and mutual help in the workplace have become inadequate (Cabinet Office, 2007). This seems to have an impact on the mental health of employees: the perceived lack of communication in the workplace correlates with an increase in mental health problems, especially among younger employees (Japan Productivity Center, 2019).

4 Experience of Stress and Insecurity in Face of "New" Inequality

Overall, these developments have dismantled the robust "protective cocoon" (Giddens, 1990: 129) of institutional embeddedness formerly provided by family, local community, and company, which functioned to make daily life manageable and the future foreseeable (Chiavacci, 2006; Hommerich, 2012; Hommerich et al., 2021). As a result, feelings of vulnerability and socioeconomic precariousness are by no means confined to the lower ranks of society but cut across all social strata (Hommerich, 2017a). According to the annual Public Opinion Survey on the Life of the People (Cabinet Office, 2019a), the number of respondents who experienced worry or anxiety in their daily lives increased sharply over the course of the 1990s and up until the late 2000s (from 46.8% in 1991 to a peak of 70.8% in 2008) and remained high at 63.2% in 2019 (Fig. 3). Among these respondents, the proportion concerned about their current income or livelihood in old age has increased over the past 30 years. While this is, in part, related to the increasing share of elderly, it also implies that social risks are perceived not only as something that is applicable to others, but also as a direct threat to one's own livelihood. Increasing numbers of Japanese feel a "nagging sense of insecurity" (Genda, 2005) and the "social evaluative threat" (Wilkinson & Pickett, 2009: 37) of not being able to keep up with the rest of society.

Social risks have undoubtedly increased in Japan over the past two decades, although it is arguable whether these strong anxieties reflect actual risks and contingencies in all cases. It is highly likely that for some, these fears stem from a precarious employment situation with low pay and an uncertain future, or a recent experience of financial distress due to reduced wages or bonus payments. For others, however, it might merely be an exaggerated reaction to the rather sudden change in societal self-image that has increased awareness of social disparities and risk of status decline.

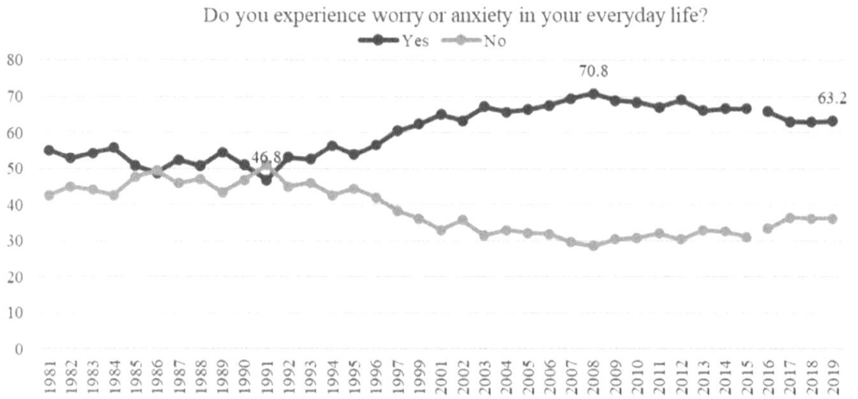

Fig. 3 Experience of worry or anxiety in everyday life, 1981–2019. *Source* Assembled by the author from the Public Opinion Survey on the Life of the People carried out annually by the Cabinet Office (2019a). Shares of respondents who answered "satisfied" or "rather satisfied" are shown. *Note* Until 2015, respondents were aged $\geq$ 20 years. From 2016 onwards, respondents were aged $\geq$ 18 years. The survey for 2020 was cancelled due to the pandemic, and the answer categories were changed from 2021 which makes comparison beyond 2019 difficult

However, even the mere perception of social inequality as a social problem, independent of a personal experience of being disadvantaged, is enough to reduce individual subjective well-being and increase anxieties (Hommerich, 2017a). This kindles fears of not fully belonging to society, a feeling that is of specific relevance for subjective well-being in Japan (Hommerich & Tiefenbach, 2018a)

This change in perception is mirrored in the stratification type selected to best describe society by Japanese respondents in the International Social Survey Program (ISSP).[7] In 1999, the highest share saw their own society as diamond-shaped, with most people in the middle strata of society (35.2%) (Fig. 4, Type D). By 2009, this figure had fallen to 20.1%. Meanwhile, the proportion of respondents who describe Japanese society as a pyramid (Type B)—with a small elite at the top, more people in the middle, and most at the bottom—increased from 31.8% in 1999 to 38.1% in 2009. Similarly, the proportion who perceive Japanese society as a strongly disparate society—with a small elite at the top, few people in the middle, and most citizens at the bottom (type A)—also increased. In 2019, the shares selecting these more extreme disparity types dropped slightly, while the share seeing Japan as stratification type C—a pyramid but with only a few people at the bottom—increased. Overall, from 2009 onwards, half of the respondents described Japanese society as unequal. This development bears witness to the declining resonance of the mass middle-class model in the lives of the Japanese, as discussed by Chiavacci (2008), and is in line with

[7] The ISSP surveys for Japan include respondents from 16 to 97 years of age. Here, Waves III (1999), IV (2009), and V (2019) of the Social Inequality Module are used. The data is available at www.issp.org.

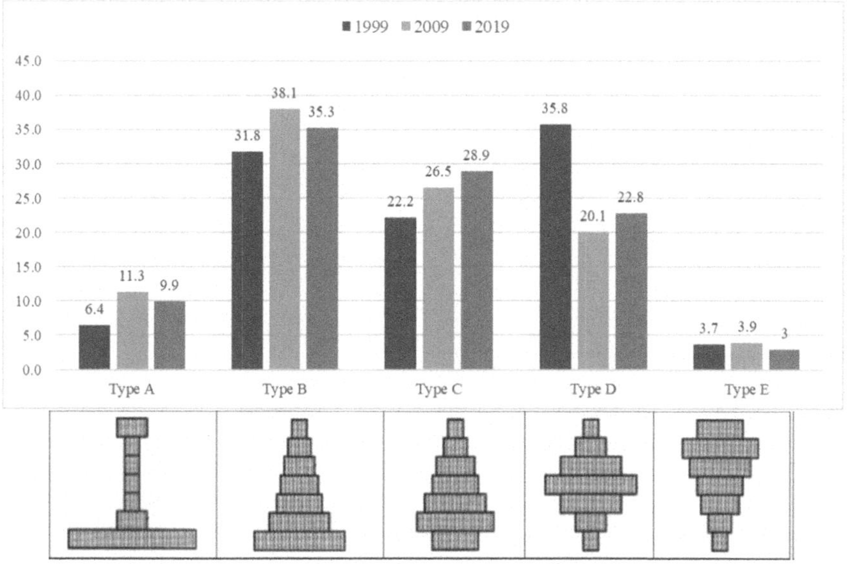

Fig. 4 Perceived type of society, 1999, 2009, 2019. *Source* ISSP 1999, 2009, 2019 (assembled by the author from ISSP data)

academic research that asserts perceptions of Japan's stratification structure to have become more realistic by the mid-2010s (Hommerich & Kikkawa, 2019).

However, nostalgia for the supposedly "good old times" remains, with more than half of the respondents naming the diamond-shaped middle-class model as the most desirable stratification model in 2019 (Fig. 5). This implies that for large parts of the population, what they perceive as social reality does not match their ideal image of how it should be.

Taken together, these developments hint at why Japan's subjective well-being may not be as high as expected if we consider only its level of development in comparison with other nations.

5 Japan's "Happy Youth"? Are Ideas of "The Good Life" Changing?

One group often focused on as especially affected by Japan's much-quoted "lost decades" is the younger generation, who never actually experienced the "good old times" (Hommerich, 2017b: 72–73). Growing up during the economic downturn and subsequent stagnation, they face insecure employment and cannot rely on the institutionalized networks that were available to their parents to give structure and meaning to their lives, let alone achieve financial independence (Yamada, 2013). Looking to the future, the younger generation can expect to shoulder the financial

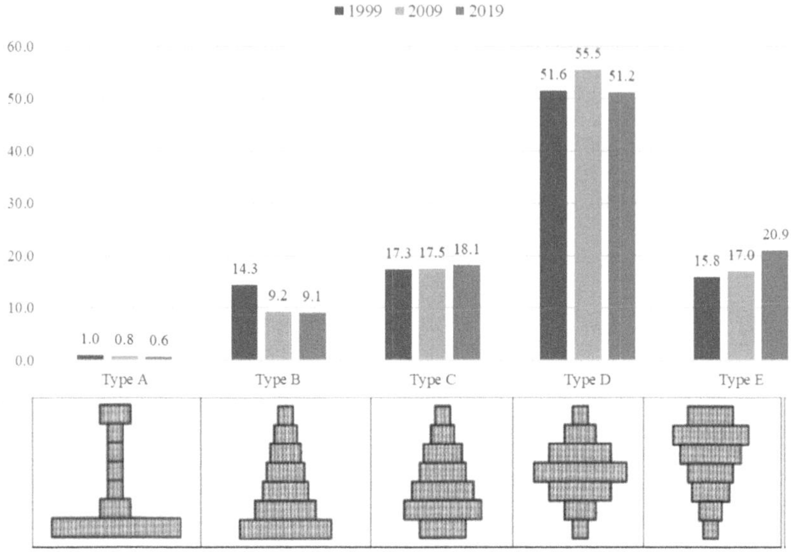

Fig. 5 Desired type of society, 1999, 2009, 2019. *Source* ISSP 1999, 2009, 2019 (assembled by the author from ISSP data)

burden associated with the demographic aging of Japanese society, while facing insecurity about whether their own livelihoods in old age will be covered by the current pension system (Hommerich, 2013). Many experience economic and social uncertainty and struggle to find their place in society (Miyamoto, 2012).

The many uncertainties that Japan's young adults face seem to be taking their toll. Various surveys indicate that young people feel highly anxious and vulnerable and have higher stress levels than older generations (MHLW, 2014). The fragility of their mental health seems to be further demonstrated by increasing cases of social withdrawal (*hikikomori*), depression, and suicide among the younger generation (Zielenziger, 2006). These are not simply typical symptoms of a certain stage in the life course, as a comparison of Japan's youth with their international peers makes clear: Japan's 13–29-year-olds have lower self-esteem than young people from the U.S., the U.K., France, Germany, Sweden, or South Korea (Cabinet Office, 2014, 2019c). At the same time, they suffer from high levels of anxiety about finding a job, their current job, or the future in general.[8]

Just as the academic discourse on the rather gloomy situation of Japan's youth was reaching its peak, young sociologist Furuichi (2011) published his book *The Happy Youth of a Desperate Country*, which caused quite a stir. Quoting data from the Cabinet Office's Public Opinion Survey on the Life of the People, he makes the rather provocative claim that Japan's youth are happier than ever, despite all the

[8] In the 2018 survey, young respondents from South Korea overtook Japanese respondents regarding anxieties about employment and the future.

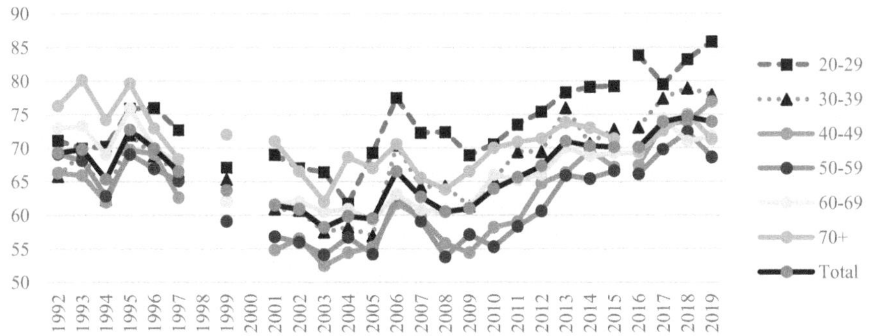

Fig. 6 Life satisfaction across age groups, 1992–2019. *Note* Assembled by the author from the Public Opinion Survey on the Life of the People, carried out annually by the Cabinet Office (2019a). Shares of respondents who answered "satisfied" or "rather satisfied" are shown. From 2016, the sample population was broadened, with the youngest age group now including 18–29-year-olds. Therefore, shares were not comparable beyond 2015

negative aspects mentioned above.[9] At the start of the 2010s, their life satisfaction appears to be higher than that of any other age group (Fig. 6), and thus, he claims that they are also more satisfied with their lives than their peers were during the economic boom years of the 1970s. This unexpected finding did not fit into the discourse on crisis-ridden youth. A heated debate ensued as to whether this should be considered a valid result and, if so, how the high life satisfaction of young people could be explained (Asano, 2016: 19–22).

However, it needs to be pointed out that the figures Furuichi uses to make his main argument (that Japanese in their twenties today are happier today than their counterparts in the 1970s and 1980s) are based on data that cannot be compared. The wording of the question on life satisfaction (what Furuichi calls "happiness") used in the Public Opinion Survey on the Life of the People has been changed since 1992. Previously, it was asked in a manner that invited a response bias toward dissatisfaction, especially among young respondents (Todoroki, 2018: 175ff.). Nevertheless, looking at the data from 1992 onward, Furuichi's argument seems to hold for the part of the data shown here.

The data indeed show that by the end of the 2010s, a larger share of 20–39-year-olds were satisfied with their lives than in older age groups. They also appeared to be more satisfied than their peers in the early 1990s, just before the bubble economy burst. However, this trend is not continuous. We see a lot of movement: a drop in satisfaction after the economic crisis of the 1990s, some recovery, another drop after the Lehman shock, and a somewhat continuous upward trend. Since the mid-2000s, the youngest group (20–29-year-olds) has shown the highest level of satisfaction, and in recent years, the 30–39-year-olds have followed in second place. This means that even several years after the publication of Furuichi's book (2011), an overall upward

[9] Furuichi is not the first to point this out. He quotes Toyoizumi (2010) and Ōsawa (2011), who both discuss this seemingly puzzling data.

trend in life satisfaction among the two youngest age groups has continued. Therefore, even if a comparison with the 1970s is not possible (as Furuichi erroneously did), it appears that Japan's young people are more satisfied with their lives than their counterparts in the early 2000s and older age groups.

Other longitudinal surveys have provided similar results. For example, the five waves of the Survey on the Life and Attitudes of Middle and High School Students carried out by public broadcaster NHK (2013) show a stark increase in the share of middle and high school students who report being "very happy" from 1982 to 2012. Although this seems to indicate that the high subjective well-being of Japan's youth discussed by Furuichi and others is not a statistical artifact, it definitely contradicts the numerous reports on the fragile mental well-being of young people, as evidenced by the increasing number of depression, social withdrawals, and even suicides. Yoshino (2015: 13) points out that this may be the result of a change in response behavior rather than an actual increase in subjective well-being. As response rates to public surveys have steadily declined over the past few decades, especially among younger age groups, he suggests that it is highly likely that respondents who feel unhappy or isolated will not participate, thereby creating an overall bias.

Nevertheless, it is worth considering why large segments of the younger generation are satisfied with their lives despite the many threats to their social standing. For Furuichi (2011: 14), the high subjective well-being of the younger generation results from their experience of what he calls an "odd stability" (*kimyō na antei*). They evaluate their lives positively at a point in time, when they are still able to enjoy a relatively prosperous and carefree life, supported and protected by their parents. At the same time, they see a rather bleak future hanging over their heads like the sword of Damocles, foreshadowing a not-so-distant time when they will have to shoulder the costs of caring for an ever-increasing proportion of the elderly, as well as the country's growing debt. Furuichi notes that young Japanese are aware of this and are feeling anxiety and dissatisfaction with the society in which they live—a countertrend to their high subjective well-being. However, instead of letting this affect them, they are content to live in the "here and now" (*ima, koko*) and prioritize their friends. Furuichi calls this attitude "consummatory," which he uses to denote "something close to self-satisfied" or "self-contained" (Furuichi, 2011: 104–105), based on Toyoizumi (2010), who also draws on this term that originates from Talcott Parsons.

This could also indicate that what they consider important for their own well-being might differ from previous generations. Some support for this assumption is given by Hommerich and Tiefenbach (2018b), who find that the structure of what is considered important, as well as what actually impacts life satisfaction, differs across age groups.[10] The clearest difference between generational groups existed for

---

[10] As Hommerich and Tiefenbach (2018b) compare between age groups, it cannot be assumed that the found differences are necessarily generational differences.

materialistic values. In contrast to the three older age groups included in the analysis,[11] it was only among the 15–29-year-olds—which Hommerich and Tiefenbach call the "Heisei generation," born and raised in times of economic stagnation—that satisfaction with their financial situation had no significant relationship with happiness. Although this seems to point to an emancipation from a lifestyle centered on materialistic desires, with more importance placed on family and friends, it could simply be a feature of a generation that has adapted to a new economic reality.[12] The non-materialistic attitudes of the young are probably born out of necessity, rather than an idealistic life choice of simplicity over abundance. Nevertheless, as the young set different priorities when evaluating their life, they achieve higher levels of life satisfaction than older generations who cling to the past. Not always yearning for "higher, faster, better," especially in a material sense, might be positive, as the expectation of constant growth is not a sustainable idea of a "good life" (Rosa & Henning, 2018). Thus, the fact that a large part of the younger generation seems to have adapted to Japan's new social reality can be interpreted as a form of resilience that enables them to be happy with less, at least for now.

However, whether this type of happiness can last is questionable. This "resilient" or "realistic" approach to life can also be interpreted as a young generation having "given up" and being in danger of feeling complacent in a seemingly comfortable present but ill-equipped to cope with future risks. Furthermore, when this means not actively claiming basic rights (adequate working conditions, coverage of minimum needs, equal opportunities for women to work or for men to stay at home and take care of children), then this kind of "happiness" becomes problematic. As many young Japanese do not feel that they can make a difference in their society, they are reluctant to get involved. Eventually, this will backfire, as they will have to take over the steering wheel at some point. This generally indicates that high levels of happiness or life satisfaction do not mean that policymakers can cross the young generation off their policy list; in fact, it could mean quite the opposite. Moreover, an increasing number of young people seem to have fallen through the cracks, feeling left behind by society and struggling to find their place, as evidenced by the aforementioned growing instances of clinical depression, social withdrawal, and suicide.

6 Looking Ahead

Overall, Japanese society has undergone fundamental societal changes over the past three decades, which necessitate adapting to a new social reality. At least a part of the younger generation has grown accustomed to economic inequality and insecurity

[11] Age groups were formed as follows, based on theoretical assumptions about generational differences: 15–29-year-olds, 30–44-year-olds, 45–64-year-olds, 65–80-year-olds.

[12] As Hommerich and Tiefenbach (2018b) rely on cross-sectional data for their analysis, it remains unclear whether this is an actual effect of generational location (*cohort effect*) or a difference that is based on different stages in the life course (*age effect*).

as inherent societal problems, and there seems to be more awareness of existing and growing inequalities overall. Nevertheless, there is still a yearning for times gone by when everyone seemed to be equally safely embedded in society. Although this is probably only a romanticization of a past that was never really true, it is likely to affect how people value their lives today, creating status anxiety among those whose livelihoods are still relatively stable.

For an increasing part of the population, however, socioeconomic problems have become more than a mere threat, but a lived reality of struggling to secure enough income to get by, with any unforeseen expense potentially pushing the household below the poverty line. The COVID-19 pandemic has made these precarious situations more visible, as its economic impact exacerbates pre-existing socioeconomic inequalities by disproportionately affecting socially vulnerable groups (Kanbayashi et al., 2021; Slater, 2020). This social gradient of experiencing income loss or even job loss is also reflected in the social gradient of mental well-being. Based on panel data collected from June to December 2020, Kanbayashi et al. (2021) show that while life satisfaction and mental health have deteriorated overall, this effect is especially large for lower status groups. These findings support the call for strengthening social security legislation and public welfare that targets and protects the most vulnerable. As this is unlikely to be compatible with calls for further economic growth, Japan's ruling party might need to ponder the sustainability of its vision for the future.

Acknowledgements This work was supported by a Grant-in-Aid for Scientific Research by the Japan Society for the Promotion of Science (Grant Number 19H00609) as part of the SSP Project (http://ssp.hus.osaka-u.ac.jp/).

References

Allison, A. (2013). *Precarious Japan*. Duke University Press.

Asano, T. (2016). Seishōnen kenkyūkai no chōsa to wakamonoron no kyō no kadai [Survey of the youth research group and current topics of discourses on youth]. In M. Fujimura, T. Asano, & I. Habuchi (Eds.), *Gendai wakamono no kōfuku—fuankan shakai o ikiru* [*The happiness of today's youth. Living in a society of uncertainty*] (pp. 1–23). Kōseisha Kōseikaku.

Cabinet Office. (2007). Heisei 19 nen-han kokumin seikatsu hakusho: Tsunagari ga kizuku yutakana kokumin seikatsu [White paper on the national lifestyle 2007: A comfortable way of life for the Japanese people, founded on personal relationships]. Retrieved December 15, 2023, from https://warp.da.ndl.go.jp/info:ndljp/pid/9990748/www5.cao.go.jp/seikatsu/whitepaper/h19/01_honpen/index.html

Cabinet Office. (2014). Heisei 25-nendo wagakuni to shogaikoku no wakamono no ishiki ni kansuru chōsa [International survey of youth attitudes 2013]. Retrieved December 15, 2023, from https://warp.da.ndl.go.jp/info:ndljp/pid/12927443/www8.cao.go.jp/youth/english/survey/2013/pdf_index.html

Cabinet Office. (2019a). Kokumin seikatsu ni kan suru yoron chōsa [Public opinion survey on the life of the people]. Retrieved December 15, 2023, from http://survey.gov-online.go.jp/index-ko.html

Cabinet Office. (2019b). Heisei 30-nendo shoushika shakai taisaku hakusho [White paper on measures for a low fertility society 2018]. Retrieved December 15, 2023, from https://www8.cao.go.jp/shoushi/shoushika/whitepaper/measures/w-2018/30webhonpen/index.html

Cabinet Office. (2019c). Heisei 30-nendo wagakuni to shogaikoku no wakamono no ishiki ni kansuru chōsa [International survey of youth attitudes 2018]. Retrieved December 15, 2023, from https://warp.da.ndl.go.jp/info:ndljp/pid/12927443/www8.cao.go.jp/youth/english/survey/2018/pdf_index.html

Chiavacci, D. (2006). The general middle class model under pressure: Mainstream Japan at a turning point? In H. Helfrich, M. Zillekens, & E. Höltner (Eds.), *Culture and development in Japan and Germany* (pp. 59–82). Daedalus Verlag.

Chiavacci, D. (2008). From class struggle to general middle-class society to divided society: Societal models of inequality in postwar Japan. *Social Science Japan Journal, 11*(1), 5–27.

Chiavacci, D., & Hommerich, C. (Eds.). (2017). *Social inequality in post-growth Japan: Transformation during economic and demographic stagnation.* Routledge.

Commission on Measuring Well-being. (2011). Measuring national well-being—Proposed well-being indicators. Retrieved December 15, 2023, from https://www5.cao.go.jp/keizai2/koufukudo/pdf/koufukudosian_english.pdf

Coulmas, F., Conrad, H., Schad-Seifert, A., & Vogt, G. (Eds.). (2008). *The demographic challenge: A handbook about Japan.* Brill.

Furuichi, N. (2011). *Zetsubō no kuni no kōfuku na wakamonotachi* [*The happy youth of a desperate country*]. Kōdansha.

Genda, Y. (2005). *A nagging sense of insecurity: The new reality facing Japanese youth* (J. C. Hoff, Trans.). LTCB International Library Trust, International House of Japan.

Genda, Y. (2013). *Koritsu mugyô: SNEP* [*Solitary non-employed persons*]. Nihon Keizai Shinbun Shuppansha.

Giddens, A. (1990). *The consequences of modernity.* Polity Press.

Hara, J., & Seiyama, K. (2005). *Inequality amid affluence: Social stratification in Japan.* Trans Pacific Press.

Heinrich, S. (2013). *Patterns of dualisation: Coordinated capitalism and the politics of flexible labour markets in Germany and Japan, 1990–2010* [Ph.D. thesis]. Ruprecht-Karls University, Heidelberg.

Helliwell, J. F., Layard, R., Sachs, J. D., De Neve, J.-E., Aknin, L. B., & Wang, S. (Eds.). (2023). *World happiness report 2023.* Sustainable Development Solutions Network.

Holthus, B., & Manzenreiter, W. (Eds.). (2017). *Life course, happiness and well-being in Japan.* Routledge.

Hommerich, C. (2012). The advent of vulnerability: Japan's free fall through its porous safety net. *Japan Forum, 24*(2), 205–232.

Hommerich, C. (2013). Adapting to risk, learning to trust: Socioeconomic insecurities and feelings of disconnectedness in contemporary Japan. *Asiatische Studien/Etudes Asiatiques, 67*(2), 429–455.

Hommerich, C. (2015). Feeling disconnected: Exploring the relationship between different forms of social capital and civic engagement in Japan. *VOLUNTAS: International Journal of Voluntary and Nonprofit Organizations, 26*, 45–68.

Hommerich, C. (2017a). The gap as threat: Status anxiety in the "middle." In D. Chiavacci & C. Hommerich (Eds.), *Social inequality in post-growth Japan: Transformation during economic and demographic stagnation* (pp. 37–53). Routledge.

Hommerich, C. (2017b). Anxious, stressed, and yet satisfied? The puzzle of subjective well-being among young adults in Japan. In B. Holthus & W. Manzenreiter (Eds.), *Life course, happiness and well-being in Japan* (pp. 72–93). Routledge.

Hommerich, C., & Kikkawa, T. (2019). Movement behind the scenes: The quiet transformation of status identification in Japan. *Social Science Japan Journal, 22*(1), 11–24. https://doi.org/10.1093/ssjj/jyy041

Hommerich, C., Sudo, N., & Kikkawa, T. (Eds.). (2021). *Social change in Japan, 1989–2019: Social status, social consciousness, attitudes and values*. Routledge.

Hommerich, C., & Tiefenbach, T. (2018a). Analyzing the relationship between social capital and subjective well-being: The mediating role of social affiliation. *Journal of Happiness Studies, 19*(4), 1091–1114. https://doi.org/10.1007/s10902-017-9859-9

Hommerich, C., & Tiefenbach, T. (2018b). The structure of happiness: Why young Japanese might be happy after all. In P. Heinrich & C. Galan (Eds.), *Being young and resilient in super-aged Japan* (pp. 132–149). Routledge.

Ishida, H. (2001). Industrialization, class structure, and social mobility in postwar Japan. *British Journal of Sociology, 52*(4), 579–604.

Ishida, H., et al. (2007). Japan: Educational expansion and inequality in access to higher education. In Y. Shavit (Ed.), *Stratification in higher education: A comparative study* (pp. 63–86). Stanford University Press.

Ishida, H., & Miwa, S. (2009). Kaisō Idō kara mita Nihon Shakai: Chōkiteki Sūsei to Kokusai Hikaku [Intergenerational class mobility and Japanese society: Long-term trends and cross-national comparisons]. *Shakaigaku Hyōron, 59*(4), 648–662.

Ishida, H., & Slater, D. H. (2010). *Social class in contemporary Japan: Structures, sorting and strategies*. Routledge.

Ishida, M. (2011). *Koritsu no shakaigaku. Muen shakai no shohôsen* [*Sociology of isolation. A recipe for a society without bonds*]. Keisôshobô.

Japan Productivity Center. (2019). Dai-9-kai mentaru herusu no torikumi ni kan suru kigyou ankeeto chousa kekka [Survey results of 9th company survey on employees' mental health]. Retrieved December 15, 2023, from https://www.jpc-net.jp/research/assets/pdf/R4attached.pdf

Kanbayashi, H., Hommerich, C., & Sudo, N. (2021). Impact of COVID-19 pandemic on household income and mental well-being: Evidence from a panel survey in Japan. *Riron to Hôhô, 36*(2), 260–278.

Kankonsôsaigojokyôkai, Z. (2012). *Muen shakai kara yûen shakai he* [*From a society without bonds towards a society with bonds*]. Suiyôsha.

Kariya, T. (2001). *Kaisōka Nihon to kyōiku kiki: Fubyōdō saiseisan kara iyoku kakusa shakai he* [*Educational crisis of stratified Japan: From reproduction of inequality to social disparity (incentive divide)*]. Yūshindō.

Kawano, S., Roberts, G. S., & Long, S. O. (2014). *Capturing contemporary Japan: Differentiation and uncertainty*. University of Hawaii Press.

MHLW (Ministry of Health Labor and Welfare). (2014). *Heisei 26-nenban kōsei rōdo hakusho* [*White paper on health, labour and welfare*]. MHLW.

MHLW (Ministry of Health Labor and Welfare). (2020). Summary report of comprehensive survey of living conditions 2019. Retrieved July 20, 2021, from https://www.mhlw.go.jp/english/database/db-hss/dl/report_gaikyo_2019.pdf

MIAC (Ministry of Internal Affairs and Communications). (1984–2017). *Statistical handbook of Japan*. MIAC.

MIAC (Ministry of Internal Affairs and Communications). (2017). *Labour force survey*. MIAC.

Miura, A. (2005). *Karyū Shakai: Aratana Kaisō Shūdan no Shutsugen* [*Low-stream society: The emergence of a new class formation*]. Kōbunsha.

Miyamoto, M. (2012). *Wakamono ga muenka suru. Shigoto, fukushi, komyuniti de tsunagu* [*The youth are losing their bonds. Connecting through work, social security and the community*]. Chikuma shobô.

Musikanski, L., Phillips, R., & Crowder, J. (2019). *The happiness policy handbook. How to make happiness and well-being the purpose of your government*. New Society Publishers.

NHK. (2010). *Muen shakai. "Muenshi" 32.000 nin no shougeki* [*Society without bonds. Unnoticed deaths: The shocking number of 32.000 people*]. NHK "Muen shakai purojekuto" shuzaihan. Bungei Shunjû.

NHK Hōsō Bunka Kenkyūjo. (2013). *NHK chūgakusei, kōkōsei no seikatsu to ishiki chōsa 2012. Ushinawareta 20-nen ga unda "shiawase" na jūdai* [*NHK survey of middle school and high

school students 2012. The "happy" teens who were born in Japan's two lost decades]. NHK Shuppan.
NIPSSR. (2018). Household projections for Japan (outline of results and methods). Retrieved September 15, 2021, from http://www.ipss.go.jp/pp-ajsetai/e/hhprj2018/t-page_e.asp
OECD. (2008). *Growing unequal? Income distribution and poverty in OECD countries*. OECD.
OECD. (2023). Better life index. Retrieved December 15, 2023, from www.oecdbetterlifeindex.org
Ōsawa, M. (2011). Kanō ni naru kakumei dai ikkai. 'Kōfuku da' to kotaeru wakamonotachi no jidai [A possible revolution, part 1. The age of a youth who states 'I am happy']. *At Plus*, 114–127.
Ōtake, F. (2005). *Nihon no Fubyōdō: Kakusa Shakai no Gensō to Mirai*. Nihon Keizai Shinbunsha.
Rosa, H., & Henning, C. (Eds.). (2018). *The good life beyond growth: New perspectives*. Routledge.
Satō, T. (2000). *Fubyōdō shakai Nihon: Sayōnara sōchūryū* [*Japan as unequal society: A farewell to mass middle class society*]. Chūō Kōron Shinsha.
Sato, Y. (2007). *Deciphering stratification and inequality: Japan and beyond*. Trans Pacific Press.
Sato, Y., & Imai, J. (Eds.). (2011). *Japan's new inequality: Intersection of employment reforms and welfare arrangements*. Trans Pacific Press.
Shirahase, S. (2014). *Social inequality in Japan*. Routledge.
Slater, D. (2020). Vulnerable populations under COVID-19 in Japan: A lull in the storm? *The Asia Pacific Journal, 18*(18), 2. https://apjjf.org/2020/18/Slater.html
Tachibanaki, T. (1998). *Nihon no keizai kakusa: Shotoku to shisan kara kangaeru*. Iwanami Shoten.
Tachibanaki, T. (2005). *Confronting income inequality in Japan: A comparative analysis of causes, consequences, and reform*. The MIT Press.
Tachibanaki, T. (2011). *Muen shakai no shôtai—ketsuen, chien, shaen wa ika ni hôkai shita ka* [*The reality of a society without bonds—Have blood relations, regional relations, social relations been lost?*]. PHP Kenkyûjo.
Todoroki, M. (2018). Seikatsumanzokudo kara miru gendai no wakamono to kōkōsei no sugata [Looking at current high school students via their life satisfaction]. In: F. Oshima & S. Aramaki (Eds.), *Kōkōseitachi no yukue: Gakkō paneru chōsa kara mita shinrō to seikatsu no 30-nen* [*Where high school students are headed: Looking at career choices and lifestyle over the course of 30 years based on a panel survey of high school students*]. Sekaishishōsha.
Tsai, M.-C., & Iwai, N. (Eds.). (2020). *Quality of life in Japan: Contemporary perspectives on happiness*. Springer.
Toyoizumi, S. (2010). *Wakamono no tame no shakaigaku. Kibō ni ashiba o kakeru* [*A sociology for the youth. Giving a foothold to hope*]. Haruka Shobō.
UNDP. (2022). *Human development report 2021/22. Uncertain times, unsettled lives: Shaping our future in a transforming world*. UNDP. Retrieved December 15, 2023, from https://hdr.undp.org/system/files/documents/global-report-document/hdr2021-22pdf_1.pdf
Wilkinson, R., & Pickett, K. (2009). *The spirit level. Why more equal societies almost always do better*. Penguin.
World Bank. (1993). *The East Asian miracle: Economic growth and public policy*. World Bank.
Yamada, M. (2004). *Kibô Kakusa Shakai—"Makegumi" no zetsubôkan ga nihon wo hikisaku* [*Society of split hopes—The despair of Japan's "losers" pulls Japan apart*]. Chikuma Shobô.
Yamada, M. (2013). *Naze Nihon wa wakamono ni reikoku na no ka? Soshite kakō idō shakai ga tōrai suru* [*Why is Japan so heartless towards its youth? The coming of a society of downward mobility*]. Tōyō Keizai Shinpōsha.
Yoshino, R. (2015). Chōsa kagaku risaachi commonzu no sōzō [The creation of empirical research commons]. *Ichiba Chousa, 296*, 4–31.
Zielenziger, M. (2006). *Shutting out the sun. How Japan created its own lost generation*. Vintage Departures.

Carola Hommerich is Professor of Sociology at Sophia University, Tokyo (Japan). Her research focuses on well-being and social inequality, particularly on the interrelation of experiences of precariousness, status anxiety and feelings of exclusion.

Beyond the Paradox of Affluence: The Korean Experience

Jaeyeol Yee

Abstract Despite its remarkable economic growth and successful democratization, Korea suffers from the paradox of affluence and democratization. Like other East Asian countries that have achieved high growth, there is a noticeable tendency for citizens' happiness to decline despite economic growth. This is because the marginal utility of expanding the supply of material goods has gradually declined, while competition for positional goods has intensified. In this scenario, social quality is crucial. Empirical analysis shows that people's happiness is highly correlated with social quality, particularly the capacity of civil society. When controlling for social quality, the impact of income on happiness vanishes. In Korea, due to the low quality of society, passive risk aversion, excessive competition for positional goods, and winner-take-all tendencies are prevalent. To increase happiness, it is urgent to improve social quality through promoting fairness and transparency.

Keywords Positional goods · Paradox of affluence · Paradox of democratization · Social quality · Transparency · Fairness

1 Has Economic Growth Brought Happiness and Sustainability?

Korea, after decades of successful industrialization and democratization, now faces significant sustainability risks. These risks include a low fertility rate, dissolution of family and community, paradox of prosperity, severe trust deficit, and declining country competitiveness (Yee, 2019a: 120–134; Yee, 2019b).

This chapter is based on research financially supported by the National Research Foundation of Korea (NRF-2020S1A5A2A03045598).

J. Yee (✉)
Department of Sociology, Seoul National University, Seoul, Republic of Korea
e-mail: jyyee@snu.ac.kr

J. Yee et al. (eds.), *Social Well-Being, Development, and Multiple Modernities in Asia*,
https://doi.org/10.1007/978-981-97-3866-3_8

The low total fertility rate poses a direct and fundamental threat to population sustainability. In 1970, one million babies were born annually. However, the number of births has declined from 1 million in 1990 to 400,000 in 2002, followed by a further reduction to approximately 249,000 in 2022. The total fertility rate (TFR), which represents the expected number of births per woman during her lifetime, was recorded at 0.78 in 2022, making it the first in the world to fall below 1.0. The TFR should ideally be above 2.1 to maintain population levels. However, the average TFR of OECD countries is only 1.68. During its high-growth period, South Korea experienced a population boom, but now faces a population burden. The number of economically active taxpayers is decreasing rapidly, while the elderly population in need of support is increasing quickly. An aging population reduces social vibrancy and lowers real growth rates. The low birthrate poses a serious sustainability challenge for South Korea.

The second challenge is the breakdown of family and community. Studies reveal that the definition of family has narrowed down to spouses and children, with grandparents no longer being considered as part of the family by the younger generation. The divorce rate increased after the 1997 financial crisis, although it has slowly reduced in recent times. Additionally, divorce rates have increased among elderly couples. The proportion of households headed by women has increased due to divorce and non-marriage, whereas bereavement was previously the primary contributing factor. Additionally, there has been a significant rise in single-person households, which accounted for 27% of all households in 2015, totaling 5.2 million, up from 2.22 million in 2000. Demographers predict that the number of single-person households will continue to increase, reaching 7.6 million by 2035, which will represent one-third of all households. The dissolution of community has led to a rise in isolated individuals. It is worth noting that the percentage of socially isolated people in Korea is substantially greater than that of European countries, which were initially believed to be more individualistic. The increasing number of single-person households indicates a lack of familial, communal, or social support. Furthermore, there is evidence of the breakdown of traditional communities. More than half of Korea's population lives in densely populated, communal housing such as apartments and villas, which often lack a sense of community. Consequently, residents tend to lead isolated and segmented lifestyles (Yee, 2019b: 49–56).

Despite the growth of Korea's GDP, the happiness of the Korean people has continued to decline. In 2022, Korea's per capita gross national income was $32,661, which is 7.7% lower than in 2021. Although Korea's per capita gross national income first reached the $30,000 range in 2017, it declined for two consecutive years starting in 2019. Currently, South Korea's per capita income is comparable to that of Japan, Taiwan, and Italy. However, South Korea's ranking in the United Nations Happiness Report has declined from 43rd in 2013 to 55th and 57th in 2017 and 2018, respectively (Helliwell et al., 2017). Additionally, Korea has the highest suicide rate among OECD countries, which illustrates the 'Easterlin paradox' that suggests that as income rises, happiness may decline (Easterlin, 1974). In the 1980s, when GDP per capita was between $2000 and $3000, rising living standards led to an increase in happiness. This phenomenon can be described as a 'tidal wave' effect, as even the most underprivileged individuals were able to benefit from economic growth. Despite political repression in the 1970s and 1980s, Koreans remained optimistic about the economy. During this period, there was a widespread tendency to consider oneself part of the middle class, accompanied by a belief that the future would bring improvement. The resilient middle-class identity, fostered by this optimistic outlook on the future, resulted in the active participation of the empowered middle class in the democratization movement (Yee, 2015a: 3–6).

The fourth issue concerns the lack of trust (Kim, 2018: 101–127). Although democratization is undoubtedly a significant achievement, there is a notable level of cynicism toward politics. Institutional politics in Korea face intense criticism, yet political participation is less popular, with Koreans having the lowest voter turnout among all OECD countries. The candlelight vigils that led to the impeachment of President Park in 2016 can be seen as a manifestation of widespread dissatisfaction with institutional politics. Essentially, the dysfunction of the political process brought people to the streets and led to the removal of an irresponsible president. This highlights the paradox of democratization. During the 1970s and 1980s, under authoritarian governments, there was a high level of institutional and general trust. After the democratization process, a 'trust deficit' emerged. This deficit is most evident in the serious lack of trust in the legislative, judicial, and executive bodies responsible for creating, enforcing, and protecting social rules. This mistrust has significant social costs, as it prevents individuals from accepting the decisions of the arbiters. As a result, social conflicts remain unresolved, and the tragedy of the commons is all too common (Fig. 1).

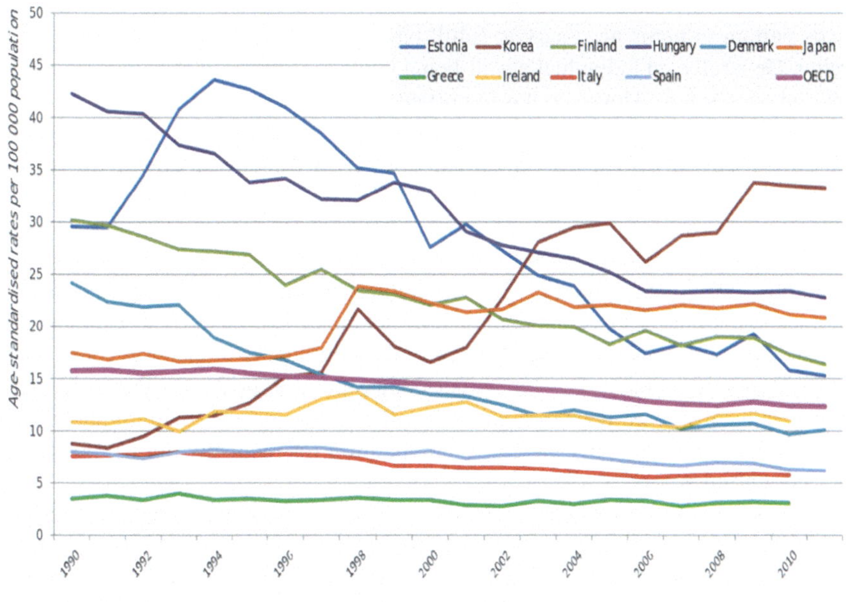

Fig. 1 Trends in suicide rates in selected OECD countries: 1990–2011

The decline in South Korea's national competitiveness has been identified as a significant issue (Yee, 2018: 362–265). According to the World Economic Forum (WEF), South Korea's national competitiveness peaked at 11th place in 2007 but has since fallen, ranking 26th out of 137 countries in 2017. In Asia, South Korea's national competitiveness ranks behind Singapore, Hong Kong, Japan, Taiwan, and Malaysia. The report identifies areas of relative competitiveness, including infrastructure, tertiary enrollment, number of patents, and broadband penetration. On the other hand, labor relations, corporate governance, transparency in government policymaking, quality of government regulation, banking soundness, and political trust are identified as the least competitive areas. In summary, the report suggests that quantitative inputs and hardware are strengths, while software and institutions are weaknesses. The report also notes that Korea has a 'high investment, low efficiency' system. Table 1 displays the comparative rankings of Korea among OECD countries. Korea ranks particularly low in fertility, aging, unemployment insurance, elderly poverty rate, public welfare spending, suicide rate, health care spending, life satisfaction, trust, anxiety about the future, social relationships, and loneliness.

2 From Material Goods to Positional Goods

The sustainability crisis underscores several issues that cannot be resolved by merely increasing supply through economic growth. In his book, *The Social Limits of Growth*, British economist Fred Hirsch explained the paradox of affluence. Hirsch (1976) introduced the differentiation between material goods and positional goods. Material goods pertain to items necessary to fulfill basic needs, such as food, clothing, and shelter. Generally, an individual's well-being tends to increase as they acquire more material possessions. However, it is important to note that the satisfaction or value of positional goods is dependent on the existence of alternatives or the needs of others.

In the 1970s, British society experienced a period of material prosperity due to rapid economic growth following World War II. However, social discontent increased as demands for economic distribution grew and personal tastes and sexual orientations became more individualistic. It is important to note that in the early stages of economic development, material goods play a significant role in increasing satisfaction and happiness. Once national income per capita exceeds $10,000, intangible goods become increasingly important. Expanding the supply of material goods may reduce competition, but it does not reduce competition for positional goods. In fact, competition for limited positional goods tends to be more intense in affluent societies. Even when the supply increases, competition for relatively limited positions does not diminish.

Typical examples of positional goods are a prestigious college degree and a decent job. In the 1980s, the authoritarian government of Korea expanded higher education to address a legitimacy deficit. In the 1990s, the civilian government removed restrictions on the establishment of universities. Consequently, the availability of higher education increased rapidly, leading to Korea's world-leading enrollment

Table 1 Korean society at a glance (2016, OECD)

Variables		Ranking
General	Household income	17/35
	Fertility rate	35/35
	Aging	35/35
Work	Employment	20/36
	Unemployment rate	3/35
	Unemployment insurance	28/35
Equality and welfare	Income inequality	18/35
	Relative poverty rate	26/35
	Elderly poverty rate	35/35
	Support for unemployed	25/32
	Welfare expenditure (% among GDP)	34/35
Health	Life expectancy	10/35
	Perception on health	34/34
	Suicide rate	35/35
	Expenditure on health	26/35
	Smoking/drinking	15–20/35
Social integration	Life satisfaction	28/35
	Trust on strangers	23/35
	Trust on government	29/33
	Anxiety for future	14/15
	Crime rate	18/35
	Social relation	28/34
	Loneliness of 50s	34/34

rates. Unfortunately, the number of jobs suitable for university graduates, such as professional, administrative, and white-collar positions, has not increased proportionally. This has led to fierce competition for these positions, resulting in a surplus of graduates seeking employment while manual labor positions remain unfilled. According to the Bank of Korea's report, there are approximately 5 million high-quality job opportunities available, including professional and clerical positions, while the number of college graduates has reached 10 million (Jang et al., 2011; Yee, 2019b; 77–79). Additionally, there are millions of people estimated to be not in employment, education, or training (NEET). A comparison between the baby boom generation (born between 1955 and 1963) and the echo boom generation (born between 1979 and 1992) reveals the contrasting effects of the rapid expansion of higher education. The baby boomers reached adulthood during a time of political authoritarianism and low income, which limited their access to higher education. Despite this, they maintained a strong middle-class identity and held high aspirations for the future. The generation known as echo boomers came of age in a prosperous and democratic society, with many of them obtaining a college degree. However, they face challenges in finding employment, purchasing a home, and starting a family. While economic growth is evident, competition is also increasing. This phenomenon is known as the paradox of affluence.

The question is how to interpret this change. The most direct and persuasive interpretation of why the effect on happiness declines as economic growth and incomes increase comes from Fred Hirsch (Hirsch, 1976). The society he was interested in was England in the 1970s. Although it had become a materially affluent society after the war, demands for distribution and equality were growing, and sexual and esthetic tastes showed a tendency toward extreme individualism. In terms of economic policy, it is closely associated with collectivism, which calls for strong national regulation.

Hirsch distinguished between material goods and positional goods. Material goods are goods needed to satisfy basic needs for food, clothing, and shelter, while positional goods are goods or services that are relatively scarce and whose relative value is determined by the existence of substitutes or the needs of others. Representative examples include the environment, transportation, education, and employment.

Hirsch argues that in the early stages of economic growth, increasing the supply of material goods can enhance people's satisfaction and happiness. However, once economic growth surpasses a certain level, the importance of positional goods gradually increases, which cannot be resolved by simply increasing the supply of material goods. This leads to the 'paradox of affluence' where dissatisfaction accumulates. Competition for material goods can be reduced by increasing the supply. However, competition for positional goods always has the characteristics of a zero-sum game, at least in the short run, because relative ranking is crucial. Additionally, positional goods are equivalent to economic rent or quasi-rent.

Looking back, it can be concluded that Korea's rapid growth was primarily focused on expanding material goods. The benefits of this growth had a significant impact on a generation that had experienced hunger and war. Even those who were previously impoverished and malnourished now have access to an abundance of food and clothing and reside in comfortable homes. The fruits of growth have had a positive impact on the lives of even the most disadvantaged, providing hope for a better tomorrow.

As the period of rapid growth came to an end and the desire for material goods reached saturation, the demand for better college education, improved job opportunities, comfortable housing, and a pleasant environment increased. It is important to note that the utility of positional goods is always relative, as comparison with others is more significant than absolute possession. For instance, in a society with low car ownership, people can drive comfortably even on narrow roads. Therefore, the utility of self-driving cars is very high. However, once cars become widely available, traffic volume will increase rapidly, leading to traffic congestion. Environmental comfort is a prime example. Suburban areas with a small population can maintain a pleasant environment. However, as the number of residents increases due to high-density development, it becomes impossible to enjoy comfort. Over the past few decades, as the desire for material goods has been satisfied, competition for status goods has intensified, leading to various problems.

Using Korea's college enrollment rate as an example, it is noteworthy that the college entrance rate for high school graduates has increased from 25 to 85% in the past 30 years. This is an unprecedented college enrollment rate worldwide. However, until the early 1990s, Korea's increase in college entrance rate was not particularly noticeable compared to other Asian countries or the USA. After the policy of increasing the supply of higher education was implemented in the early 1990s through the liberalization of university establishment, the college entrance rate continued to increase and reached the highest level in the world (Noriko, 2011). Although college admission became easier, competition for admission to prestigious universities became unimaginably fierce. Competition for prior learning has had a ripple effect, impacting not only high schools but also middle schools.

The issue persists beyond the competition for entrance exams. The mass production of college graduates has made it increasingly challenging to secure desirable office jobs in large companies or the public sector. Consequently, there is a significant rate of unemployment among young college graduates. However, it is frequently reported that finding low-skilled production workers is challenging, leading to intense competition among small and medium business owners to hire foreign workers. This situation exemplifies the economics of positional goods, where the expansion of supply has worsened the problem instead of resolving it. If the supply of education exceeds the institutionally optimized level without a corresponding increase in decent jobs, it leads to overeducation. This, in turn, increases overall labor market inefficiency. College graduates are now performing jobs that were previously done by high school graduates.

Housing is considered a status good. Although the housing penetration rate has reached 110% nationwide, it is still challenging for young people to purchase their own homes, especially in Seoul. This passage exemplifies incidental scarcity. In essence, satisfaction is determined by the level of competition, which is the number of other individuals seeking the same good or service. If traffic jams represent physical congestion, then excessive competition for desirable jobs or admission to prestigious universities represents social congestion.

Despite rapid economic growth and democratization, the public's sense of happiness has declined, and there has been a deepening of distrust toward institutions and political parties, leading to more serious social conflicts. This illustrates the paradox of affluence, as Korea, once a hungry society, has become an angry society (Jeon, 2008). The symptoms of this anger take various forms, such as mistrust, dissatisfaction, and fear.

A stronger tendency to compare oneself with others can contribute to economic performance, but if this tendency is stronger than the optimal level, it can lower happiness and life satisfaction. Upward comparison tends to be dysfunctional rather than a catalyst for self-development, especially when fair competition is not possible. In summary, the more individuals tend to compare themselves to others, the more they experience a sense of relative deprivation, which in turn leads to lower levels of happiness (Kim & Ohtake, 2014).

As the number of people in poor relative positions increases, social anger will intensify. For instance, in Korea, the proportion of low-wage workers is 25.7%, which is much higher than the OECD average of 16.3%. The distinction between regular and irregular workers is not only a difference in working hours but also extends to status discrimination. The poverty rate among the elderly is 45.1%, which is three times the OECD average of 13.5%. Four out of every 100 seniors live on less than $600 per month. Korea's suicide rate is 31 per 100,000 people, which is nearly three times the OECD average of 13. Additionally, Korea's recent voter turnout was the lowest in the OECD at 46%. In 1987, the push for democratization through direct elections created a new framework for political democratization. However, this resulted in widespread cynicism and distrust in politics, leading to what can be called the 'paradox of democratization.' Individuals in their 20s may experience uncertainty regarding employment and career paths, while those in their 30s may be concerned about housing plans. Individuals in their 40s and 50s may have concerns about retirement plans.

When examining Korea's modern history, it becomes evident that there has been a general and unspoken consensus among members of society regarding the values and societal goals to be pursued during each era. In the 1970s, the economic value of 'living well' was dominant during the high-growth period. Following 1987, the focus shifted to 'democratization.' However, it is difficult to identify a clear *zeitgeist* after the 2000s, even though national income has exceeded $20,000. Some propose growth as a solution, while others suggest democratization. However, it is important to note that these may not fully address the current era of mistrust, dissatisfaction, and anxiety.

3 Happiness and Social Quality

If the paradox of affluence is true, we must question the true meaning of development. Kim Kyong-dong has conceptually specified the core values of development that cannot be solved by economic growth alone (Kim, 2002: 92–94). He presents two values that make up a good society: improving the quality of life and expanding life opportunities. Improving the quality of life involves two dimensions: enhancing objective conditions for physical well-being and promoting good psychological and mental health. Objective conditions refer to the minimum material resources and the economic margin required to support them. Subjectively, a good life is characterized by spiritual abundance and happiness. Furthermore, the expansion of life opportunities is directly related to the distribution of resources. Life opportunities can be divided into two aspects: social justice related to distributive justice, which includes social inequality, exclusion, and discrimination, and the basic freedoms and choices that every human being should enjoy. Kim's development value focuses on both institutional and constructivist aspects, as well as macro- and micro-aspects, to create a good society.

Studies on qualitative development and social quality can be divided into two types: those that measure the level of society by the sum of development at the individual level, and those that focus on the societal level, which is somewhat independent of the individual level. One representative study that falls under the former category is the 'quality of life' approach. The latter category can be further divided into two approaches: one that deals with specific social characteristics, such as social cohesion, exclusion, or social capital, and another that measures the nature of society more broadly, such as sustainability, human development, and social quality (Noll, 2002).Social quality, which is of particular interest here, refers to the degree to which each individual can participate in the life of the socioeconomic and cultural public sphere under conditions that can enhance his or her well-being or personal potential (Beck et al, 1997). According to Beck and his colleagues, who first defined social quality, it is a multidimensional concept that encompasses both objective and structural dimensions, as well as macro- and micro-dimensions, like Kim Kyeong-dong's critical awareness.

Social quality refers to the characteristics of relationships at the societal level, as opposed to the quality of life at the individual level. The balance between the centrifugal force of individual self-realization and the centripetal force of collective identity expressed in the social context determines the quality of society. Individual life development and social development must complement each other to improve the quality of society. It is argued that maintaining the tension and balance between the organized formality of the system and the axis dividing the intimate informal world is crucial for improving the quality of society. Thus, the level of social conditions in each domain can be assessed by dividing the domain into the individual and society and the system and the lifeworld, and evaluating the degree to which they are met (Beck et al., 2001; van der Maesen and Walker, 2005; Yee, 2007; Yee et al., 2015). The quality of society is based on four components that form the basis of social relations: resources, solidarity, access, and participation, as well as capabilities. The conditions that affect each component can be categorized into indicators based on the following principles.

(1) Socioeconomic safety, which shows how people have access to material and environmental resources.
(2) Social cohesion, which shows how social relationships are based on shared identity and value norms
(3) Social inclusion, which shows how accessible people are to the various institutions and social relationships that make up their daily lives.
(4) Social empowerment, which shows the extent to which an individual's skills and abilities are enhanced by social relationships.

By combining the indicators of these four dimensions, it will be possible to index the quality of society as a new measure of community. A good society is one with high social quality. It is a 'safe society' rather than a 'dangerous society,' a 'trusting society' rather than a 'suspicious society,' and an 'inclusive society' rather than an 'exclusive society' and is characterized by a 'vital society' rather than a 'lethargic society.'

Socioeconomic security measures whether material and environmental resources for human life are adequately secured at the societal level. A society in which basic needs are met is considered safe, while one in which they are not met is considered a risk society.

Social cohesion is a crucial measure of solidarity and shared identity among individuals. A society that maintains cohesion is often referred to as a 'trust society,' while a disorganized society with no shared values, inconsistent social norms, and selfish competition between groups is defined as a 'distrust society.'

Social inclusion is an objective measure of accessibility to institutions and social relationships in everyday life. It is based on the normative principle that all members of society should have equal access to opportunity structures, regardless of their color, gender, age, values, or beliefs. The society that is the opposite of an 'inclusive society' is referred to as an 'exclusionary society.'

Empowerment is an indicator of whether a society is structured, so that individuals can develop their capabilities and participate in important decisions about their destiny. A society in which individuals can develop their capabilities and participate well politically can be defined as a 'vital society,' and the opposite can be defined as a 'lethargic society.'

European scholars have identified 95 indicators across four domains to measure social quality (van der Maesen and Walker, 2005). However, the European scholars' approach to social quality has some issues (Yee and Chang, 2011). One of these issues is caused by an excessive focus on theory. The strong tendency to pursue consistency at the level of concepts and theories has led to neglect of the correspondence of the analytical framework with reality. Empirical research on multidimensionality should be supported by multilevel concepts and methods. However, studies such as those by van der Maesen and Walker (2005) do not explicitly indicate the level of analysis. As a result, the same variables are sometimes used as overlapping indicators to measure different domains and levels.

The concept of social quality has a European bias, as European countries have already achieved a high level of social quality compared to the global average. This leads to a tendency to assume that the rule of law, which is the foundation of social quality, is a given. In other words, there is a tendency to take for granted a high level of national income, a well-functioning democracy, and a high degree of transparency and rule of law. However, many developing countries and East Asian nations face significant challenges with issues that European countries consider routine. Transparency and the rule of law are the most critical factors.

To conduct an empirical study on social quality in an international context, it is essential to establish a macro-level framework for analysis. Additionally, it is crucial to reframe social quality from a developmental perspective. Social quality can serve as a conceptual measure of how advanced or successful a society is. It is particularly useful in understanding the reasons behind social conflicts, mistrust, and unhappiness despite economic growth and democratization.

To achieve this goal, it is important to ensure the one-dimensionality and simplicity of the concept for successful comparative empirical analysis. To measure social quality at the societal level, indicators must be measured at the macro-social level, and the concept of social quality must be reformulated as a realistic implication for social policy.

The author defines social quality as the sum of a society's institutional and civic capacities that enable it to cope with various social risks. The ability to cope with social risks is divided into two functions: providing social protection, which is usually mediated by macro-level and institutional processes, and promoting individual resilience, which usually results in the expression of individual capabilities. The revised components of social quality prepared in this way are given in Table 2.

The public system's capacity lies in its ability to provide social protection through the welfare system, as well as education and employment opportunities that can enhance individual resilience. The study used various variables to measure the capacity of the welfare system, including the relative poverty rate, public social spending, union density, and public pension replacement rate. Additionally, the study used indicators such as employment rates for men and women, public education spending, and higher education enrollment rates to measure the capacity to provide education and jobs.

Civil society capacity is determined by social cohesion, which measures the extent to which members of society feel that they belong to common rules and are united with each other, and the extent to which they participate politically to solve their own problems. Variables for cohesion include press freedom, government effectiveness, Internet usage, transparency, awareness of rights, gender equality, and general trust.

Table 2 Revised components of social quality

	Providing social protection		
Public system capacity	**Welfare protection** • Relative poverty • Public social expenditure • Trade union density • Gross pension replacement rate (public)	**Social cohesion** • Freedom of the press • Government effectiveness • Percent of internet users • Corruption perception index • Average rights • Gender empowerment • General trust	Civil society capacity
	Resilience by education and employment • Female employment rate• Male employment rate • Public expenditure on education • Gross enrollment rate in upper secondary education	**Political empowerment** • Institutional trust • Voter turnout • Total organizational participation • Democracy	
	Improving individual resilience		

The elements that constitute participation are trust in the system, voter turnout in various elections, participation in associations, and the level of democracy (Yee & Chang, 2011).

4 Structural Conditions for Social Quality

The data used to measure social quality in OECD countries was obtained from the OECD for representative macro-indicators and from the World Values Survey or barometer survey data. The following procedures were used to construct the quality of society. The quality of society for each country was determined by entering and standardizing indicators, with a maximum value of 100 and a minimum value of 0 for each variable. Subsector scores were calculated by taking the arithmetic mean of relevant variables to produce a score for each category. The social quality index was constructed by taking the arithmetic mean of all subsector scores.

Based on the results, Denmark has the highest social quality among OECD countries, followed by Iceland, Sweden, Norway, and Finland. The Nordic countries are leading in this aspect. Germany ranks 14th, while Italy ranks 22nd and Greece ranks 26th.

Korea ranks 28th out of 30 OECD countries in terms of social quality. While the country performs relatively well in providing education and jobs, ranking 18th, it falls behind in social cohesion, ranking 23rd. Additionally, both welfare capacity and civic political participation are at the bottom, ranking 29th. The capacity of the public system ranks 28th, and civil society ranks 27th.

What is the relationship between social quality and happiness? Based on the correlation analysis, it can be observed that both GDP per capita and social quality have a strong positive correlation with happiness (see Table 3). The correlation coefficient for GDP per capita was 0.7466, while for social quality it was 0.6745. However, when examining the correlation between social quality and happiness by dividing its sub-elements, the results showed a correlation coefficient of 0.5034 with public system capacity and 0.7642 with civil society capacity. This indicates that civil society capacity has a stronger correlation with happiness than the public system. After breaking down these sectors into sub-sectors and analyzing them, it was found that public system capabilities had a relatively high correlation of 0.5886, while welfare capabilities had an insignificant relationship of 0.2845. In contrast, civil society capabilities, which include social cohesion and political competence, had a very high correlation with happiness at 0.7316 and 0.7124, respectively.

Table 4 displays the results of the regression analysis conducted to examine the factors that affect happiness. Due to the limited scope of the study to OECD countries, several variables could not be included due to the small number of cases. The analysis confirmed a significant positive effect of GDP per capita. However, when we introduced the capacity of the public system as a control variable responsible for resilience and welfare, the additional effect was minimal, and the adjusted explanatory power was poor. Conversely, when we added civil society capacity as a control

Table 3 Correlation between social quality components and happiness

Variables	Correlation coefficients
Log (GNI)	0.7466**
Social quality	0.6745**
System capacity	0.5034**
• Resilience	0.5886**
• Welfare	0.2845
Civil society capacity	0.7642**
• Social cohesion	0.7316**
• Political empowerment	0.7124**

** Significant at .01

variable, the effect of income disappeared. The impact of civil society capacity was significant in explaining the high levels of happiness in high-income advanced countries. Specifically, the effect of political empowerment within civil society capacity was more pronounced than that of social cohesion.

How do the elements of social quality relate to competition and happiness? Let us start by examining the intersection of protection (welfare) and resilience (education and jobs), which make up the capacity of the public system. Although Korea is weak in protecting against social risks, it is considered a relatively good model for enhancing individual resilience through education and jobs. Nordic countries, including Denmark, Iceland, Norway, Finland, and Sweden, are often cited as examples of balanced development with excellent protection and resilience capacities. In contrast, Turkey, Mexico, Poland, and Slovakia are considered deficient in both protection and resilience capacities. In contrast, Southern European countries like Greece and Italy are 'overprotective' as they have lower resilience capacities but higher levels of protection through welfare. On the other hand, the USA, Japan, the

Table 4 Income and social quality influencing happiness (Regression analysis)

	(1)	(2)	(3)	(4)	(5)
GDP (PPP)	1.081***	1.094***	0.506	0.654	0.702*
Public system capacity		– 0.0006			
Civil society capacity			0.018**		
• Social cohesion				0.012	
• Political empowerment					0.014^
Constant	– 4.382**	– 4.478	0.457	– 0.816	– 1.155
Observations	29	29	29	29	29
Adj R-squared	0.541	0.523	0.589	0.555	0.586

Note ^: Significant at the 0.1 level, *: Significant at the 0.05 level, **: At the 0.01 level, ***: Significant at the 0.001 level

United Kingdom, Australia, and New Zealand have lower levels of protection but higher levels of resilience, which is indicative of a typical 'neoliberal' market system.

How does this qualitative difference affect competition? In Denmark, which has an excellent social welfare system and offers many educational and job opportunities, there are many chances for those who have failed to try again. This is why young people are brave enough to take on creative challenges. In contrast, young people in Korea, which has a weak social welfare system, are overly competitive but eager to avoid risks. Innovative entrepreneurship is discouraged because failure is not tolerated. In Korea, the low rate of youth entrepreneurship confirms a pattern of passive and risk-averse competition. Another symptom is the phenomenon of individuals gravitating toward stable employment opportunities, such as civil service or public enterprise positions.

A possible typology exists at the intersection of social cohesion and political empowerment, which together form civil society capacity. In countries like Denmark or Sweden, where social cohesion and civic participation are high, citizens are more willing to solve common problems, and institutional politics for problem-solving works well. This leads to competition in capabilities at a socially appropriate level. However, Korea's institutions and systems suffer from low transparency and high levels of distrust. As distrust in fair and reasonable rules is pronounced, it is important to emphasize the negative effects of excessive competition for signaling games that focus solely on objective and quantifiable evaluations. It is crucial to avoid subjective evaluations unless they are clearly marked as such.

Advocates of the market often extol the benefits of competition, but they tend to overlook the social costs. An instance of excessive competition is peacock tail competition, where male peacocks grow long and beautiful tails to compete for females. However, the tail is cumbersome and serves no purpose other than to attract mates, which ultimately hinders protection from attacks by other animals. If competition in a society is too high, the waste resulting from competition for its own sake, such as peacocking, may outweigh its benefits (Seo, 2011: 16). The private education battle for admission to prestigious universities is a prime example of this extreme hyper-competition. As previously stated, entrance exams for prestigious universities are a competition for positional goods. Therefore, the competition is likely to intensify even with an increase in the enrollment rate for higher education. Additionally, once a certain income level is achieved, relative income and income inequality have a greater impact on individuals' life satisfaction and happiness.

Price and value are two distinct concepts. While price is easily observable, value is an intrinsic attribute that is not always apparent. Price may reflect value, but not always accurately. Measuring value correctly requires time and effort to obtain the right information. For instance, companies aim to hire the most talented individuals, and universities seek to admit the best students. However, evaluating a candidate's ability requires a long-term assessment of their performance. According to Gary Becker, a Nobel laureate economist, wages reflect an individual's traits related to human capital, such as years of schooling and tenure. Empirical data from various countries supports his theory, showing that approximately 30% of wages can be explained by human capital variables, such as education and experience. In the

Korean labor market, the human capital model has an explanatory power of over 60%. When limited to a single firm, it often exceeds 90%. However, this result is not due to a perfect market economy, but rather a bureaucratically operated compensation system based on gender, age, and education level. The uniform signaling game has become strong due to external fairness. During entrance examinations, students are selected based on numerical grades to ensure fairness. A letter of recommendation provides additional information about a candidate's personality and abilities to aid in their selection. This method is effective in a culture where the recommender's fairness and ability are trusted. However, in the absence of such trust, various compensations and school grades must be quantified uniformly based on numerical scores.

Peer evaluation based on professional ethics of the expert group can more accurately reflect the value of an expert's skills as their level of expertise increases. However, weaker expert groups may not establish professional ethics properly. The presence of external signals can dampen the effect of internal values.

A growth-oriented strategy may not be a viable option since growth without employment is often prevalent. Extreme competition on a uniform scale is also not a feasible alternative as it does not bring any benefits to society. The problem of competition based on prior learning can be solved overnight if all parents and students agree not to participate in private tutoring. However, this solution cannot be implemented due to the lack of trust in the social institution.

Harmonious coexistence can be achieved in a society with high social quality, where inequality is low and trust among members is high. However, in Korea, where relative inequality and mistrust are high, a winner-take-all system is prevalent.

Comparative research on social quality clearly shows qualitative differences in the way social risks are managed in welfare policies among countries. Countries with strong social programs and ample educational and employment opportunities can offer more chances for those who have experienced failure to try again. However, in Korea, where welfare protection is lacking, young people are hesitant to take risks. The fear of failure discourages innovative entrepreneurship. Additionally, countries with high levels of transparency provide equitable universal welfare, even if it requires significant investment in social programs. Korea currently has low transparency and welfare spending. To prevent Korea's welfare spending growth from following the path of the unfair dual welfare system in Southern Europe, transparency must be dramatically improved. A society with high social quality allows for harmonious win–win development due to low inequality and high trust among members. However, in Korea, where relative inequality and mistrust are high, the system is closer to a winner-takes-all approach.

Developed countries had a high level of civil society capacity even when their income levels were much lower than Korea's today. When per capita income exceeded \$20,000, Sweden achieved this in 1988 and Germany in 1991, while Korea did so in 2007. A comparison of the quality of Korea's society with that of Sweden or Germany at that time shows that Sweden already had 5.7 times the welfare and protection capacity of Korea. Germany had 3.1 times the welfare and protection capacity of Korea. The income tax burden in Sweden was eight times higher than in Korea, and in Germany, it was four times higher. However, Korea's resilience status is not inferior to that of Sweden or Germany at that time, and its college entrance rate is much higher. In terms of civic capacity, Korea falls behind Sweden and Germany, especially in regard to press freedom, government effectiveness, transparency, general trust, political participation, and voter turnout.

5 Conclusion

In this chapter, the results of a regression analysis on the major social factors that impact happiness in over 80 countries are presented. The analysis reveals significant differences in happiness levels even among countries with similar income levels. When comparing the happiness levels of East Asian countries, such as Korea, China, and Japan, with Southeast Asian countries, such as Vietnam, Indonesia, Pakistan, and Bangladesh, which have a per capita income of less than $10,000, it is observed that East Asian countries have relatively lower happiness scores, even when income levels are controlled.

Low social quality is a significant factor in reducing happiness in international comparisons. Social quality refers to the level of social interactions that determine the nature and content of relationships surrounding individuals. The implications of this finding are significant. In economically developed Korea, where incomes exceed $30,000, there is a level of distrust and low transparency that is not appropriate. The variation in happiness levels between Nordic and Asian countries can be attributed to the level of social quality that supports open democracy and a welfare state.

When compared to other OECD countries, the competition in Korea is passive and risk-averse, rather than bold and creative. Furthermore, there is an excessive emphasis on selecting winners based on signals rather than promoting socially optimized meritocratic competition. One of the reasons for the decline in happiness in Korea is the winner-takes-all competition, which impedes harmony and symbiosis. The decline in happiness is closely related to the recent trend of increased competition for positional goods, as opposed to the past few decades of high growth when life satisfaction was achieved by increasing the supply of material goods. Therefore, despite economic growth, Koreans are experiencing the paradox of affluence. From the perspective of long-term systemic transformation, Korea is currently in a transitional phase. The society is transitioning away from its past as a hierarchical and authoritarian society that combined high levels of trust with low levels of transparency. Currently, trust is declining without significant improvement in transparency, while positional goods, which require fairness and transparency, are becoming increasingly important.

The traditional system is being dismantled rapidly due to digital transformation and deindustrialization, while the formation of a high-quality alternative system is progressing slowly. To increase people's happiness, national-level reforms are necessary to improve social quality by providing moral resources beyond the paradigm of industrialization and democratization. The core task is to improve fairness and transparency.

References

Beck, W., van der Maesen, L. J. G., & Walker, A. (1997). Theorizing social quality: The concept's validity. In W. Beck, L. J. G. van der Maesen, & A. Walker (Eds.), *The social quality of Europe*. Kluwer Law International.

Beck, W., van der Maesen, L. J. G., Thomese, F., & Walker, A. (Eds.). (2001). *Social quality: A vision for Europe*. Kluwer Law International.

Easterlin, R. A. (1974). Does economic growth improve the human lot? In P. A. David & M. W. Reder (Eds.), *Nations and Households in economic growth: Essays in honor of Moses Abramovitz*. Academic Press.

Helliwell, J., Layard, R., & Sachs, J. (Eds.). (2017). *World happiness report 2017*. Sustainable Development Solutions Network.

Hirsch, F. (1976). *Social limits to growth*. Harvard University Press.

Jang, G., Im, J., & Kim, S.-H. (2011). *Situation of supply and demand for quality jobs and policy directions. Bank of Korea Economic Brief* (in Korean).

Jeon, S. (2008). Social conflict and social integration in the angry era. *Philosophy and Reality. Philosophy and Culture Research Institute. No. 76*, 30–40 (in Korean).

Kim, B. (2018). The economic importance of social capital. In: M. Park & J. Yee (Eds.), *Social value and social innovation: For a sustainable harmonious community*. Hanul Academy (in Korean).

Kim, K. (2002). *Korean social development theory*. Jipmundang (in Korean).

Kim, H. S., & Ohtake, F. (2014). *Status race and happiness: What experimental survey tell us*. Korea Development Institute Policy Study Report.

Noll, H. (2002). Towards a European system of social indicators: Theoretical framework and system architecture. *Social Indicators Research, 58*, 47–87.

Noriko, K. (2011). Why does Korea's college entrance rate continue to rise? Korea's passion for education seen through case comparison with Japan. [Ph.D. thesis], Department of Sociology, Seoul National University (in Korean).

Seo, S. (2011). *Infinite competition is encroaching on the Republic of Korea*. Jiho. (in Korean).

van der Maesen, L. J. G., & Walker, A. (2005). Indicators of social quality: Outcomes of the European Scientific Network. *European Journal of Social Quality, 5*(1/2)

Yee, J. (2007). 10 years after the foreign exchange crisis, to what level has the quality of Korean society improved? In U. Chung & H. Cho (Eds.), *10 years after the foreign exchange crisis, how much has Korean society changed?* Seoul National University Press (in Korean).

Yee, J., & Chang, D. (2011). Social quality as a measure for social progress. *Development and Society, 40*(2)

Yee, J. (2015). Social quality, competition, and happiness. *Asia Review, 4*(2) (in Korean).

Yee, J. et al. (2015). *Quality of Korean Society: From theory to application*. Hanul Academy (in Korean).

Yee, J. (2018). Social transformation and social value. In M.-K. Park & J. Yee (Eds.), *Social value and social innovation: For a sustainable harmonious community*. Hanul Academy (in Korean).

Yee, J. (2019a). The quality of society and the role of corporate citizenship. In H.-G. Song, J.-M. Cho, J. Yee, J.-G. Yoon, & J. Han (Eds.), *The road to corporate citizenship: Becoming and making*. Nanam (in Korean).

Yee, J. (2019b). *If you were born again, would you live in Korea: from the miracle of the Han River to Hell Joseon*. 21st Century Books (in Korean).

Jaeyeol Yee is a professor of sociology at Seoul National University and an international project member of the Center for Social Well-being Stud-ies, Institute for the Development of Social Intelligence, Senshu University. He has contributed to the harmonization of social well-being surveys in Asia as director of the Korea Social Science Data Archives. His research interests include social quality, social well-being, social capital, disaster and safety issues, and sociological theory construction.

When Economic Growth is Gone: The Global Generation and Disparities in Happiness in Taiwan

Ming-Chang Tsai and Liang-Wei Chen

Abstract This chapter analyzes the prospective optimism and subjective well-being of Taiwanese people, with a special research aim to test the global generation hypothesis that predicts a lower level of life satisfaction among younger cohorts due to their distinctive experience with global economic transformations. On the basis of three recent national survey datasets from Taiwan, this study performs an age–period–cohort analysis and obtains findings opposite to the global generation perspective. Younger cohorts are found to hold a prospective optimism which in turn leads to higher life satisfaction and happiness in Taiwan. This paper discusses inter-generational disparity as plausible explanatory factor and calls for comparative designs in future research for young cohorts across societies.

Keywords Happiness · Cohort analysis · Youths · Subjective well-being

1 When Economic Growth is Gone: The Global Generation and Disparities in Happiness in Taiwan

Youths in today's Taiwan have been described as a "collapsed generation," to highlight their economic predicaments and a gloomy future throughout their life course (Lin et al., 2011). This cohort, born in the 1980s, grew up to enter a neoliberal, market-dominated economy in Taiwan. Their economic life and well-being were gravely impacted by massive capital flight out of the country and declining manufacturing production. Job instability, low wages, and long working hours are now features of their working conditions. Indeed, many young entrants were only able to compete in a slack labor market in which most jobs paid no more than US$1000 per month (Tsai, 2023). Real estate speculation clearly added fuel to the fire, as housing prices became unaffordable for young couples, most of whom decided to have only one child. As a result, the societal fertility rate has declined to a super-low level. As

M.-C. Tsai (✉) · L.-W. Chen
Research Center for Humanities and Social Sciences, Academia Sinica, Taipei, Taiwan
e-mail: mtsai304@gate.sinica.edu.tw

J. Yee et al. (eds.), *Social Well-Being, Development, and Multiple Modernities in Asia*,
https://doi.org/10.1007/978-981-97-3866-3_9

the number of future generations decreases, the tax revenue of the government is projected to dwindle, and the national health insurance and the pension system will soon be in crisis. The young cannot afford to support both themselves and a swelling aging population. They would not be happy under these dire circumstances.

This pessimistic view of the young cohort seems to echo many other studies in Asia, as well as in Western societies (Brinton, 2011; Furlong et al., 2018; Guerrero, 2001; Newman, 2012). Yet this descriptive analysis does not provide empirical evidence that younger cohorts in Taiwan are negatively affected in terms of well-being, and instead merely assumes that they are experiencing a private toll of the macro-economic recession. First of all, Taiwanese in general stay at a higher level of happiness. In the most recent World Happiness Report (Helliwell et al., 2021), Taiwanese ranked the top in the world (19th) in terms of life evaluation on a Cantril ladder as of 2020, and remarkably outperformed other Asian countries (Japan is 40th and South Korea is 50th) (p.19). Previous studies using panel data tracking teenagers until they were in their early 20 s showed that they were not unhappy. They even became happier as they matured and entered the labor market (Huang & Chien, 2013). This phenomenon of sustained happiness sits at the opposite side of the Easterlin Paradox, which states that higher income does not lead to higher level of happiness (Easterlin, 1995; Easterlin et al., 2010). However, this does not mean that young people and others are equally happy, as there is comparable evidence for different age groups. In fact, inequality in happiness between age groups or across generations has long been observed in Western societies (Clark et al., 2018; Diener et al., 2010; Frey, 2008; Yang, 2008).

This study attempts to provide new evidence on cohort differences in economic security and subjective well-being using recent national survey data from Taiwan. Young people in Taiwan, like those in many other societies, have been impacted gravely by economic globalization regarding their working conditions, family life, and social mobility. It has been argued that their prospective life situations have become less favorable over time. This study reviews recent debates on youth as a global generation and conducts an empirical analysis of their subjective well-being (SWB) using a new technique of age–period–cohort (APC) model. Data are drawn from the Taiwan Social Change Survey, a national survey project that has provided adequate data on adult social values and behaviors for three decades. This study provides evidence which challenges the basic argument of the global generation and proposes new research directions to better understand the current young cohort navigating a changing global environment.

1.1 The Global Generation, Prospective Optimism, and Happiness

Young cohorts have conventionally played a marginal role in social science research agenda in Taiwan. Existing studies focus on their occupational attainment and earnings, sense of fairness, their support for confrontational politics, or their improvised involvement in emerging social movements (Ho, 2019; Kuan et al., 2020; Tsai, 1998; Zheng et al., 2020). How they perceive their economic conditions and how their perceptions affect their well-being and happiness has not been fully explored.

Indeed, the description of a collapsed generation in fact is not quintessentially different from how the *global generation* has been described in rich countries (Beck & Beck-Gernsheim, 2009; Edmunds & Turner, 2005). It appears that as globalization deepens, young people across countries increasingly share strikingly similar life experiences, not because they are biologically alike, but because they are concurrently embedded in a highly globalized economy. This unique experience of living in a highly globalized world makes them a global generation (Beck & Beck-Gernsheim, 2009). Despite their better educational opportunities and familiarity with online communication and media use techniques, this generation is also a generation *at-risk*. They are entering a labor market that offers lower-end jobs with working conditions characterized by instability, short-term contracts, and insufficient pay. Moreover, their educational credentials are devalued by the global expansion of education. It is argued that the escalation and dominance of a market economy in fact incurs more fear, uncertainty and anxiety than a feeling of meaning and solidarity (Giddens, 1991). This risk society perspective locates the sources of youth precariousness, individualization, and disconnections in the changing social structures that surround them, rather than in some psycho-developmental crisis in the adolescent phase (Cahill, 2015). While these youths endeavor to generate stronger social capital in the community, society, and even the wider world outside of their own countries, these efforts are often in vain, further reinforcing distress and discontent that seem to have no cause.

Do the young people in Taiwan express discontent and a lower level of well-being as a result, when compared to other, older generations? Before answering this question, it is necessary to clarify what constitutes a generation. Alwin and McCammon (2003) contend that the mere fact that a group of people are born at the same time, while being a necessary condition, is not sufficient to form a generation. They have to share a distinctive culture or a self-conscious identity by virtue of having experienced the same historical events in their lives. This sufficient condition deserves to be highlighted in order to understand how a global generation forms a tangible collectivity and becomes a group of "actors," rather than a statistical category, so that they collectively respond to the outside world in a manner different from that of other cohorts.

Another approach to youths and their risks pursues an in-depth understanding of their personal troubles from a micro-biographical angle. Shildrick and MacDonald (2008) contend that socially disadvantaged and economically marginal positions of young people can be better understood through a detailed analysis of their critical transitions over the course of their lives. They highlight several critical transitions, including school-to-work, family, housing, or delinquency, etc. The young generation indeed is more likely to have experienced one or more *poor* transitions than older cohorts. These critical transitions can be spurs to negative pathways and undesirable outcomes, such as feeling unsuccessful, deprived or less happy. Yet caution is needed for evaluating this hypothesis. The close-up, biographical methods used in youth studies have often drawn samples from poor neighborhoods (Shildrick & MacDonald, 2008), where a low-wage market is the only source of income for them and their families (Newman, 2006). This has implications for theorizing about the observed generational gap in well-being. It is a result of socio-economic resources rather than a difference between age groups. Moreover, the gap might be reduced as young people grow up and become better equipped with human capital. There do not appear to be any available studies on this issue in Taiwan. But this inquiry raises the fundamental question of how to disentangle the intricate relationships between age and cohort influences. In addition, it is likely that the decline in well-being predicted by global generation theory also occurs among other generations. It could a phenomenon due to a specific time period, rather than the influence of age or cohort. The influences of age, generation, and period are intermingled. I will specify an APC model to effectively disentangle the mixture of age, generation, and period differences in subjective well-being.

In addition to this major concern of the APC framework, this study also examines the influences of background characteristics on perceived well-being as an outcome. There are important mediating mechanisms that require further explanation in this pursuit. It is likely that income does not have a strong direct correlation with happiness for youth in Taiwan, because their income gap is unlikely to be substantial or because they still receive financial support from their parents (Tsai & Wang, 2019). This does not mean that income or other material factors do not matter. Those with higher incomes may have better well-being through certain mediating factors, such as having stable family relationships, better health care, better housing, peaceful neighborhoods, and so on. These relationships or material conditions may then translate into an optimistic evaluation of life conditions. That is, socio-economic differences affect the level of prospective optimism, which in turn incurs a favorable evaluation of one's life condition and positive affect. This mediating hypothesis is tested using empirical data from Taiwan. The previous discussion can be summarized in two proposed hypotheses.

H1: The younger cohort tends to have lower subjective well-being, compared to the older cohorts (the global generation hypothesis).

H2: The effect of socio-economic status on subjective well-being (SWB) is mediated by prospective optimism, i.e., the perception that future life conditions will improve. Generations may also operate through this mechanism to generate their potential influence on SWB (the prospective mediation hypothesis).

With these two proposed hypotheses in mind, we now turn to the specifications of the APC analysis.

1.2 Disparity in Perceived Well-Being: APC Models

The main interest of this study is to see whether younger generations, particularly the global generation, are less satisfied with life conditions. It is assumed that there are disparities between generations, that is, between the youngest cohort and those who are older. The global generation encounters a historical moment of deepening of the liberal market economy and shares an experience of job precariousness, being born at the same time and reacting similarly to this changing external world. This specific embeddedness in a historical moment is a central feature of the typical lives of the cohort born after the 1980s. Conceptually, this cohort effect differs from age effects, which are changes that occur with chronological aging. Age effects refer primarily to changes due to physiological maturing and aging. They also include influences derived from the accumulation of social experiences, social roles, and status changes over the life course (Elder & Johnson, 2003; Yang & Land, 2013). In the context of cross-sectional data, age effects are highly confounded with cohort effects, because an identified age group also belongs to a certain cohort. This confounding has been termed the conundrum of APC analysis (Glenn, 2005). What needs to be asserted in APC analysis is that cohort effects are distinguished from age effects. That is, the global generation continues to have its higher level of dissatisfaction even as it moves to the next stage of life course. This cohort effect, established in their youth, is fixed and remains with them throughout their life course. It is plausible that the unhappiness of the global generation is actually more a consequence of a specific *historical time* in which globalization deepened and the world economy generated huge impacts on their well-being as well as that of others. In other words, these effects may not only have affected the global generation, but may also have had a negative impact on other generations' perceptions of life. Thus, this *period* effect, which subsumes a historical economic restructuring and represents a drastic change in living conditions, coincides with the age and cohort effects mentioned above, making it very difficult to estimate disparities in happiness among young people and other social groups.

The extremely high correlation among age, period, and cohort effects is called the identification problem because of the perfect correlation between them, which can be shown in the expression: Period (P) − Age (A) = Cohort (C). Specification errors in conventional regression models occur when the A, P, and C factors are estimated in the same equation. Even a detour strategy of estimating any two of them simultaneously does not yield satisfactory results (Yang & Land, 2013). In this study, a new estimation technique called the intrinsic estimator (IE) is used to generate more efficient estimates. The IE method uses a set of analysis-of-variance type constraints such that the sums of the respective A, P, and C coefficients equal zero, which is similar to the effect coding procedure. To obtain the effect coefficient, the orthonormal transformation of a principal components regression is performed (Yang & Land, 2013: 79). The IE model can be seen as a special case of the ridge regression estimator (Hoerl & Kennard, 1970) because it limits the shrinkage penalty to zero. The central feature of the IE is to remove the influence of the design matrix (the matrix of values of explanatory variables) on the coefficient estimates to obtain unbiased and efficient estimation (Yang et al., 2008).

1.3 Data and Measurement

The data are drawn from the Taiwan Social Change Survey (TSCS). TSCS is a social survey project that was established in 1985 and has since collected various information on social values, family behaviors, religious practices, political participation, etc., through direct face-to-face interviews with the mass public in Taiwan on an annual basis. It is supervised by the Institute of Sociology, Academia Sinica, Taiwan, and is available to the public (www2.ios.sinica.edu.tw/sc/cht/home.php). The current study uses data collected in 2005, 2010, and 2015, with sample sizes of 2146, 1895, and 2034, respectively. The sampling frames were Taiwanese citizens aged 18 years and above, whose addresses were obtained from the household registration information provided by the government. The sampling method is probability proportional to size (the PPS). The first stage of sampling selected towns and cities from 7 large regions with different levels of urbanization. In the second stage, about 70 city districts, villages, or settlements were selected from the towns and cities chosen in the first stage. In the third phase, 25–30 adults were interviewed, depending on the number of residents from their administrative units. The response rate was just under 50%.

The current study focuses on their perceived well-being, with an interest in comparing the global generation, defined as those born in the 1980s and after, to older people. In pooling three waves of cross-sectional data, we have excluded those aged 65, who are mostly retired from the labor market. Household workers and students are not included because they are not in the labor market. However, the unemployed are included because it is important to understand how unfavorably they perceive their life situation compared to those who have a job (Böckerman & Ilmakunnas, 2006).

In measuring SWB, two commonly used indicators are chosen. The first one is: "Are you satisfied with your overall quality of life?", and the second: "In general, do you feel happy or unhappy these days?" In the 2005 and 2015 surveys, both questions are on a four-point scale. In the 2010 survey, half of the respondents were asked on a four-point scale and the other half were asked on a five-point scale. For consistent measurement, I recoded the midpoint score on a five-point scale ("neither happy nor unhappy") as 2.5; the other four responses—very happy, happy, unhappy, very unhappy—are coded from 4 to 1. Higher scores indicate better SWB.

The focal mediating and outcome variable is prospective optimism. Two proxies for prospective optimism are used: (1) "Is your (or you and your spouse's) income enough to live on?" There are five response options: very much enough, fair enough, roughly make even, not enough, not enough at all (coded from 5 to 1). (2) "Will your living condition get better or worse in the next five years?" There are five response options on a five-point scale: will become "much better," "a little better," "same as now," "a little worse than now," and "much worse than now" (coded from 5 to 1). While the first indicator refers to the current financial situation, the second clearly solicits personal forecast of future living conditions.

For the APC analysis, the age, period, and cohort groupings are designed as follows. The age group is differentiated by five years, resulting in 9 categories in this design: 20–24, 25–29, ... 60–64. Periods refer to three survey years: 2005, 2010, and 2015. There are 11 cohorts generated, with birth years ranging from 1941–1945, 1946–1950, and so on, to 1991–1995.

A range of demographical backgrounds and socio-economic status levels are included in the analysis. To compare differences between genders, males are coded as 1, with females as the reference. Ethnic background is differentiated by a conventional typology that separates Taiwanese into Hoklo and Hakka (both are ethnic Chinese who arrived on the island one or two centuries ago), Mainlanders (Chinese who arrived after the 1950s), and the aboriginals. Occupational status is grouped into five strata according to skill level: (1) managerial and professional, (2) assistant professional and technician, (3) clerical, (4) semi-skilled, and (5) unskilled. In addition, the unemployed are included in this dummy design for comparison. Income is measured in terms of personal earnings per month. Additional consideration is given to an individual's subjective evaluation of social status, which in the original design has ten levels (from the highest = 10 to the lowest = 1) for self-placement on a hierarchical status ladder.

1.4 Analysis and Results

The analysis begins by examining the differences among age groups from the pooled cross-sectional data. Figure 1a shows the age 20–24 group on the far left and the 60–64 age group on the far right. There is a downward trend in the feeling of having enough income and a better future, with younger people reporting higher scores than older people, although the latter remain above the middle point on a five-point scale. For two SWB indicators measured on a four-point scale, the happiness level is higher for people under 30. There is an upward trend after the age of 35–39. Figure 1b shows the period effects, in which all but the happiness indicator increases substantially.

The cohort differences shown in Fig. 1c are an important finding of the current study. Both the evaluation of income sufficiency and the forecasting of future condition appear to be favorable, especially for the younger cohort, as the upward slopes for both are quite observable. In addition, the younger, "generation cohort" seems to report slightly better SWB. This result is clearly contrary to what is predicted by the global generation hypothesis (H1).

These gross disparity relevant to age, period, and cohort may, as argued earlier, be affected by confounding relationships among them. For instance, the higher levels of happiness among younger people may reflect period effects, as they enter the sample in 2010 and 2015. The most recent cohorts in the analysis, those born in 1981–1985, 1986–1990 and 1991–1995, may in fact coincide with younger age groups

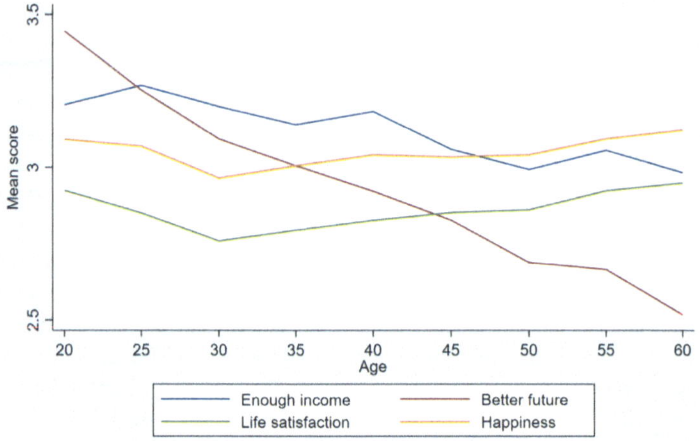

a (Age)

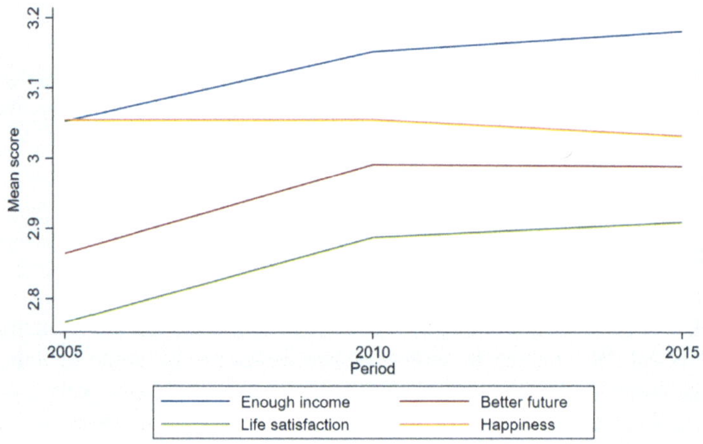

b (Period)

Fig. 1 Gross age, period, and cohort effects of prospective optimism and subjective well-being

in terms of high life satisfaction. It is difficult to disentangle these intermingled relationships without an appropriate model that can simultaneously estimate the distinctive influences of age, period, and cohort. This intricate relationship justifies our use of the APC-IE model to provide efficient estimates in the following analysis.

Table 1 displays the results from the APC-IE model for perception of income sufficiency and future life conditions. In column 1, males are less likely to report that their income is sufficient. It has been suggested that males in Taiwan are expected to take the role of family provider, and this identity may account for their lower perceived insufficiency in meeting their family's economic needs (Hori & Kamo,

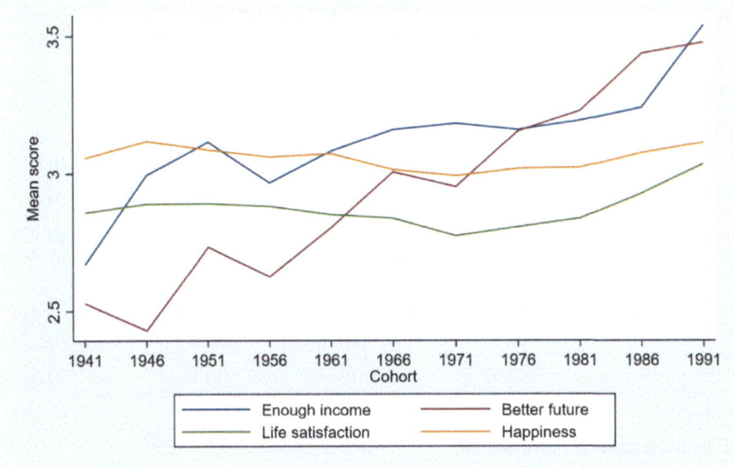

c (Cohort)

Fig. 1 (continued)

2018). While ethnic groups do not differ from each other, all socio-economic status factors have significant effects. The more educated respondents report a stronger sense of having sufficient income than those with less education. Compared to the managerial/professional class, all other less-skilled occupational groups show lower levels of perceived income sufficiency. Not surprisingly, the unemployed also report a high level of concern about having insufficient income. Personal income has a notable positive effect. Subjective class status is also a strong predictor in the equation.

The differences among age groups appear trivial, as none of them reach statistical significance on the first model for "income is enough." In the APC-IE estimation, the sums of the effect coefficients for the age, period, and cohort groups are constrained to zero. This is more evident for the three period effects. The year 2010 shows a higher level for all respondents, revealing that there is no linear trend for the observed period. With regard to cohort effects, the 1941–45 cohort reports a lower level of sufficiency. One interpretation is that members of this cohort, if they are still working for an income, have a high sense of economic insecurity, probably due to their early experiences of poverty immediately after the war in Taiwan. In contrast, the 1951–55 cohort reports a higher level of income sufficiency. This may be an effect of the baby boomers, who benefited greatly from rapid economic growth when they first entered the labor market in the 1970s. The youngest cohort reports that they feel their earning is sufficient—a finding that is the opposite of what the global generational perspective predicts.

The second equation in Table 1 shows the result of the perception of living conditions in the future. Gender and ethnic backgrounds have little influence. As for education, it is only those with a master's degree or higher that expect a better future. There is no appreciable difference between those working with different skill

Table 1 Perception of income and life conditions—APC model

	Income enough		Future life better	
Male (ref: Female)	– 0.07*	(0.03)	– 0.03	(0.03)
Ethnic group (ref: Hoklo)				
Hakka	0.05	(0.04)	0.01	(0.05)
Mainlander	– 0.03	(0.05)	– 0.02	(0.06)
Aboriginal	– 0.20	(0.14)	0.08	(0.15)
Edu (ref: Elementary or less)				
Junior h	0.17*	(0.07)	0.05	(0.07)
Senior h	0.31**	(0.06)	0.10	(0.07)
College	0.52**	(0.07)	0.14	(0.07)
Master or higher	0.58**	(0.10)	0.21*	(0.10)
Occ. (ref: Managerial and professional)				
Assistant professional	– 0.14*	(0.06)	0.09	(0.07)
Clerical	– 0.14*	(0.06)	0.07	(0.06)
Technician-skilled	– 0.19***	(0.06)	– 0.01	(0.06)
Non-skilled	– 0.36**	(0.08)	0.09	(0.09)
Unemployed	– 0.32**	(0.08)	0.20*	(0.08)
Income (in 10,000 TD)	0.07**	(0.01)	0.03**	(0.01)
Subjective social status	0.10**	(0.01)	0.08**	(0.01)
Age effect				
20–24	0.00	(0.06)	0.38**	(0.07)
25–29	0.08	(0.05)	0.15***	(0.05)
30–34	– 0.01	(0.05)	0.05	(0.05)
35–39	– 0.07	(0.05)	– 0.03	(0.06)
40–44	– 0.02	(0.05)	– 0.05	(0.06)
45–49	– 0.06	(0.05)	– 0.05	(0.06)
50–54	– 0.06	(0.05)	– 0.13*	(0.05)
55–59	0.01	(0.05)	– 0.10	(0.05)
60–64	0.12	(0.06)	– 0.22***	(0.07)
Period effect				
2005	– 0.03	(0.02)	– 0.04	(0.03)
2010	0.05*	(0.02)	0.06*	(0.02)
2015	– 0.02	(0.02)	– 0.01	(0.02)
Cohort effect				
1941–1945	– 0.20*	(0.10)	0.00	(0.11)
1946–1950	– 0.01	(0.07)	– 0.26**	(0.07)
1951–1955	0.13***	(0.05)	– 0.00	(0.05)
1956–1960	– 0.05	(0.06)	– 0.20**	(0.06)

(continued)

Table 1 (continued)

	Income enough		Future life better	
1961–1965	– 0.04	(0.06)	– 0.08	(0.06)
1966–1970	– 0.03	(0.06)	0.06	(0.06)
1971–1975	– 0.07	(0.06)	– 0.04	(0.06)
1976–1980	– 0.09	(0.05)	0.11*	(0.05)
1981–1985	– 0.04	(0.04)	0.07	(0.05)
1986–1990	– 0.01	(0.06)	0.19***	(0.06)
1991–1995	0.40**	(0.10)	0.14	(0.11)
Constant	2.27**	(0.09)	2.32**	(0.10)
Observations	4011		4011	
AIC	11,076.59		11,633.95	
BIC	11,296.98		11,854.34	

Standard errors in parenthesis
* $p < 0.05$, ** $p < 0.001$, *** $p < 0.01$

levels. The unemployed, however, believe that their future conditions will improve, revealing an optimism rarely reported in previous research. Both income and subjective social status remain significant predictors as observed in the estimation of income sufficiency.

Younger people tend to see a better future, as the two youngest age groups register positive coefficients. Not surprisingly, the oldest age group is quite pessimistic about their life conditions to come, especially the oldest group in the table. The results for the period effect again show that 2010 is a time featuring a stronger belief in a better future. Those born in 1986–1990, a typical global generation, show high optimism that good times will come. The 1976–1980 cohort, while not typically considered a global generation, is as positive about the future. In contrast, the 1946–1950 and 1956–1960 cohorts are particularly worried about their future. The cohort in between these two (that is, the 1951–1955 cohort) does not feel discouraged.

The APC analysis of two important indicators of SWB is presented in Table 2. The first equation estimates life satisfaction. Males are less satisfied with life conditions, replicating recent research findings (Hori & Kamo, 2018; Hsu et al., 2015; Tsai, 2016). Despite their relatively disadvantaged situation in terms of socio-economic resources, aboriginals report higher levels of life satisfaction than the *Han* (Chinese) people. Education, occupation, and income, three basic indicators of social stratification, do not generate differences here. Subjective social status remains a crucial predictor. Having enough income and perceiving a better future both are positively correlated with life satisfaction, implying that these two indicators serve as mediating factors for an individual's socio-economic status in affecting life satisfaction (supporting H2).

Estimates of the age effect reveal that it is the young adults in their 30 s who are most likely to have lower life satisfaction. This pattern is a replication of previous

Table 2 Life satisfaction and happiness—APC model

	Life satisfaction		Happiness	
Male (ref: Female)	– 0.09*	(0.02)	– 0.07*	(0.02)
Ethnic group (ref: Hoklo)				
Hakka	0.02	(0.03)	0.02	(0.03)
Mainlander	– 0.04	(0.03)	– 0.06	(0.03)
Aboriginal	0.22**	(0.09)	0.24***	(0.08)
Edu. (ref: Elementary or less)				
Junior h	– 0.01	(0.04)	– 0.04	(0.04)
Senior h	– 0.05	(0.04)	– 0.06	(0.04)
College	– 0.07	(0.04)	– 0.07	(0.04)
Master or higher	– 0.11	(0.06)	– 0.06	(0.06)
Occ. (ref: managerial and professional)				
Assistant professional	– 0.02	(0.04)	0.04	(0.04)
Clerical	0.02	(0.04)	0.03	(0.03)
Technician– skilled	0.04	(0.04)	0.05	(0.04)
Non– skilled	– 0.01	(0.05)	0.04	(0.05)
Unemployed	– 0.10	(0.05)	– 0.17*	(0.05)
Income (in 10,000 TD)	– 0.00	(0.00)	0.00	(0.00)
Subjective social status	0.05*	(0.01)	0.04*	(0.01)
Income sufficient	0.19*	(0.01)	0.13*	(0.01)
Future life better	0.06*	(0.01)	0.06*	(0.01)
Age effect				
20–24	0.06	(0.04)	0.06	(0.04)
25–29	– 0.04	(0.03)	0.00	(0.03)
30–34	– 0.11*	(0.03)	– 0.09***	(0.03)
35–39	– 0.06**	(0.03)	– 0.05	(0.03)
40–44	– 0.04	(0.03)	– 0.03	(0.03)
45–49	– 0.02	(0.03)	– 0.05	(0.03)
50–54	0.03	(0.03)	– 0.02	(0.03)
55–59	0.06**	(0.03)	0.04	(0.03)
60–64	0.12***	(0.04)	0.13*	(0.04)
Period effect				
2005	– 0.09*	(0.01)	0.01	(0.01)
2010	0.04***	(0.01)	0.01	(0.01)
2015	0.05*	(0.01)	– 0.02	(0.01)
Cohort effect				
1941–1945	0.04	(0.06)	– 0.08	(0.06)
1946–1950	– 0.01	(0.04)	0.01	(0.04)

(continued)

Table 2 (continued)

	Life satisfaction		Happiness	
1951–1955	– 0.02	(0.03)	0.00	(0.03)
1956–1960	0.05	(0.03)	0.07**	(0.03)
1961–1965	– 0.00	(0.04)	0.07**	(0.03)
1966–1970	0.01	(0.04)	0.01	(0.04)
1971–1975	– 0.04	(0.04)	– 0.01	(0.03)
1976–1980	0.01	(0.03)	– 0.00	(0.03)
1981–1985	– 0.01	(0.03)	– 0.02	(0.03)
1986–1990	– 0.01	(0.03)	– 0.01	(0.03)
1991–1995	– 0.02	(0.06)	– 0.04	(0.06)
Constant	1.94*	(0.06)	2.37*	(0.06)
Observations	4,011		4,011	
AIC	7234.59		6946.46	
BIC	7467.57		7179.44	

Standard errors in parenthesis
* $p < 0.001$, ** $p < 0.05$, *** $p < 0.01$

research on the U-shaped curve of SWB when comparing different age groups in the East Asian region (Hori & Kamo, 2018; Shin & Inoguchi, 2009). However, the lowest points of the U-shaped curve might differ across societies, depending on the resources, responsibilities, and constraints encountered over the life course, which clearly needs further exploration. Life satisfaction observed in 2010 and 2015 is on average much higher than in 2005 (compared to Fig. 1b), indicating an upward trend of life satisfaction in Taiwan. However, cohort effects are limited, in that there are no observable differences among generations.

The second equation in Table 1 shows the estimates of happiness. Males continue to report a lower levels of happiness than females, when major covariates are controlled. Aboriginals again respond that they are happier. Education does not produce notable influence. Nor does a better occupational status lead to more happiness. Yet those who are unemployed are actually less happy than those who have a job. Subjective status identification is positively correlated with happiness. Income sufficiency and the perception of the future life again generate a strong positive influence on the estimation of happiness.

The pattern of the age effect shows that the 30–34 age group has the lowest level of happiness, and the oldest group (age 60–64) is the happiest. The findings as such show a U-shaped influence similar to that of life satisfaction. The period effects, however, are much attenuated. The two cohorts of 1956–1960 and 1961–1965 reveal a slightly happier feeling than all others, a result not found for their life satisfaction.

1.5 Concluding Remarks

The global generation is a central focus of social science research because it is the generation of the future. They represent the future society that is yet to come, but which can already be gauged by their expectations of economic security and life conditions in broad terms. Researchers adopting a global generation perspective have forecast a dismal fate for the younger cohort, predicting that in a neoliberal economy, their growing pains will certainly be acute and they will not be as satisfied with how life is going as their parents were. The main responsible causes are devalued educational credentials, a slack labor market, lack of permanent jobs, low wages, weak state regulation, widespread social inequality, and so on. These structural barriers are supposed to have unfavorable impact on their lives. But is the global generation really unhappy?

The evidence gathered from Taiwan does not confirm the global generation thesis (disfavoring H1). Rather, the evidence suggests that the young people are able to take an optimistic view of their economic situations (particularly the cohort born in 1991–1995) and future conditions (particularly the cohort born in 1986–1990) (supporting H2), which in turn helps to keep their perceived well-being at the level of other, older cohorts. On the basis of the APC models, which effectively disentangle the cohort effect from the confounding influences of age and period effects, this study shows that the younger cohorts tend to be optimistic about their current economic situation and future life conditions. They are neither unhappy nor dissatisfied with life compared to earlier cohorts. They appear to remain in good spirits despite a series of global economic impacts that have been perceived to be operating against them.

In the global generation argument, the young cohorts are seen as a culturally distinct entity with their own identity, which even their parents find hard to understand. In this view, the global generation appears to be in conflict with parents or older cohorts. But this viewpoint might not hold as a rule. In the Taiwanese context, there remains a strong link between "generations" (in the sense of familial lineage). Parents pay for education, allowing young people to prolong their "stay" in the parental home before they graduate from college, enter the labor market when many of them earn no more than a meager entry-level salary. Later in the life course, parents may plausibly provide financial support for the down-payment on a first housing at marriage, and later they may help care for grandchildren so that young couples can avoid work–family conflicts. Perhaps it is this kind of family support that keeps the global generation optimistic and spirited. In a preliminary analysis, we tested whether living with parents improves the perceived well-being of younger cohorts, but there is not much evidence to support this. Speculatively, it is likely that other aspects of inter-generational relationships provide needed social support for the global generation. We suggest that social support or social capital in the surrounding relationships or environments should be taken into consideration in future research designs to better understand the global generation. The bottom line is that it is fruitful from investigating their ties and connections with relatives, friends, or intimate others in understanding their life satisfaction.

There are other limitations to the research. First, the APC ideally analyzes a large number of waves of cross-sectional observations so that the younger cohorts are increased in number and the estimation can be more stable (Yang & Land, 2013). This study utilizes only three pooled datasets due to the lack of information on the mediating factors analyzed in other TSCS surveys. Future design should incorporate more waves of the TSCS, and this practice will also allow a finer comparison of within-group differences, to see whether all (newcomer) cohorts born after 1980 behave similarly to each other. Second, the TSCS provides limited information on working conditions or company benefits. These details, if added, would help to understand the characteristics of the firms in which the global generation currently works and their influence on personal well-being. Other studies also suggest inclusion of religious affiliation, familial life, and health status (Hori & Kamo, 2018; Jou, 2013; Shin & Inoguchi, 2009). These factors deserve to be tested the analyses of the Taiwanese case. Third, to better understand the well-being of the young generation, longitudinal panel data can provide stronger and more conclusive evidence (Yang, 2008). Some panel projects in Taiwan, such as the Taiwan Youth Project (http://www.typ.sinica.edu.tw), have endeavored to collect panel data for youths (Tsai, 2023; Yi et al., 2009). This different research design allows for the analysis of the trajectory of a global generation to see how they respond to both local and global economies and how their well-being evolves over time. From this perspective, the global generation in fact is a local happening. How each local experience unfolds and concludes should be investigated with suitable designs, while attempting to generalize across different societies. At any case, comparative observations of the global generations in cross-national designs will surely promise a fruitful understanding of young cohorts in Taiwan and elsewhere.

References

Alwin, D. F., & McCammon, R. J. (2003). Generations, cohorts, and social change. In J. T. Mortimer & M. J. Shanahan (Eds.), *Handbook of the life course* (pp. 23–49). Kluwer.

Beck, U., & Beck-Gernsheim, E. (2009). Global generations and the trap of methodological nationalism for a cosmopolitan in the sociology of youth and generation. *European Sociological Review, 25*, 25–36.

Böckerman, P., & Ilmakunnas, P. (2006). Elusive effects of unemployment on happiness. *Social Indicators Research, 79*, 159–169.

Brinton, M. C. (2011). *Lost in transition: youth, work, and instability in postindustrial Japan.* Cambridge University Press.

Cahill, H. (2015). Approaches to understanding youth well-being. In J. Wyn, & H. Cahill (Eds.), *Handbook of children and youth studies* (pp. 95–113). Springer.

Clark, A. E., Flèche, S., Layard, R., Powdthavee, N., & Ward, G. (2018). *The origins of Happiness: The science of well-being over the life course.* Princeton University Press.

Diener, E., Helliwell, J. F., & Kahneman, D. (Eds.). (2010). *International differences in well-being.* Oxford University Press.

Easterlin, R. A. (1995). Will raising the incomes of all increase the happiness of all? *Journal of Economic Behavior and Organization, 27*, 35–47.

Easterlin, R. A., McVey, L. A., Switek, M., Sawangfa, O., & Zweig, J. S. (2010). The happiness–income paradox revisited. *PNAS, 107*(52), 22463–22468.
Edmunds, J., & Turner, B. S. (2005). Global generations: Social change in the twentieth century. *British Journal of Sociology, 56*, 559–577.
Elder, G. H. Jr., & Johnson, M. K. (2003). The life course and aging: Challenges, lessons, and new directions. In R. Setterstem, & A. Jr. Amityville (Eds.), *Invitation to the life course: Toward new understandings of later life* (pp. 49–81), Baywood.
Frey, B. S. (2008). *Happiness: A revolution in economics*. MIT Press.
Furlong, A., Goodwin, J., O'Connor, H., Hadfield, S., Hall, S., Lowden, K., & Plugor, R. (2018). *Young people in the labour market: Past, present, future*. Routledge.
Giddens, A. (1991). *Modernity and self-identity*. Polity.
Glenn, N. D. (2005). *Cohort analysis* (2nd ed.). Sage.
Guerrero, T. J. (2001). *Youth in transition: Housing, employment, social policies and families in France and Spain*. Ashgate.
Helliwell, J. F., Layard, R., Sachs, J., & De Neve, J.-E. (Eds.). (2021). *World happiness report 2021*. Sustainable Development Solutions Network.
Ho, M.-S. (2019). *Challenging Beijing's mandate of heaven: Taiwan's Sunflower movement and Hong Kong's umbrella movement*. Temple University Press.
Hoerl, A. E., & Kennard, R. W. (1970). Ridge regression: Applications to nonorthogonal problems. *Technometrics, 12*, 69–82.
Hori, M., & Kamo, Y. (2018). Gender differences in happiness: The effects of marriage, social roles, and social support in East Asia. *Applied Research Quality Life, 13*, 839–857.
Hsu, H.-C., Chang, W.-C., Chong, W.-S., & An, J. S. (2015). Happiness and social determinants across age cohorts in Taiwan. *Journal of Health Psychology, 21*, 1828–1839.
Huang, F. -M., & Chien, Y. -N. (2013). Working, schooling, and psychological well-being: Evidence from longitudinal data for Taiwanese youth. In Yi, C. –C. (Eds.), *The psychological well-being of East Asian Youth* (pp. 185–207). Springer.
Jou, Y. -H. (2013). Family relationship quality and its psychological effects among Taiwanese adolescents. In Yi, C. -C. (Eds.), *The psychological well-being of east Asian Youth* (pp. 69–88), Springer.
Kuan, P. -Y., Peng, S. -C., & Choi, S. (2020). Does college degree still pay? A causal analysis of the impact of college expansion on earnings and occupational Prestige in Taiwan. *Journal of Social Sciences and Philosophy*.
Lin, T. -H., et al. (2011). *A collapsed generation*. Taiwan Labor Front.
Newman, K. S. (2006). *Chutes and ladders: Navigating the low-wage labor market*. Russell Sage Foundation.
Newman, K. S. (2012). *The accordion family: Boomerang kids, anxious parents, and the private toll of global competition*. Beacon.
Shildrick, T., & MacDonald, R. (2008). Understanding youth exclusion: Critical moments, social networks and social capital. *Youth and Policy, 99*, 43–54.
Shin, D. C., & Inoguchi, T. (2009). Avowed happiness in Confucian Asia: Ascertaining its distribution, patterns, and sources. *Social Indicators Research, 92*, 405–427.
Tsai, M.-C., & Wang, Y.-T. (2019). Intergenerational exchange in East Asia: A new look at financial transfers. *Comparative Sociology, 18*, 173–203.
Tsai, S. -L. (1998). The transition from school to work in Taiwan. In Y. Shavit, W. Müller (Eds.) *From school to work: A comparative study of educational qualifications and occupational destinations* (pp. 443–470). Clarendon.
Tsai, M. -C. (2016). Happiness and sociability in a nonrecursive model: The US and Taiwan Compared. In F. Maggino (Ed.), *A life devoted to quality of life—festschrift in honor of Alex C. Michalos* (pp. 297–314). Springer.
Tsai, M. -C. (2023). Landing a middle class position: College degree, occupational status and income of young adults in Taiwan. In Yi, C. -C., & Tsai, M. -C. (Eds.), *Journey to adulthood: East Asian perspectives* (pp. 126–151). Sage.

Yang, Y. (2008). Social inequalities in happiness in the United states, 1972 to 2004: An age-period-cohort analysis. *American Sociological Review, 73*, 204–226.
Yang, Y., & Land, K. C. (2013). *Age-period-cohort analysis: New models, methods, and empirical applications*. CRC Press.
Yang, Y., Schulhofer-Wohl, S., Fu, W. J., & Land, K. C. (2008). The intrinsic estimator for age-period-cohort analysis: What it is and how to use it. *American Journal of Sociology, 113*, 1697–1736.
Yi, C.-C., Wu, C.-Y., Chang, Y.-H., & Chang, M.-Y. (2009). The psychological well-being of Taiwanese youth: School versus family context from early to late adolescence. *International Sociology, 24*, 397–429.
Zheng, V., Hsiao, H.-H.M., Wan, P.-S., & Wong, K. (2020). Young people's sense of fairness and social action: A survey analysis of Taiwan, Hong Kong, and Macao. *Asian Journal of Comparative Politics, 5*, 270–287.

Diverse Mechanisms of Social Well-Being

Introduction to Part Three

Masayuki Kanai

Part 3 comprises eight chapters that investigate a variety of mechanisms contributing to social well-being in Asian societies. The analyses employ a quantitative methodology and utilize international comparative survey data, including the Social Well-Being Survey in Asia (SoWSA).

As outlined in the introductory sections, the idea of social well-being encompasses the assessment of social quality through the personal evaluations of individuals with respect to their personal, relational, and societal realms. Although social well-being can be measured objectively, such as through GDP and Gini coefficients, it primarily hinges on subjective appraisals by the members of society. These subjective evaluations can focus on personal life, like subjective well-being, relational life, like satisfaction with family, friends, and communities, and societal aspects, such as perceived inequality. All of these aspects are inherently interconnected. The impact of physical, psychological, and demographic characteristics, as well as socioeconomic status, on individual perception has been explored by the extensive literature on subjective well-being. The primary objective of social well-being studies is to examine the intricate relationship between objective circumstances and subjective measurements at the micro-, meso-, and macro-levels in order to obtain a comprehensive understanding of society at a particular point in time. Although various research designs can be employed to achieve this, the most commonly used approach is to investigate the mechanisms of subjective well-being using multivariate analysis, as is the case in most of the chapters in this part.

Social well-being studies offer a promising perspective in that they acknowledge the inherent diversity and heterogeneity of the quality of society and its underlying mechanisms. Rather than following a single path, development or modernization occurs along multiple paths. As Part 2 chapters revealed, each society in East and

M. Kanai (✉)
School of Human Sciences, Senshu University, Kawasaki, Japan
e-mail: mkanai@senshu-u.jp

J. Yee et al. (eds.), *Social Well-Being, Development, and Multiple Modernities in Asia*,
https://doi.org/10.1007/978-981-97-3866-3_10

Southeast Asia has its own unique historical, socioeconomic, and cultural context, which shapes a specific institutional setting of society at a particular time. The aim of social well-being studies is to describe these institutional settings through narratives. While Part 2 achieved this through longitudinal/historical description of each society, Part 3 will conduct cross-sectional and comparative analysis of cross-national survey data. Although historical/longitudinal studies of a society can provide valuable insights into its persistent characteristics over time, cross-national analyses are better equipped to uncover both commonalities and differences in the mechanisms of social well-being across societies.

Part 3 commences with Chapter "Inequality of Well-Being in Asia: A Comparative Analysis of Happiness in Eight Countries," which conducted primary analyses of the Social Well-Being Survey in Asia (SoWSA) in seven Asian societies and an equivalent survey in Mongolia. The authors geographically divided these societies into East Asia, comprising Japan, South Korea, Taiwan, Mongolia, and Southeast Asia, including Indonesia, the Philippines, Thailand, and Vietnam. They initially compared the means and variances of subjective well-being between the two groups and discovered that East Asian societies had low means and high variances, while Southeast Asian societies had high means and low variances. They subsequently conducted regression analyses of subjective well-being in relation to demographic and socioeconomic traits, such as education, employment, income, and marital status, among others. Again, there is a striking contrast in the factors that promote subjective well-being between the two regions; that is, East Asia shares common factors such as income and marriage, while Southeast Asia does not.

Chapter "Determinants of Happiness and Life Satisfaction in Four Asian Countries" investigated the factors that influence subjective well-being in two East Asian countries (Japan and Korea) and two Southeast Asian countries (Indonesia and Thailand). In addition to individual traits, as explored in the previous chapter, this chapter examined subnational macroeconomic conditions, such as gross regional domestic product (GRDP) per capita. The mixed effects ordered logit model revealed that personal traits had similar effects as in the previous chapter, while subnational macroeconomic conditions had no significant impact or even inverse effects in Thailand. Specifically, the worse the regional economic conditions, the higher the residents' subjective well-being. This finding suggests a counterintuitive relationship between macro-level conditions and micro-level well-being, similar to the cross-national trend that the average level of happiness is low in affluent East Asian societies but high in developing Southeast Asian societies.

Chapter "Comparative Analysis of Income and Happiness in Japan and Korea" examined the complex relationship between income and happiness through the lens of the relative income hypothesis in economics. The relative income hypothesis posits that a higher relative income will decrease a person's well-being in an immobile environment due to feelings of envy, while it will increase it in a mobile environment as a signal of a bright future. The authors applied this theory to the Asian societies of Japan and Korea and found that relative income has a negative impact on well-being in later life respondents but no significant effects in early-life samples. Japan and Korea are relatively immobile societies compared to Western societies, and the environment is less mobile in later life than in earlier life. These findings underscore the importance of considering contextual factors, such as the degree of mobility, when attempting to understand the mechanisms of social well-being.

Chapter "Trust in Strangers and Well-Being: A Comparison in Asian Societies" demonstrated a contextual effect in the relationship between well-being and trust, which is a crucial meso-level factor of social well-being, similar to the comparison with others in the relative income hypothesis. Trust is one of the essential measures of social capital, and the literature has analyzed trust in various types of others, such as trust in family, trust in neighbors, and trust in general others, referred to as generalized trust. The author focused on trust in strangers and compared its effect on subjective well-being with that of generalized trust. The results revealed that trust in strangers had a positive impact on well-being in Southeast Asia with strong social ties and fewer strangers, but had no significant effects in East Asia with weak ties and more strangers. Conversely, the impact of generalized trust was positive in East Asia, but harmful in Southeast Asia. These findings also illustrate the diverse mechanisms between well-being and its determinants in different social contexts.

Chapter "War Experience, Fear of War, and Social Unrest" investigated macro-level factors that contribute to social well-being. War, whether between states or within a state, is a significant event that can have a profound impact on the lives of citizens. It can result in devastating personal and relational consequences, which could lead to a decrease in happiness for those who have experienced it compared to those who have not. Even for those who have not personally experienced war, the fear of it can erode trust in the government, cause social unrest, and provoke a threat of war (security dilemma). In this chapter, the author examined the complex relationship between war experience, happiness, fear of war, trust in the government, and other related factors using multiple data sources from around the world. Unfortunately, the results were not conclusive, largely due to the small sample size of individuals who had experienced war. Despite this limitation, the chapter highlights the importance of considering macro-level factors in understanding social well-being.

Chapter "Politics of Belonging and Citizenship: Relational Well-Being Based on Gender and Religious Identities in Indonesia and South Korea" examined the macro-level societal structure, specifically the potential for social divisions based on gender and religious identities within nation-states. The authors utilized an intersectional approach to analyze the concurrent effects of these two factors on relational well-being in Indonesia and South Korea, which have distinct historical, political, and cultural contexts pertaining to the two factors. The findings indicated separate effects of gender and religious identities on relational well-being, but no interaction effects in either country. Nonetheless, this chapter underscores the significance of political and cultural structures in influencing social well-being.

Chapter "Religious Association and Relational Well-Being: A Comparative Study Between Indonesia and Japan" delved deeper into the role of religion in social well-being within the context of resacralization in contemporary society. Resacralization is a phenomenon observed in diverse societies, including religious ones like Indonesia and non-religious ones like Japan. The authors employed three indicators—religious fairness, religious activities, and religious organization—to measure the concept of "religious association" and examined the bivariate relationship between religious association and relational well-being across different religious identities. While the authors' descriptive findings were both multifaceted and thought-provoking, it is challenging to provide a succinct summary of their results. However, it is clear that religious identity plays a crucial role in social well-being in Asian societies, which are characterized by diverse religious traditions.

Chapter "Multiple Ways to Improve Life Satisfaction in Asian Countries," effectively concludes this book by presenting a comprehensive overview of social well-being mechanisms across various societies and the implications of these mechanisms for policymaking. Through the use of Bayesian network analysis, a leading statistical model for exploring causal relationships, the authors examined the SoWSA dataset, which included numerous variables categorized into socioeconomic variables, subjective life conditions, relational well-being, societal well-being, and overall personal well-being. The results of the analysis revealed that the network of factors is denser in East Asia than in Southeast Asia, indicating that the factors are strongly correlated with each other in East Asia, but not in Southeast Asia, which aligns with the findings of other chapters in Part 3. The second significant finding is that there are two separate paths from income to life satisfaction in East Asia: satisfaction with income and social capital. To explain these findings, the authors propose the "compensatory mechanism hypothesis" in East Asian societies, suggesting that both satisfaction with income and social capital compensate for low-level baseline well-being to result in a higher variance of well-being in these societies. This chapter showcases a promising research design for analyzing the intricate and interdependent structure of social well-being to understand the unique characteristics of a society at a specific time using international comparative survey data.

Masayuki Kanai is a Professor of Sociology at Senshu University. His research interests include subjective well-being, social capital, and social inequality.

Inequality of Well-Being in Asia: A Comparative Analysis of Happiness in Eight Countries

Jun Kobayashi and Dolgion Aldar

Abstract This chapter poses the research question of whether well-being inequalities exist in East and Southeast Asian countries. Layard (*Happiness: Lessons from a new science*, Penguin Press, 2005) proposes the "big seven" drivers of subjective happiness, but Asia may have more complicated and diverse mechanisms. We therefore compare eight countries in East and Southeast Asia using a case study approach and hypothesize differentiated levels, variances, and drivers of happiness between the two regions. Data are collected via a survey ($N = 8166$). Happiness is measured by Cantril's ladder of life. Key findings include, first, that there are well-being inequalities among East and Southeast Asian countries because East Asia experiences relatively low and unequal happiness. Second, East Asia shares happiness determinants such as marriage and income, while Southeast Asia has no such common drivers. This reveals that there are geographical, rather than economic differences in happiness in Asia. Such findings can be obtained only by comparing countries using an integrated perspective. Perhaps this chapter's most important contribution is that we can draw no single picture of happiness in Asia, but must develop potential Asian models of well-being.

Keywords Well-being · Happiness · Asia · Inequality · Comparative analyses

This chapter is based on Jun Kobayashi and Dolgion Aldar, 2018, "Inequality of Well-being in Asia: A Comparative Analysis of Happiness in Eight Countries," *The Senshu Social Well-being Review* 5: 75–82. Its editorial board allowed us to revise the paper and publish it for this volume.

J. Kobayashi (✉)
Department of Contemporary Societies, Seikei University, Tokyo, Japan
e-mail: jun.kobayashi@fh.seikei.ac.jp

D. Aldar
Independent Research Institute of Mongolia, Ulaanbaatar, Mongolia
e-mail: dolgion@irim.mn

J. Yee et al. (eds.), *Social Well-Being, Development, and Multiple Modernities in Asia*,
https://doi.org/10.1007/978-981-97-3866-3_11

1 Introduction

1.1 Research Question

It remains an challenging question whether there are inequalities in well-being (well-being inequality) across countries and whether determinants of well-being are shared between countries or differ by region. Focusing on East and Southeast Asia as a case study, this chapter considers the following research questions.

Research question. Are there any well-being inequalities among East and Southeast Asian countries? If so, do these countries have different or shared determinants of well-being?

This chapter compares happiness in eight countries, divided into two regional groups: Japan (JP), South Korea (KR), Taiwan (TW), and Mongolia (MN) in East Asia; the Philippines (PH), Indonesia (IN), Vietnam (VN), and Thailand (TH) in Southeast Asia. These countries have sufficient diversity—and similarities—to represent these two parts of Asia well.

People may need differentiated supports in different regions. Leaving these questions unresolved may mean that we fail to support those in need.

1.2 Literature

Research on subjective well-being (such as happiness and satisfaction) has mainly focused on Western societies. Layard (2005), for instance, argues that subjective happiness is subject to the "big seven" drivers. These seven drivers are, from strongest to least effective: family, income, employment, community and friends, health, individual freedom, and philosophy of life (for other determinants, see Blanchflower & Oswald, 2004; Bonke et al., 2009; Clark et al., 2008; Diener et al., 1993; Di Tella et al., 2001; Ferrante, 2009; Frey & Stutzer, 2002; Stutzer, 2004; Thoits & Hewitt, 2001; Tsang et al., 2003; Winkelmann & Winkelmann, 1998).

There is no guarantee, however, that these findings hold true in regions other than the West, such as in Asia. Rather, Asian countries may have other unique mechanisms of happiness than Europe and North America. If this difference is ignored, it is possible that we may be overlooking rich and diverse implications for well-being.

1.3 Hypotheses: Economy or Geography?

To hypothesize the similarities and differences in the eight countries, we must first consider how much happiness people feel. Easterlin (1974) shows that a country's

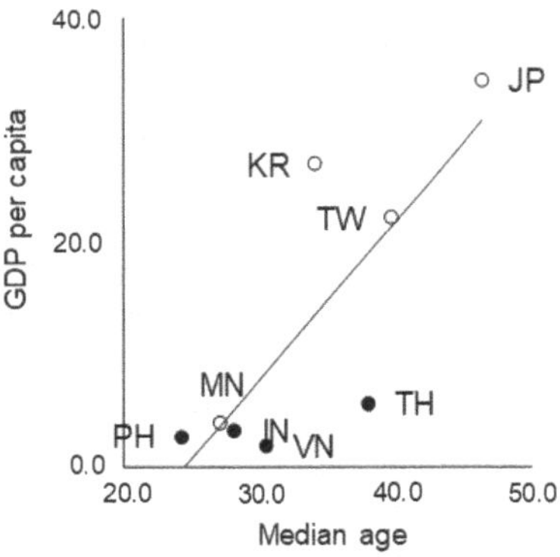

Fig. 1 Median Age and Gross Domestic Product per Capita in Eight Countries in 2015. *Source* United Nations for age, World Bank for GDP. *Note* White dots denote East Asian countries. Black dots denote Southeast Asian countries. The line shows a regression line

economic level frames people's happiness levels in the area. So it is possible that the country's gross domestic product (GDP) will predict its residents' happiness.

Figure 1 highlights the median age and per capita GDP in 2015 for the eight countries studied. This clarifies how old and rich, on average, each country is. The results clearly differentiate two distinct archipelagos: the older and wealthier countries, such as Japan, South Korea, and Taiwan, and the remaining countries, which are less rich, but younger.

Note that Mongolia is located among the poorer countries—generally associated with Southeast Asia. A map, however, indicates that it is a part of East Asia and cannot be grouped geographically elsewhere. Thus, Mongolia functions as a litmus test of whether the economy or geography influences happiness more.

Let us assume that geography (and therefore culture) matters more than economy. Although they are intertwined with each other, each region has followed a distinctive historical, cultural, and social trajectory, which may have an impact on forming residents' happiness (see Hommerich & Klien, 2012). If so, the levels and varieties of happiness can be predicted as follows.

Hypothesis 1. The levels and varieties of happiness in each country will be different between the East and Southeast Asia countries and similar within each regional group (East Asia and Southeast Asia).

We must then consider the determinants of happiness. If geography matters, drivers can be shared in each regional group but differ across groups as follows.

Hypothesis 2. The determinants of happiness in each country will be different between East and Southeast Asia countries and similar within each regional group (East Asia and Southeast Asia).

2 Data and Methods

2.1 Data

Quantitative data were collected by survey. The International Comparative Surveys on Lifestyle and Values (SWB Survey) provides data for the seven countries other than Mongolia. The 2016 survey measuring subjective well-being gives information on Mongolia. All the surveys were conducted in 2015–2017. In Japan, South Korea, and Taiwan, surveys were conducted online. In the other five countries, face-to-face interviews were conducted on nationally representative samples (only Java and Bali were included in Indonesia). The sample sizes ranged from 2000 to 10,000 for the three online surveys and from 800 to 1200 in the remaining field surveys. To equalize sample sizes, we resampled Japan, South Korea, and Taiwan so that $N = 1050$.

2.2 Measures

Happiness, as the dependent variable, is measured as described below, following the Gallup World Poll known as "Cantril's ladder of life" (hereafter called "happiness").

Question. Please imagine a ladder with steps numbered from 0 at the bottom to 10 at the top. Suppose we say that the top of the ladder represents the best possible life for you and the bottom of the ladder represents the worst possible life for you. On which step of the ladder would you say you personally feel you stand at this time, assuming that the higher the step the better you feel about your life, and the lower the step the worse you feel about it? Which step comes closest to the way you feel?

Worst life	←				.				→	Best life
0	1	2	3	4	5	6	7	8	9	10

The independent variables consisted of standard socioeconomic status, including education (measured as years of education), employment (as employed dummy), and income (as equivalent income). The controlling variables included gender (as male dummy), age, marital status (as currently married dummy and currently widowed/divorced dummy, with a baseline being never married), and household (as the number of members in the household). The analytical subsample consisted of respondents with no missing values aged 20 or older ($N = 8166$). The descriptive statistics for the samples in each country are outlined in Table 1.

Table 1 Means and proportions of samples in eight countries

		N	Male (%)	Age	Married (%)	Widowed/ Divorced (%)	Number of household	Years of education	Employed (%)	Equivalent income
East Asia	JP	1050	50.0	46.1	67.0	5.0	2.8	14.7	69.0	0.0
	KR	1050	52.0	43.0	63.0	7.0	3.1	15.2	77.0	0.0
	TW	1050	50.0	40.8	51.0	5.0	3.6	15.3	85.0	0.0
	MN	698	50.0	38.9	64.0	10.0	3.8	13.2	61.0	0.0
Southeast Asia	PH	1082	50.0	43.4	73.0	11.0	5.1	11.5	65.0	0.0
	IN	1179	50.0	39.2	73.0	7.0	5.2	11.0	64.0	0.0
	VN	1063	49.0	39.9	72.0	7.0	4.4	10.0	85.0	0.0
	TH	994	47.0	48.6	63.0	15.0	3.9	10.0	80.0	0.0

Note Samples are limited to those aged 20 or older. Japan, South Korea, and Taiwan are resampled to $N = 1050$. Equivalent income is standardized in each country

Table 2 Mean, standard deviation, and Gini coefficient of happiness

		Mean	Standard deviation	Gini coefficient
East Asia	JP	5.8	1.9	0.18
	KR	5.6	2.0	0.20
	TW	5.5	1.8	0.18
	MN	5.6	2.0	0.20
Southeast Asia	PH	6.7	1.8	0.15
	IN	6.9	1.5	0.12
	VN	7.0	1.6	0.12
	TH	7.3	1.7	0.13

Note Happiness is measured by Cantril's ladder of life

3 Results

3.1 Means and Gini Coefficients

Compare the distributions of happiness: they were mostly single-peaked, with two two-peaked exceptions (Japan and the Philippines). Means are reported in Table 2. All of the East Asian countries ranged between five and six points, while the Southeast Asian countries were concentrated around seven points. An ANOVA test revealed that the differences between East and Southeast Asia are significant ($p < 0.001$). On average, Southeast Asia was found to be happier than East Asia. Within each region, however, countries had significantly different levels of happiness ($p < 0.05$ in East Asia and $p < 0.001$ in Southeast Asia).

We next compared happiness across countries. The standard deviations may have suffered from a ceiling effect, so we chose to calculate the Gini coefficients of happiness for each country. The higher a Gini coefficient was, the more skewed and thus unequal the happiness distribution was. Note that calculating Gini coefficients implied the allocation of happiness to people in a country (rather like withdrawing individual happiness from a central happiness bank).

Table 2 and Fig. 2 show the means and Gini coefficients of the eight countries, and these reveal two archipelagos of countries, with the East Asian countries generally having low and unequal happiness, while the Southeast Asian countries, in contrast, mostly having higher and more equal happiness (Fig. 2 can be called a "happiness map").

3.2 Means by Groups

When mean happiness was compared by socioeconomic status groups, education was divided into three groups (primary, secondary, and tertiary), employment was

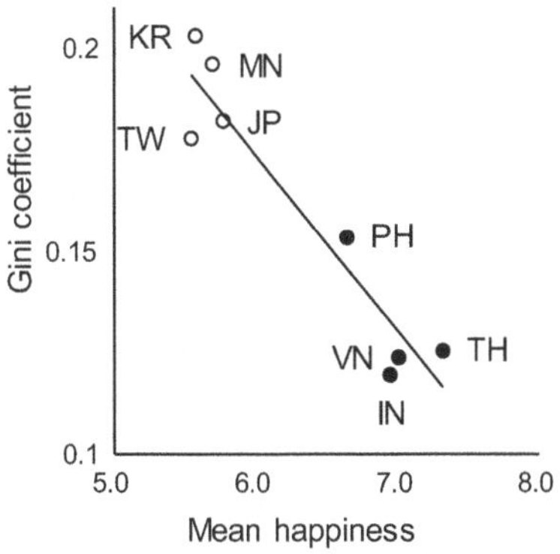

Fig. 2 Mean Happiness and Gini Coefficient of Eight Countries (Happiness Map). *Note* Values are reported in Table 2. Happiness is measured by Cantril's ladder of life. White dots stand for East Asian countries. Black dots stand for Southeast Asian countries. The line shows a regression line

coded into two groups (employed and not employed), and equivalent income was grouped into four (first, second, third, and fourth quartiles). Figure 3 illustrates the happiness levels by these groups in each country. In most countries, we observed a clear indication that higher levels of education resulted in higher levels of happiness. ANOVA tests revealed that these differences were significant, with the exception of Mongolia.

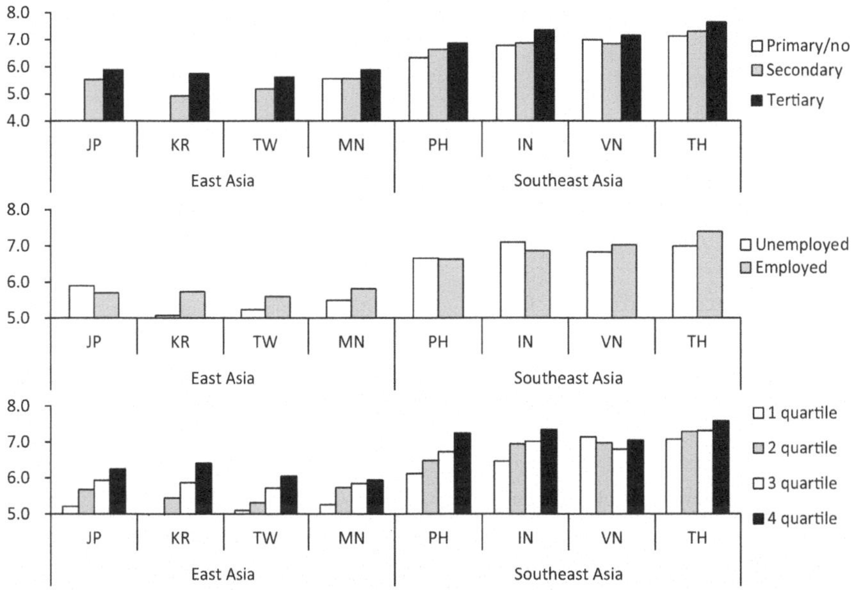

Fig. 3 Mean Happiness by Education, Employment, and Equivalent Income. *Note* See Table 1 for *N*. Happiness is measured by Cantril's ladder of life. No respondents with primary education in Japan and Taiwan; only one respondent with primary education in South Korea was ignored. Income is divided into four quartiles

Employment yielded mixed effects. In South Korea, Mongolia, Indonesia, and Thailand, employment created significant differences in happiness levels. By contrast (but like education), higher levels of income made people happier; these effects were significant except in Vietnam.

3.3 Regression Analyses

Table 3 reports regression results in each country.

In the East Asian countries, marriage and income commonly had significant positive effects on happiness. In the Southeast Asian countries, by contrast, we found no effects of marriage and limited ones of income (limited to the Philippines and Indonesia). These results confirm most of the trends shown in Fig. 3.

As a check on robustness, we added general happiness, life satisfaction, and health satisfaction as control variables and obtained the same results. Education became significant when income was subtracted.

Table 3 Regression results on happiness

	East Asia				Southeast Asia			
	JP	KR	TW	MN	PH	IN	VN	TH
Male	-0.055^{a}	-0.031	-0.010	-0.095^{b}	-0.073^{b}	-0.080^{b}	-0.022	-0.057^{a}
Age	0.024	-0.039	0.054	0.261^{c}	0.026	-0.032	-0.078^{a}	-0.014
Married	0.255^{c}	0.179^{c}	0.109^{d}	0.006	0.011	0.068^{a}	-0.049	0.076^{a}
Widowed/divorced	0.087^{d}	0.013	0.039	-0.147^{d}	-0.018	-0.072^{a}	-0.157^{c}	0.060
#Household	0.003	0.032	0.064^{b}	-0.025	-0.012	0.003	0.032	-0.015
Years of education	0.044	0.094^{d}	0.151^{c}	0.024	0.088^{d}	0.078^{b}	-0.072^{a}	0.125^{d}
Employed	-0.049	0.069^{b}	0.048	0.100^{b}	0.011	-0.059^{a}	0.038	0.080^{b}
Income	0.191^{c}	0.271^{c}	0.098^{d}	0.137^{d}	0.143^{c}	0.122^{c}	0.045	0.063^{a}
R^2	0.115	0.147	0.061	0.074	0.040	0.053	0.034	0.033
N	1,050	1,050	1,050	698	1,082	1,179	1,063	994

Note Happiness is measured by Cantril's ladder of life. ^{a} $p < 0.10$, ^{b} $p < 0.05$, ^{c} $p < 0.001$, ^{d} $p < 0.01$

4 Conclusions

4.1 Summary: Geography Matters

Geography was found to make a difference to happiness levels in both regions. The East Asian countries shared lower and more unequal happiness, as well as the common drivers of happiness: marriage and income. Southeast Asian countries enjoyed higher and more equal happiness, but shared no common drivers (Table 4). Figure 4 summarizes the causal relationships, and these findings generally support both hypotheses stated above.

We can now give an answer to our research question by comparing the countries from an integrated perspective.

Answer to research question. There are inequalities in well-being across East and Southeast Asian countries because East Asia, compared to Southeast Asia, experiences relatively low and unequal happiness. East Asia shares marriage and income as happiness determinants, while Southeast Asia has no such common drivers.

As shown in Fig. 2, this answer implies that Mongolia's happiness belongs among the East Asian countries. This suggests that geography matters more than economy does; in Asia, we observed geographical rather than economic differences in happiness. One possible explanation may be that geographical proximity has led to psychological proximity through religious, cultural, and political interactions; in particular, the Chinese dynasties are likely to have had varying degrees of influence in East Asian countries.

Table 4 Comparisons of East and Southeast Asia on happiness

	Happiness level	Happiness variety	Happiness driver
East Asia	Lower	More unequal	Shared (marriage, income)
Southeast Asia	Higher	More equal	Not shared

Note Happiness is measured by Cantril's ladder of life

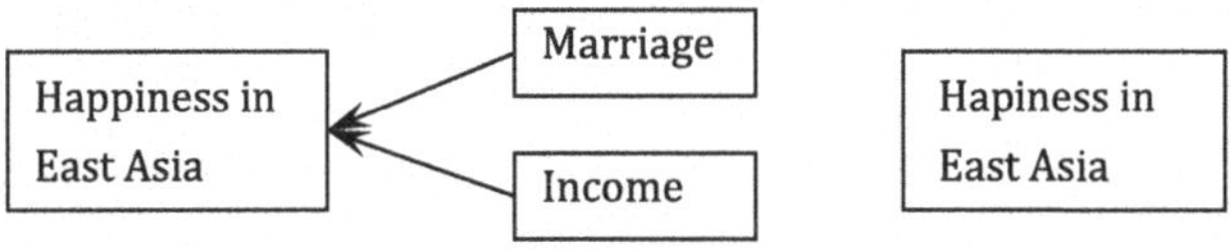

Fig. 4 Summary of Results. *Note* Arrows denote causal relationships of happiness (no arrows mean no causality)

4.2 Toward Asian Models of Well-Being

In contrast to Layard's (2005) prediction, it seems we cannot draw a single picture of happiness in Asia, but have to admit its diversity. Further research should scrutinize the causal mechanisms of well-being to develop potential Asian models of happiness. This would, in turn, enrich the big picture of what well-being implies for the world (for a model on Japan, see Kobayashi & Hommerich, 2017).

Acknowledgements The authors thank Masayuki Kanai and Kenji Kawabata for their comments. This work was supported by the MEXT-Supported Program for the Strategic Research Foundation at Private Universities of Japan, 2014–2018 (S1491003). "International Comparative Surveys on Lifestyle and Values" were designed and conducted by the Center for Social Well-being Studies, Institute for the Development of Social Intelligence, Senshu University, Japan, in collaboration with Social Well-being Research Consortium in Asia. Mongolian data were collected by the Independent Research Institute of Mongolia (IRIM)'s Social Cohesion and Subjective Well-Being Survey. This work was supported by JSPS KAKENHI Grant Number JP15H01969.

References

Blanchflower, D. G., & Oswald, A. J. (2004). Well-being over Time in Britain and the USA. *Journal of Public Economics, 88*, 1359–1386.

Bonke, J., Deding, M., & Lausten, M. (2009). Time and money, a simultaneous analysis of men's and women's domain satisfactions. *Journal of Happiness Studies, 10*(2), 113–131.

Clark, A. E., Fritjers, P., & Schield, M. A. (2008). Relative income, happiness, and utility: An explanation for the Easterlin paradox and other puzzles. *Journal of Economic Literature, 46*(1), 95–144.

Diener, E., Sandvid, E., Seidlitz, L., & Diener, M. (1993). The relationship between income and subjective well-being: Relative or absolute? *Social Indicators Research, 28*(3), 195–233.

Easterlin, R. A. (1974). Does economic growth improve the human lot? Some empirical evidence. In P. A. David & M. W. Reder (Eds.), *Nations and households in economic growth: Essays in honor of Moses Abramovitz* (pp. 89–125). Academic Press.

Easterlin, R. A., McVey, L. A., Switek, M., Sawangfa, O., & Zweig, J. S. (2010). The happiness: Income paradox revisited. *Proceedings of the National Academy of Sciences, 107*(52), 22463–22468.

Ferrante, F. (2009). Education, aspirations and life satisfaction. *Kyklos, 62*(4), 542–562.

Frey, B. S., & Stutzer, A. (2002). *Happiness and economics: How the economy and institutions affect well-being*. Princeton University Press.

Hommerich, C., & Klien, S. (2012). Happiness: Does culture matter? *International Journal of Wellbeing, 2*(4), 292–298.

Kobayashi, J., & Hommerich, C. (2017). Are happiness and unhappiness two sides of the same coin? An analysis of happiness and unhappiness. *Sociological Theory and Methods, 32*(1), 49–63.

Layard, R. (2005). *Happiness: Lessons from a new science*. Penguin Press.

Stutzer, A. (2004). The role of income aspirations in individual happiness. *Journal of Economic Behaviour and Organisation, 54*, 89–109.

Tella, R. D., MacCulloch, R. J., & Oswald, A. J. (2001). Preferences over inflation and unemployment: Evidence from surveys of happiness. *American Economic Review, 91*(1), 335–341.

Thoits, P. A., & Hewitt, L. N. (2001). Volunteer work and well-being. *Journal of Health and Social Behavior, 42*, 115–131.

Tsang, L. L. W., Harvey, C. H., Duncan, K. A., & Sommer, R. (2003). The effects of children, dual earner status, sex role traditionalism, and marital structure on marital happiness over time. *Journal of Family and Economic Issues, 24*(1), 5–26.

Winkelmann, L., & Winkelmann, R. (1998). Why are the unemployed so unhappy? Evidence from panel data. *Economica, 65*(257), 1–15.

Jun Kobayashi is Professor of Sociology at Seikei University and the Director of Seikei Institute for Social Research. He studies social inequality and family.

Dolgion Aldar is a Board Member and Consultant of the Independent Research Institute of Mongolia (IRIM). Her research focuses on social well-being and social cohesion.

Determinants of Happiness and Life Satisfaction in Four Asian Countries

Indera Ratna Irawati Pattinasarany

Abstract This study examined the determinants of perceived happiness and life satisfaction in four Asian countries: Indonesia, Thailand, Japan, and South Korea. Aside from controlling for standard individual traits and household characteristics, this study also controls for subnational macroeconomic conditions. The research relied on data from the Social Well-Being Survey in Asia 2015–2017 and employed the multilevel mixed-effects ordered logistic method to analyze the findings. The findings indicate factors associated with increased likelihood of experiencing happiness and life satisfaction. These factors encompass being female (in contrast to being male), possessing a higher level of education, enjoying a greater household income, and owning one's residence. Conversely, the likelihood of happiness and life satisfaction tends to decrease with age (up to a certain age), being divorced or unmarried (as opposed to being married), being in temporary or no employment (as opposed to permanent employment), and when living in households with many family members. The estimation results varied from country to country. This study found limited evidence for the role of economic activity in explaining happiness in Indonesia and South Korea. In Thailand, subnational macroeconomic indicators had a statistically significant but unexpected impact, while in Japan, they were statistically insignificant.

Keywords Happiness · Inequality · Life satisfaction · Multilevel mixed-effect ordered logit method

1 Introduction

The 2015 edition of the World Happiness Report documented happiness as a legitimate benchmark for societal development and a target within public policy (Helliwell et al., 2015). The 2019 edition of the same report claims that governments and international organizations have begun to focus their attention on the happiness

I. R. I. Pattinasarany (✉)
Department of Sociology, Universitas Indonesia, Depok, Indonesia
e-mail: indera.pattinasarany@ui.ac.id

J. Yee et al. (eds.), *Social Well-Being, Development, and Multiple Modernities in Asia*,
https://doi.org/10.1007/978-981-97-3866-3_12

or subjective well-being (SWB) of citizens[1] (Helliwell et al., 2019). Bhutan established gross national happiness (GNH) as the national goal of its constitution.[2] This was a drastic move from the traditional economic policies, which were generally focused on regular employment, price stability, economic growth, efficiency, and equity. Considering that it will still take time to include happiness as a goal of public policy, several countries have begun collecting the national level statistics pertaining to well-being.

Nonetheless, the ultimate question is "what makes people happy?" Studies on happiness and life satisfaction have been conducted by researchers across nations in various fields of study, such as psychology, economics, biology, sociology, and political science. These studies have been growing rapidly over the last twenty years, with studies ranging from discussions on subjective feelings of individuals to assessing their living conditions (Diener et al., 2009). Dolan et al. (2008), Blanchflower and Oswald (2011), Stutzer and Frey (2012), and Lee (2022) reviewed the determinants of happiness.

Research that employs a uniform statistical model and methodology to compare the factors influencing happiness and life satisfaction across different countries and subsequently presents the outcomes and associated discussions at the country level is not widely available. Two noteworthy examples are Chen's (2012) investigation into the connection between education and well-being in four East Asian nations (Japan, South Korea, China, and Taiwan) and the study by Oshio et al. (2011) that examined the correlation between relative income and happiness in China, Japan, South Korea, and the United States. The advantage of such studies is that one can closely compare the particular determining factors across countries. For example, the estimation of the age variables, which are entered in the statistical model in the quadratic form, can produce a U-shaped pattern in one country and an inverted U-shape in another country. If age estimates in both countries follow a U-shaped pattern, it is plausible that the estimates will result in a huge age difference in the turning point of such U-shaped patterns. Researchers can engage in in-depth research by examining the causes of these differences. Such comprehensive knowledge will provide guidance to those responsible for formulating public policies. This study attempted to bridge this gap.

This chapter examines the determinants of perceived happiness and life satisfaction in four Asian countries, namely Indonesia, Thailand, Japan, and South Korea by using the Social Well-Being Survey in Asia 2015–2017 (SoWSA). Seven countries participated in the SoWSA surveys; three countries other than the four that have been included in this study were the Philippines, Vietnam, and Taiwan. Indonesia and Thailand were selected from amongst the countries in the Southeast Asian region; these

[1] The report lists the Ranking of Happiness 2016–2018 in which the four countries of interest in this study occupied the following positions: Indonesia (92 out of 156 countries), Thailand (52), Japan (58), and South Korea (54).

[2] GNH is a multidimensional index that comprises nine domains and 33 indicators. These domains are psychological wellbeing, health, usage of time, education, cultural diversity and resilience, good governance, community vitality, ecological diversity and resilience, and living standards (Ura et al., 2012).

two countries are categorized as middle-income countries by the World Bank. Japan and South Korea were chosen as the representative country of the East Asian region and high-income country, respectively. Similarities and differences in the determinants of self-reported happiness and life satisfaction among these four countries were explored using the data of the SoWSA survey that was specifically designed to study lifestyles and values related to the social well-being.

A distinctive aspect of this study lies in its comprehensive examination of happiness and life satisfaction determinants. It goes beyond the typical considerations of individual traits and household characteristics by incorporating control over subnational macroeconomic indicators, as exemplified in the works of Cuñado and Gracia (2012), Oshio and Kobayashi (2009), and Sujarwoto and Tampubolon (2015). These encompass metrics like gross regional domestic product (GRDP), human development index (HDI), poverty rate, and income inequality (measured by the Gini coefficient of per capita expenditures). These indicators are known to influence SWB (Clark, 2017; Di Tella et al., 2003). As a result, this study investigates the impact of subnational-level macroeconomic factors on self-reported happiness and life satisfaction, setting it apart from most studies that mainly focus on national-level macroeconomic factors. The insights gained from this research can inform local government policy decisions aimed at enhancing the well-being and contentment of their populations.

This chapter is structured into five sections. Section 2 discusses the data used in the study. This section also compares survey data on self-reported life satisfaction in the four selected countries with data from the World Values Survey. Section 3 briefly describes the multilevel mixed-effects ordered logistic model used to estimate determinants. Section 4 presents and discusses the findings and their variations across countries, along with the influence of subnational macroeconomic factors on happiness and life satisfaction estimation. Section 5 summarizes the study's findings and proposes future research directions.

2 Data

The main data source that was analyzed was the SoWSA conducted in Indonesia (survey conducted in 2018), Thailand (2017), Japan (2015), and South Korea (2015).[3] The SoWSA was designed and conducted by the Center for Social Well-being Studies, Institute for the Development of Social Intelligence, Senshu University, Japan, in collaboration with the Social Well-Being Research Consortium in Asia.

---

[3] This work used the data version 0.5 (May 5, 2018) of the Social Well-Being Survey in Asia (SoWSA) which was formerly referred to as International Comparative Surveys on Lifestyle and Values (ICSLV). The survey was supported by Japan's Ministry of Education, Culture, Sports, Science and Technology (MEXT)-Supported Program for the Strategic Research Foundation at Private Universities of Japan, 2014–18 (S1491003), Senshu University, LabSosio Department of Sociology-Universitas Indonesia, and ROIS-DS-JOINT, 2017–18 (002RP2017 and 003RP2018).

The SoWSA explored the lifestyles and values related to the social well-being of Asian countries.

The two SWB variables of interest—levels of happiness and life satisfaction—were the ordinal variables. The data on these variables was recorded on an ordered scale of 0–10. The explanatory variables comprised three groups representing individuals, households, and regional characteristics. The individual traits consisted of binary variables: gender (male and female), educational attainment[4] (four groups, different across countries), employment status (permanent, non-permanent, and no employment), marital status (married, divorced, and unmarried), and one continuous variable: age. Household characteristics were entered into the model as binary variables: household income[5] (four groups, different across countries), endowment (proxy by living in their own house), and one continuous variable: household size. A summary of the data used in this study is illustrated in Table 5.

This study specifically targeted participants aged between 20 and 70 years to maintain consistency with self-reported levels of happiness and life satisfaction, which are known to be significantly age-dependent (Bartram, 2021; Blanchflower, 2021). The selection of the age range for this study is derived from the sample age ranges in Japan and South Korea, which have the highest number of observations within the SoWSA dataset. As such, all individuals interviewed in Japan and South

[4] The disparity in educational attainment between Indonesian and Thai respondents, on one hand, and Japanese and South Korean respondents, on the other, necessitates a differentiation in the class definition used in this study. For Indonesian and Thai respondents, the four education categories include primary education, junior secondary, senior secondary, and tertiary education. In contrast, for Japanese and South Korean respondents, the four education categories comprise secondary education, junior college, 4-year college, and graduate school.

[5] The SoWSA questionnaire features a question regarding monthly household income, and the response options are presented in the form of income categories, with varying numbers of categories in different countries. In this study, we aim to map these response options into four groups, which we have labeled "low," "lower-middle," "upper-middle," and "high" income groups. We aim to achieve an equal distribution of respondents among these income groups in each country.

For Indonesia, the available response options consist of 13 income categories, which we find incongruent with real-world income distribution, as evident from specific income groups with a disproportionately high number of respondents. The "low income" group includes individuals with a monthly household income below Indonesia Rupiah (IDR) 2 million, representing 28% of the total respondents. The "lower-middle income" category (IDR 2 to < 5 million) is occupied by 43% of respondents, while the "upper-middle income" group (IDR 5 to < 10 million) comprises 20% of respondents, and the "high income" category (IDR $\geq$ 10 million) includes 9% of respondents.

In the case of Thailand, the response options encompass six income categories. The "low income" category (Thailand Baht (THB) < 100,000) accounts for 43% of respondents, the "lower-middle income" group (THB 100,000 to < 200,000) is represented by 24%, the "upper-middle income" category (THB 200,000 to < 400,000) by 19%, and the "high income" (THB $\geq$ 400,000) group consists of 14% of respondents. In contrast, for Japan and South Korea, the questionnaire offers more than 20 income categories, allowing for a more balanced distribution of respondents across income classes. In Japan, the distribution is 23% for "low income," 27% for "lower-middle income," 23% for "upper-middle income," and 27% for "high income." Similarly, in South Korea, the percentages are 23% for "low income," 27% for "lower-middle income," 26% for "upper-middle income," and 24% for "high income." This results in a more equitable distribution of income classes in Japan and South Korea, whereas the distribution appears uneven in Indonesia and Thailand.

Korea fell within this age range. In the case of Indonesia, two respondents exceeded the age of 70. Conversely, for Thailand, there were 16 respondents under 16 years of age and 105 respondents over 70 years old. Consequently, we excluded data points from Indonesia and Thailand that did not conform to the above age criteria.

We examine the influence of subnational (i.e., provincial, district, prefectural, or regional) macroeconomic conditions on determining individuals' happiness and life satisfaction by including covariates for local indicators like GRDP per capita, HDI, poverty rate, and the Gini coefficient of household expenditures per capita. The subnational indicators selected for Indonesia were based on the Statistics Indonesia (BPS) interactive database search and publications; Thailand from the National Economic and Social Development Board (NESDB) and the United Nations Development Program (UNDP) report on Human Achievement Index (HAI); Japan from the Statistics Japan and the Cabinet Office of the Government of Japan; and South Korea from Statistics Korea. In addition, the data for Japan and South Korea is also sourced from the Global Data Lab.

2.1 Levels of Happiness and Life Satisfaction

The distribution of two main measures of SWB in this analysis, happiness [question W01][6] and life satisfaction [W02], is shown in Fig. 1. Some similarities were observed between the two distributions in some countries. The distribution of happiness and life satisfaction for Indonesia and Thailand were found to be left-skewed, implying that most individuals interviewed in these countries expressed their contentment with life in general. The level of happiness in Japan and Korea was not as high as in Indonesia and Thailand. The survey responses reflect the cultural and economic diversity (Veenhoven, 2012; Ye et al., 2015).

Indonesian adults, on average, had a marginally higher degree of happiness than their Thai counterparts (Table 1). Among the respondents from the four countries, the South Korean respondents reported the lowest degree of happiness. The average level of satisfaction with current life among the Indonesian respondents was the highest across the four countries, while that of the South Korean respondents was the lowest. Pearson's chi-squared test results show that the levels of happiness and life satisfaction across countries do not exhibit a similar distribution, suggesting that the determinants of both measures of SWB are probably country-specific.

Nevertheless, the correlation coefficient between happiness and life satisfaction was found to differ across countries. Despite Indonesia having the highest levels of happiness and life satisfaction, the correlation between the two measures of SWB among Indonesian adults was the lowest among the four countries (0.534). This

[6] Question W01 reads: "How happy are you currently?" Answer on a scale of 0–10, with 10 being "very happy" and 0 being "very unhappy." Question W02 reads: "How satisfied are you currently with your life?" Responses to W02 also follows a scale of 0–10, with 10 being "very satisfied" and 0 being "very unsatisfied."

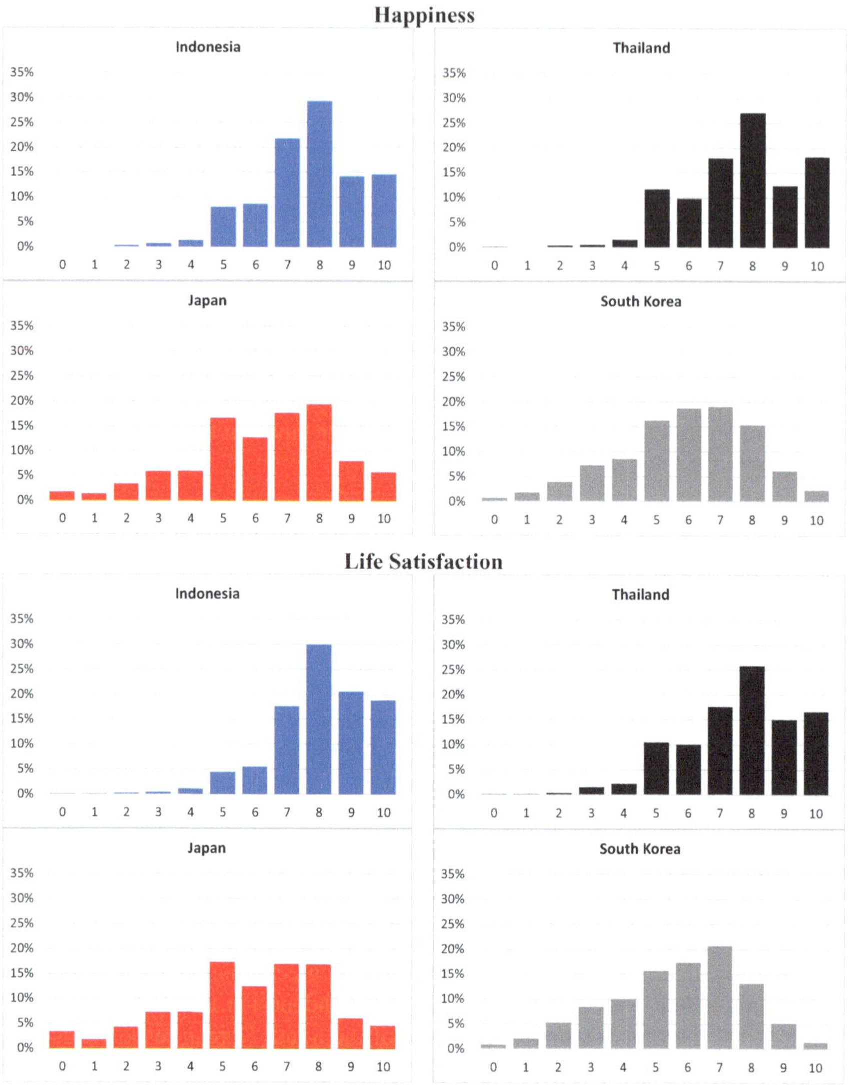

Fig. 1 Distribution of happiness and life satisfaction levels

implies that the Indonesian respondents had different perceptions of happiness and life satisfaction, at least when they responded to the survey questions. The correlation coefficients pertaining to the Thai, Japanese, and South Korean adults were 0.720, 0.836, and 0.866, respectively.

Table 1 Country comparison

Country	Happiness		Life satisfaction		Pairwise correlation
	Mean	SD	Mean	SD	
Indonesia	7.68	1.59	8.04	1.55	0.534
Thailand	7.65	1.70	7.58	1.76	0.720
Japan	6.25	2.27	5.87	2.40	0.836
South Korea	5.93	2.06	5.70	2.08	0.866
Pearson's χ^2	1080.6		1872.0		
p-value	0.000		0.000		

2.2 *Comparison with the World Value Survey*

Surveys have been conducted to explore the various measures and models for investigating the SWB, including the two analyzed in this study, one of which is the World Values Survey (WVS). The WVS has examined public values and beliefs in almost 100 countries since 1981, by conducting representative national surveys. The question on life satisfaction in WVS was comparable to that of the SoWSA.[7] Figure 2 depicts a comparison of the distribution of life satisfaction levels between the SoWSA and WVS surveys across the four countries (Indonesia, Thailand, Japan, and South Korea).[8]

The distribution scores pertaining to life satisfaction among Indonesian adults in the SoWSA survey was more skewed to the left in comparison to that of the WVS. The results may be attributed to the different ways in which the questions were presented, difference in locations, and the 12-year difference between the two surveys (WVS was conducted in 2006 and SoWSA in 2018). The distribution of scores pertaining to life satisfaction and happiness in Thailand was somewhat similar, although WVS recorded a higher percentage of respondents who were "completely satisfied." Meanwhile, the distributions of responses pertaining to life satisfaction in the two surveys were similar for Japan and South Korea.

In the context of Indonesia, we conducted a comparison between self-reported happiness data from the SoWSA dataset and the 2017 Happiness Level Measurement Survey (SPTK), a nationwide survey that periodically assesses happiness levels in Indonesia. The comparative analysis revealed a congruent distribution of happiness levels between the two sources.

[7] The question pertaining to life satisfaction in the WVS reads: "Considering all aspects, how satisfied are you with your life?" On this scale in which 1 means you are 'completely dissatisfied' and 10 means you are 'completely satisfied' what is your life-satisfaction level?

[8] A 10-point scale was used to obtain information on the level of life satisfaction in WVS while in the case of SoWSA documents a 11-rung response was used, and the lowest two responses in SoWSA (i.e., 0 and 1) were pooled into one category.

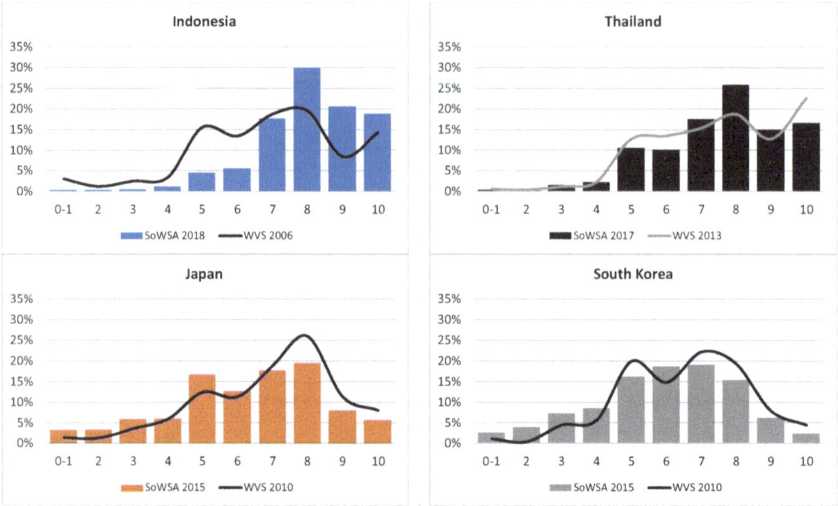

Source: World Value Survey from WVS interactive tables (http://www.worldvaluessurvey.org/WVSOnline.jsp)

Fig. 2 Life satisfaction—SoWSA versus World Value Survey. *Source* World Value Survey from WVS interactive tables (http://www.worldvaluessurvey.org/WVSOnline.jsp)

2.3 Recoding of Levels of Happiness and Life Satisfaction

To conduct an ordered logit analysis, we adjusted the distribution of happiness and life satisfaction. Since some levels of these measures had very low responses (e.g., less than 3% of survey respondents in Indonesia perceived their happiness as levels 1–4), we merged two or more adjacent responses to make the distribution more equal in size. Moreover, data recoding was carried out as per the ordered logit method, which required a cell to contain at least 3% of observations.

After the recoding, each country in the final dataset comprised 6-ring SWB measures. Table 2 shows the recoded distributions of responses pertaining to happiness and life satisfaction.

3 Methodology

This study utilizes a Multilevel Mixed-Effects Ordered Logistic model to account for nesting and the categorical nature of the dependent variables. Our observations include individuals (level 1) nested within subnational (level 2), acknowledging the hierarchical structure. We incorporate random intercepts for each subnational to account for variations in macroeconomic conditions across subnational. Additionally, we employ an ordered logit model since the dependent variables, happiness and life satisfaction levels, are ordered in nature. By employing this model, we can control for

Table 2 Recoding self-reported happiness and life satisfaction responses

After recoding	Happiness: original response (W01)				Life satisfaction: original response (W02)			
	Indonesia	Thailand	Japan	South Korea	Indonesia	Thailand	Japan	South Korea
1	0–5	0–5	0–4	0–3	0–5	0–5	0–3	0–3
2	6	6	5	4–5	6	6	4–5	4
3	7	7	6	6	7	7	6	5
4	8	8	7	7	8	8	7	6
5	9	9	8	8	9	9	8	7
6	10	10	9–10	9–10	10	10	9–10	8–10

individual and subnational-level variables to isolate the macroeconomic conditions on self-reported happiness and life satisfaction levels (Mehmetoglu & Jakobsen, 2017; Rabe-Hesketh & Skrondal, 2022).

In our empirical model we posit a latent variable to represent underlying SWB measures. We examine the association between the latent variable and individual characteristics, household characteristics, and subnational contextual variables. We specify the model as follows:

$$y_{ij}^{*} = x1_{ij}\beta 1 + x2_{j}\beta 2 + z_{ij}u_{j} + \epsilon_{ij}$$

$$y_{ij} = \begin{cases} 0 \text{ if } y_{ij}^{*} \leq \kappa_1 \\ 1 \text{ if } \kappa_1 < y_{ij}^{*} \leq \kappa_2 \\ 2 \text{ if } \kappa_2 < y_{ij}^{*} \leq \kappa_3 \\ 3 \text{ if } \kappa_3 < y_{ij}^{*} \leq \kappa_4 \\ 4 \text{ if } \kappa_4 < y_{ij}^{*} \leq \kappa_5 \\ 5 \text{ if } \kappa_5 < y_{ij}^{*} \end{cases}$$

where y_{ij}^{*} is the unobserved happiness and life satisfaction levels for individual i who resides in subnational j (latent variable); $x1_{ij}$ is the individual and household characteristics for individual i living in subnational j; $x2_j$ is the subnational macroeconomic contextual variables for subnational j; z_{ij} is the covariates corresponding to the random effects; as this model follows a random-intercept model, z_{ij} is simply the scalar 1; u_j is the random effects; and ϵ_{ij} is the errors, distributed as logistic with mean 0 and variance $\pi 2/3$ and are independent of u_j.

This study assumes that individuals residing within a specific subnational region tend to exhibit comparable patterns when reporting their levels of happiness and life satisfaction, as opposed to those living in other subnational areas. In this context, the term "subnational unit" corresponds to the location variable within the SoWSA data, "f141," which varies for each country. In Indonesia, this location variable pertains to

17 districts; in Thailand, 11 provinces; in Japan, 47 prefectures; and in South Korea, seven metropolitan cities and nine provinces.

When determining the appropriate subnational level, we consider the availability of contextual variable data at that specific level. For example, in Indonesia, all the macroeconomic data used in this study, GRDP per capita, HDI, poverty incidence, and Gini of expenditures per capita, are accessible at the district level. Similarly, in Thailand, data on Gross Provincial Product (GPP) per capita, the Human Achievement Index (HAI), and poverty levels are obtainable at the provincial level. In contrast, the situation differs for Japan and South Korea, where GNI per capita (in the case of Japan) and GRDP per capita (in the case of South Korea), as well as HDI data, are accessible at a broader regional level. This study adopts the subnational region classification of 10 regions for Japan and seven regions for South Korea, in line with the categorization provided by the Global Data Lab.

4 Analytical Results and Discussions

Table 3 displays the estimated happiness (Columns [1]–[4]) and life satisfaction (Columns [5]–[8]) levels obtained from a multilevel mixed-effects ordered logistic analysis. Intraclass Correlation Coefficient (ICC) are small, ranging from 0.001 to 0.051 (found in the second row from the bottom). An ICC for happiness level model for Indonesia (Column [1]) of 0.017 suggests that approximately 1.7% of the variance in the latent response is explained by variability between districts. Despite the small magnitude of the ICC, following Sommet and Morselli (2017), we continue to utilize a multilevel model in this study. This decision is based on the understanding that even the smallest ICC (unless it is zero) does not necessarily indicate the absence of variation in respondents' happiness levels between districts in Indonesia.

The Likelihood Ratio (LR) test, shown in the third row from the bottom, examines whether the multilevel mixed-effects ordered logistic model provides a significantly improved fit to the data compared to the simple (single-level) ordered logistic model. A p-value of 0.000 for the LR test indicates the presence of significant between-provinces variation in happiness or life satisfaction levels.

An anomaly is observed in the context of South Korea, where the p-value for the happiness model is 0.333 (Column [4]), and for the life satisfaction model, it is 0.472 (Column [8]). These values indicate no statistically significant differences between the estimates obtained from the multilevel mixed-effects ordered logistic model and the single-level ordered logistic model. The relatively low p-values, coupled with a notably low intra-class correlation (ICC) in the South Korean case, suggest that employing the multilevel model does not result in substantial improvements in estimation compared to the single-level model. We also conducted a single-level ordered logit model for the South Korean case and found that the point estimates from the single-level model share the same signs and levels of significance as those from the multilevel model. The magnitude of these point estimates is close, though not precisely identical.

Table 3 Multilevel mixed-effects ordered logit estimates for life satisfaction and happiness levels

	Happiness											
	Indonesia			Thailand			Japan			South Korea		
	[1]			[2]			[3]			[4]		
Women	0.237	(0.116)	**	0.071	(0.117)		0.476	(0.038)	***	0.292	(0.082)	***
Age	– 0.073	(0.031)	**	– 0.091	(0.033)	***	– 0.155	(0.010)	***	– 0.111	(0.026)	***
Age-squared (* 1/100)	0.070	(0.035)	**	0.092	(0.035)	***	0.164	(0.011)	***	0.116	(0.029)	***
Education: 2	– 0.011	(0.188)		0.224	(0.203)		0.133	(0.056)	**	– 0.077	(0.141)	
Education: 3	0.069	(0.157)		0.183	(0.184)		0.166	(0.038)	***	– 0.036	(0.112)	
Education: 4	0.153	(0.195)		0.353	(0.206)	*	0.276	(0.067)	***	0.390	(0.157)	**
Divorced	– 1.242	(0.233)	***	– 0.192	(0.185)		– 0.699	(0.073)	***	– 0.532	(0.189)	***
Unmarried	– 0.870	(0.175)	***	– 0.219	(0.171)		– 1.299	(0.048)	***	– 0.706	(0.120)	***
Employment: non-permanent	– 0.096	(0.170)		0.127	(0.179)		– 0.180	(0.044)	***	– 0.242	(0.098)	**
Employment: no	– 0.161	(0.189)		– 0.326	(0.219)		– 0.123	(0.047)	***	– 0.329	(0.111)	***
Household size	– 0.008	(0.018)		0.009	(0.034)		– 0.051	(0.015)	***	– 0.085	(0.039)	**
Income: 2	0.539	(0.132)	***	– 0.047	(0.147)		0.168	(0.048)	***	0.331	(0.120)	***
Income: 3	0.734	(0.165)	***	0.386	(0.164)	**	0.424	(0.052)	***	0.542	(0.125)	***
Income: 4	1.012	(0.222)	***	0.517	(0.197)	***	0.708	(0.052)	***	0.927	(0.135)	***
Lives in own house	0.140	(0.113)		0.362	(0.150)	**	0.186	(0.041)	***	0.315	(0.088)	***

(continued)

Table 3 (continued)

	Happiness											
	Indonesia			Thailand			Japan			South Korea		
	[1]			[2]			[3]			[4]		
κ1	− 3.626	(0.718)		− 3.437	(0.820)		− 4.844	(0.240)		− 4.301	(0.613)	
κ2	− 2.875	(0.715)		− 2.722	(0.817)		− 3.873	(0.238)		− 2.843	(0.610)	
κ3	− 1.713	(0.714)		− 1.815	(0.815)		− 3.274	(0.238)		− 2.029	(0.608)	
κ4	− 0.381	(0.712)		− 0.581	(0.813)		− 2.449	(0.237)		− 1.099	(0.607)	
κ5	0.520	(0.712)		0.166	(0.814)		− 1.229	(0.237)		0.161	(0.609)	
Variances: subnational (constant)	0.058	(0.037)		0.145	(0.078)		0.007	(0.005)		0.002	(0.006)	
LR test ordered logit (*p*-score)	0.000			0.000			0.007			0.333		
Intraclass correlation (ICC)	0.017			0.016			0.002			0.001		
Observations	1246			1004			11,804			2000		
	Life satisfaction											
	Indonesia			Thailand			Japan			South Korea		
	[5]			[6]			[7]			[8]		
Women	0.132	(0.116)		0.126	(0.117)		0.498	(0.038)	***	0.247	(0.082)	***
Age	− 0.068	(0.031)	**	− 0.073	(0.033)	**	− 0.164	(0.010)	***	− 0.107	(0.026)	***
Age-squared (* 1/100)	0.060	(0.035)	*	0.076	(0.036)	**	0.175	(0.011)	***	0.110	(0.029)	***
Education: 2	− 0.066	(0.185)		0.139	(0.201)		0.159	(0.056)	***	0.016	(0.141)	
Education: 3	0.056	(0.159)		0.001	(0.186)		0.238	(0.039)	***	0.062	(0.111)	
Education: 4	0.206	(0.197)		0.253	(0.204)		0.388	(0.067)	***	0.473	(0.157)	***
Divorced	− 0.909	(0.241)	***	− 0.235	(0.184)		− 0.699	(0.074)	***	− 0.687	(0.189)	***

(continued)

Table 3 (continued)

	Life satisfaction											
	Indonesia			Thailand			Japan			South Korea		
	[5]			[6]			[7]			[8]		
Unmarried	– 0.716	(0.179)	***	– 0.272	(0.172)		– 1.066	(0.048)	***	– 0.763	(0.120)	***
Employment: non-permanent	0.125	(0.174)		– 0.041	(0.178)		– 0.227	(0.044)	***	– 0.268	(0.098)	***
Employment: no	0.077	(0.194)		– 0.345	(0.220)		– 0.071	(0.048)		– 0.357	(0.111)	***
Household size	– 0.006	(0.018)		– 0.022	(0.033)		– 0.095	(0.015)	***	– 0.132	(0.040)	***
Income: 2	0.418	(0.133)	***	0.116	(0.147)		0.147	(0.049)	***	0.403	(0.119)	***
Income: 3	0.584	(0.166)	***	0.568	(0.167)	***	0.516	(0.052)	***	0.713	(0.124)	***
Income: 4	0.809	(0.226)	***	0.476	(0.199)	**	0.862	(0.053)	***	1.110	(0.134)	***
Lives in own house	0.252	(0.115)	**	0.440	(0.147)	***	0.322	(0.042)	***	0.354	(0.087)	***
$\kappa 1$	– 3.905	(0.727)		– 3.025	(0.815)		– 4.982	(0.241)		– 4.033	(0.616)	
$\kappa 2$	– 3.215	(0.723)		– 2.335	(0.812)		– 3.579	(0.238)		– 3.391	(0.615)	
$\kappa 3$	– 2.032	(0.720)		– 1.425	(0.810)		– 3.003	(0.238)		– 2.623	(0.613)	
$\kappa 4$	– 0.693	(0.718)		– 0.281	(0.809)		– 2.168	(0.237)		– 1.853	(0.612)	
$\kappa 5$	0.388	(0.718)		0.655	(0.810)		– 0.944	(0.237)		– 0.763	(0.611)	
Variances: subnational (constant)	0.084	(0.045)		0.176	(0.093)		0.007	(0.005)		0.005	(0.007)	
LR test ordered logit (*p*-score)	0.000			0.000			0.003			0.472		
Intraclass correlation (ICC)	0.025			0.051			0.002			0.001		
Observations	1232			1004			11,804			2000		

Note ***, **, * significant at the 1, 5, and 10% levels

The line labeled "Variances: Subnational (constant)" in the fourth row from the bottom represents the degree to which provinces contribute to the overall variation in happiness/life satisfaction levels among individuals. The multilevel model considers the hierarchical data structure, acknowledging that individuals within the same subnational unit may share more similarities due to common contextual factors compared to individuals in different subnational units. These contextual factors can include macroeconomic indicators, access to local infrastructure (such as healthcare and education), local norms and culture, among others. A higher value in this line signifies a more pronounced variation in self-reported happiness/life satisfaction at the subnational level, suggesting that the subnational exerts a discernible influence on individual happiness levels, which could outweigh the impact of individual-level factors.

The subsequent sections delve into the findings for each covariate in the empirical model.

4.1 Gender

In Japan and South Korea, women are more likely than men to express happiness and contentment with their lives. Meanwhile, in the case of Indonesia, women marginally report higher levels of happiness compared to men. The observation that women tend to report higher levels of happiness and life satisfaction is a recurring trend in numerous countries, including Japan (Tiefenbach & Kohlbacher, 2013), Thailand (Senasu & Singhapakdi, 2018), and Malaysia (Boo et al., 2016). However, it is worth noting that Rahayu (2016) did not identify significant differences in the way Indonesian men and women perceive their levels of happiness.

Figure 3 offers a visual representation of the estimates provided in Table 2. The figure shows predictive margins for happiness and life satisfaction levels at both ends: the lowest (i.e., life satisfaction = 1 and happiness = 1; shown in solid lines) and the highest (i.e., life satisfaction = 6 and happiness = 6; depicted with dashed lines) outcomes. We have chosen this representation to optimize space and enhance the figure's clarity. Furthermore, the figure's arrangement places the Indonesian (blue lines) and Thailand (black lines) cases in the left panels, while the Japan (red lines) and South Korea (gray lines) cases occupy the right panels.

The data presented in the graph illustrates differences in life satisfaction and happiness between men and women across various outcomes. Specifically, men tend to report higher levels of happiness and life satisfaction when the outcome is at its lowest point. In comparison, women report higher levels of happiness and life satisfaction when the outcome is at its highest. In Japan, women are 6.7% less inclined than men to assess their happiness at the lowest level (1), but they exhibit a 5.4% greater tendency than men to rate their happiness at the highest level (6). Similarly, in South Korea, women have a 3.2% reduced propensity compared to men for reporting a life satisfaction level of 1. In comparison, they show a 3.7% increased inclination to indicate a life satisfaction level of 6. The inference drawn from this image indicates

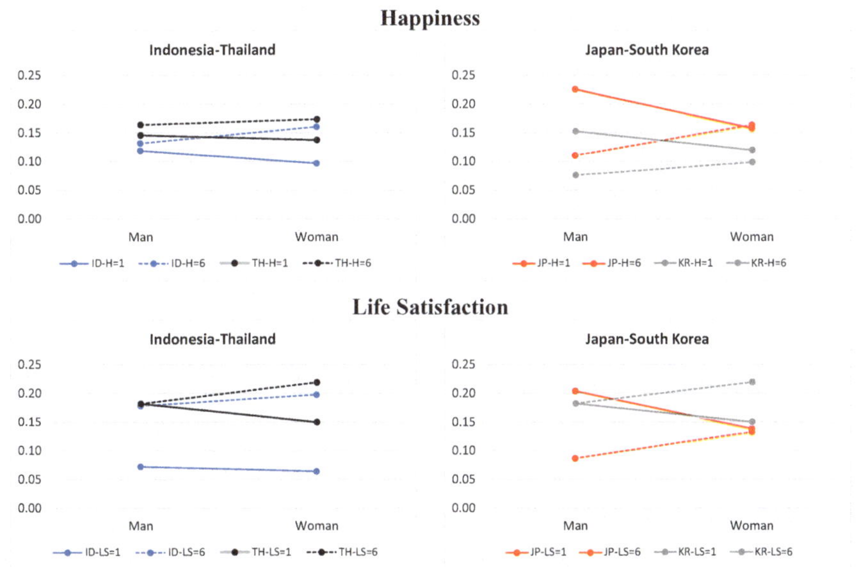

Notes: Calculated based on estimates of Table 2

Fig. 3 Predictive margins of happiness and life satisfaction levels by gender. *Note* Calculated based on estimates of Table 2

that women typically provide more favorable assessments of their happiness and life satisfaction levels.

4.2 Age

Age enters the model in quadratic terms. The estimation results reveal a U-shaped pattern in how respondents' age influences their assessments of happiness and life satisfaction. Respondents generally reported declining levels of happiness and life satisfaction with age up to a certain threshold, beyond which they started to increase. In the case of Indonesia, this turning point occurred earlier than in the other three countries, at 44 years for the happiness model and 48 years for the life satisfaction model. Conversely, for the other three countries, the turning point is within the age range of 50–53 years.

The relatively young average age of 38.9 years among respondents in Indonesia (as shown in Table 5) stands in stark contrast to the other three countries, where the average age ranges from 43.1 to 46.1 years. This significant age difference in Indonesia plays a role in the earlier occurrence of the turning point of the age covariate in the estimated levels of happiness and life satisfaction. In addition, the earlier inflection point in happiness seen in Indonesia can be attributed to a multifaceted interaction of demographic factors, societal norms, economic conditions, and health status. These factors collectively shape how individuals in each country perceive and experience happiness and life satisfaction as they age.

The U-shaped pattern of age in the happiness equation is substantiated by an extensive body of international research, as evidenced in the works of Easterlin (2004), Blanchflower (2021), and Toshkov (2022), among others. The observed U-shaped trend aligns with the concept of the "midlife dip," as emphasized by Blanchflower and Graham (2020). This phenomenon indicates that individuals often encounter a decrease in happiness during midlife, followed by a subsequent increase in later years. Additionally, Ferrer-i-Carbonell (2013) noted that people in their early adult years tend to hold high expectations that may prove challenging to fulfill. This initial gap between expectations and reality could result in decreased happiness as they age, particularly around their midlife, after which individuals tend to have more modest expectations.

4.3 Education Levels

The estimation results showed that the covariates on educational attainment did not affect the assessment of the status of the SWB of Indonesian respondents. The finding implied that the respondents who had attained junior secondary education or higher did not perceive themselves as happier or more satisfied with life than their counterparts who had attained primary education. In Fig. 4, we observe point estimates concerning education covariates in the Indonesian context, which do not display statistical significance. The predictive margins for happiness and life satisfaction levels at the lowest and highest values remain unchanging (or relatively flat). For context, individuals with tertiary education in Indonesia are only 1.4% less likely than those with primary education to report their happiness at the lowest level. It is worth noting that the disparity in predictive margins between individuals with tertiary and primary education in both the lowest and highest levels of happiness is minimal and lacks statistical significance. Our conclusion differs from the study of Landyanto et al. (2011), which found that Indonesian adults with more than nine years of basic education were more likely to be happy than those who had completed nine years or less of schooling. Furthermore, Rahayu (2016) found that happiness levels increased with higher educational attainment.

In Thailand, individuals who have achieved tertiary-level education typically report greater levels of happiness when compared to those with primary education. Conversely, in South Korea, educational factors positively correlate with SWB measures, especially among individuals with graduate-level education. A study conducted by Royo and Velazco (2006) found that in rural Thailand, the educational attainment of the household head was associated with a higher likelihood of happiness among adults. Furthermore, another study by Senasu and Singhapakdi (2017) revealed that individuals who had obtained Bachelor's and graduate-level education reported heightened levels of happiness within the Thai context. According to the findings of Oshio et al. (2011), in the context of South Korea, when controlling

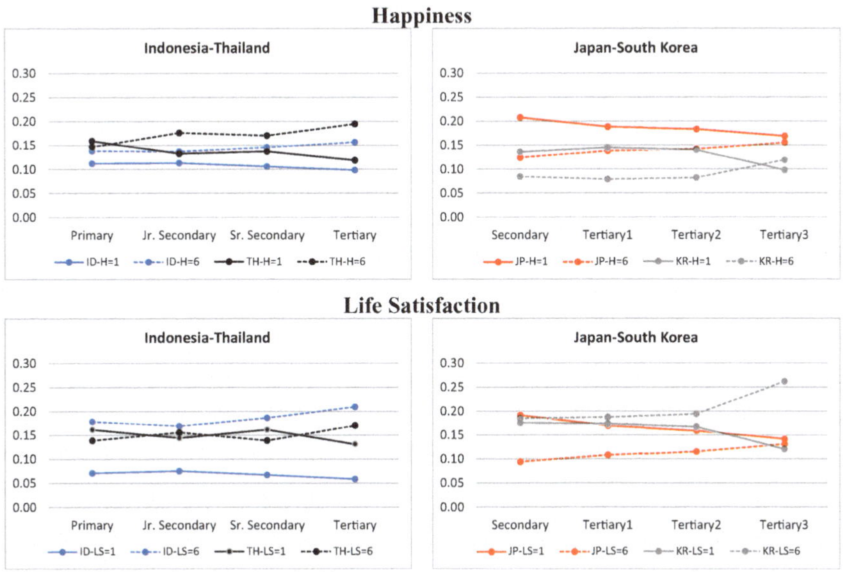

Notes: Calculated based on estimates of Table 2

Fig. 4 Predictive margins of happiness and life satisfaction levels by education. *Note* Calculated based on estimates of Table 2

for individual relative income, educational attainment exhibited no correlation with happiness. However, individuals with higher education showed a positive association with happiness when the model controlled for family relative income. Finally, in the Japanese context, our research results indicate that achieving higher levels of education is linked to reporting higher levels of happiness and life satisfaction. This finding aligns with Chen's (2012) study, which observed that more completed years of education among Japanese individuals were associated with higher happiness levels.

Regarding the link between educational achievement and happiness, Frey (2018) asserted that individuals who attain higher levels of education can enhance their capabilities and unlock a greater array of life opportunities, leading to increased life satisfaction. In a study that explored life satisfaction in 28 countries in Asia, Ngoo et al. (2015) found a positive and increasing effect of educational attainment on life satisfaction among the countries in East, South, and Southeast Asia. Di Tella et al. (2003) found similar results in the case of European countries. On the contrary, in most of the Western countries, as noted by Ferrer-i-Carbonell (2013), higher educational qualifications correlated negatively with the level of life satisfaction. This finding indicates that the positive effect exerted by the provision of opportunities associated with higher education in terms of social status and securing an exciting job is smaller than the negative effect resulting from the difficulty experienced in meeting the higher expectations that highly educated individuals may have.

4.4 Marital Status

Except for Thailand, our estimation results reveal that married individuals in Indonesia, Japan, and South Korea generally report higher levels of happiness and life satisfaction compared to those who are unmarried or divorced. Nevertheless, in Indonesia, divorced individuals tend to report lower happiness and life satisfaction than their unmarried counterparts. Conversely, in Japan and South Korea, unmarried individuals report lower happiness and life satisfaction compared to those who are married.

In Indonesia, divorce is often associated with a significant degree of social stigma and disapproval, unlike being unmarried. Societal norms in Indonesia strongly emphasize marriage and family as the ideal way of life. Divorce is frequently perceived as a failure to maintain a stable family unit, leading to social ostracism and a sense of shame. On the other hand, unmarried individuals in Indonesia may receive more social support and understanding. There is a societal recognition that some individuals have not yet found the right partner or have chosen to delay marriage for various reasons. Unmarried individuals may not face the same negative judgment or pressure to conform to marital norms.

In contrast, in Japan and South Korea, which are often considered more prosperous and advanced societies compared to Indonesia and Thailand, some individuals who have experienced unhappy or unsatisfactory marriages may view divorce as a liberating experience, fostering personal growth, independence, and enhanced happiness. However, Japanese and South Korean societies may pressure individuals to adhere to traditional marital and family norms. Consequently, being unmarried may be seen as a departure from these societal expectations, leading to feelings of social inadequacy or unhappiness. The cultural emphasis on marriage can create a sense of unfulfilled expectations for unmarried individuals in these societies.

Oshio et al. (2011) arrived at conclusions in line with our findings for Japan and South Korea, indicating that both being divorced and unmarried were linked to reduced happiness levels compared to the married population. Furthermore, their study also revealed that unmarried individuals in these countries reported even lower happiness levels than divorced individuals. Numerous studies have consolidated the divorced category with the unmarried category within the marital status variable. For instance, Rahayu (2016) observed that married adults in Indonesia reported higher levels of happiness compared to their unmarried counterparts. Ngoo et al. (2015) discovered a positive correlation between marriage and life satisfaction, with married individuals being notably happier than their unmarried counterparts across the 28 Asian countries examined. Stutzer and Frey (2006) conducted research suggesting that individuals with higher happiness levels were more inclined to enter into marriage. They also concluded that marriage not only made people happier but that happier people also had a higher probability of marrying.

4.5 Employment Status

Similar to educational attainment, employment status did not exhibit a significant correlation with increased levels of happiness and life satisfaction among respondents in Indonesia and Thailand. Conversely, in Japan and South Korea, holding a temporary job or experiencing unemployment was linked to reduced happiness compared to individuals with permanent positions. Notably, Japanese respondents who were not permanently employed did not report lower levels of happiness compared to those with no employment. In contrast, the situation among Korean adults was quite the opposite.

In Indonesia, 50.2% of respondents are involved in non-permanent (or informal) employment, while in Thailand, this figure is 64.2% (see Table 5). These percentages suggest that both countries have relatively flexible labor markets. In such adaptable work settings, individuals may not necessarily report reduced happiness when not in permanent employment, which helps explain the absence of statistical significance in the point estimates for non-permanent employment and unemployment. In contrast, Japan and South Korea likely feature more inflexible labor markets with robust safeguards for permanent employees. This situation may lead to a more pronounced connection between non-permanent employment and diminished happiness, primarily due to the comparatively lower job security and social benefits available to individuals in temporary positions.

In contrast to our observations in Indonesia and Thailand, employment status in Malaysia significantly impacts individuals' levels of happiness and life satisfaction, as demonstrated by the research of Boo et al. (2016). Similarly, Shams (2014) discovered that unemployed individuals in rural Pakistan reported lower happiness levels than their employed counterparts. Stutzer and Frey (2012) reported that being unemployed is associated with low subjective well-being, and this association persists even when accounting for the decline in income. These authors suggest that an individual's unemployment can trigger a psychological crisis from the loss of social status, self-esteem, personal relationships, and the amount of time typically devoted to the workplace.

4.6 Household Size

Our analysis reveals that the presence of an additional family member is associated with a decrease in self-reported happiness and life satisfaction in Japan and South Korea. However, in the cases of Indonesia and Thailand, this correlation lacks statistical significance. It is worth noting that Japan and South Korea have notably smaller average household sizes of 2.8 and 3.1 individuals (see Table 5), respectively, in contrast to the larger household sizes in Indonesia (5.2 individuals) and Thailand (3.9 individuals). In Japan and South Korea, the addition of an extra household member results in a decline in happiness and life satisfaction. This phenomenon could be attributed to increased crowding, resource sharing, or heightened interpersonal conflicts within larger households, which may contribute to reduced reported happiness. Conversely, the absence of statistical significance for Indonesia and Thailand suggests that variations in household size within the dataset do not strongly influence happiness levels. Other cultural or contextual factors in Indonesia may have a more dominant impact on individuals' happiness levels, thereby mitigating the influence of household size on reported happiness.

The global body of research on the connection between household size and happiness yields diverse findings. Some studies have uncovered adverse relationships in countries such as Italy (Scoppa & Ponzo, 2008), Turkey (Sönmez & Sönmez, 2018), and Germany and the United Kingdom (Katsaiti, 2012). In contrast, other investigations have indicated a positive correlation between household size and happiness, as observed in Afghanistan (Amirzai & Sönmez, 2022) and rural China (Zhu et al., 2021).

4.7 *Income*

The findings from the analysis indicate that an increase in household income positively correlates with higher levels of happiness and life satisfaction. As household income levels rise, individuals report higher subjective well-being (SWB) than those with the lowest income levels. Figure 5 reveals a discernible pattern: Individuals belonging to the high household income stratum in Japan exhibit a 9.9% lower likelihood of rating their happiness at the lowest level compared to their counterparts in the low household income category. Furthermore, this cohort of high-income individuals demonstrates an 8.0% greater propensity to articulate happiness at the highest level than low-income individuals. Analogously, in Thailand, those with high incomes manifest a 4.3% diminished likelihood of reporting the lowest level of life satisfaction and a 12.0% augmented likelihood of reporting the highest level, as opposed to their low-income counterparts.

Rahayu (2016) concluded that the absolute and the relative income positively affected the level of happiness in Indonesia. Yiengprugsawan et al. (2012) found a positive association between increasing household income and self-reported happiness among Thai adults. Studies pertaining to the determinants of happiness that have utilized household- or individual-level data, however, have found a positive relationship between income and happiness (Blanchflower & Oswald, 2011). Nevertheless, some studies have reported a positive relationship, whereas others have reported a negative relationship. The latter case has usually been found in the studies that have been conducted at the inter-country level. Easterlin (1995) claimed that a higher level of a country's gross domestic product (GDP) per capita does not have any relationship with high levels of happiness among its citizens; this is known as the "Easterlin paradox." Another stream of studies suggest that the effect of income on happiness becomes negligible once a certain level of income is achieved (Kahneman & Deaton, 2010; Muresan et al., 2020).

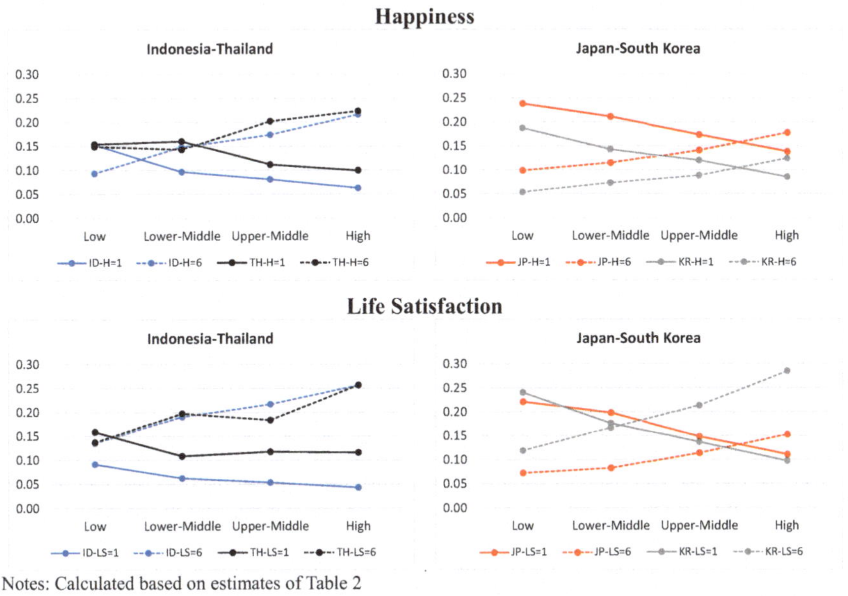

Fig. 5 Predictive margins of happiness and life satisfaction levels by income. *Note* Calculated based on estimates of Table 2

4.8 Living in Own House

Individuals who live in their own houses tend to report higher level of happiness and life satisfaction than those who live in leased houses or other arrangements. The exception takes place in happiness equation for the case of Indonesia, where the point estimate is not statistically significant. The lower proportion of respondents living in their own houses in Indonesia (54.7%; see Table 5) compared to Thailand (68.6%), Japan (69.0%), and South Korea (61.4%) may suggest that cultural norms and values regarding homeownership in Indonesia are less emphasized compared to the other three countries. The reduced cultural emphasis on homeownership in Indonesia could contribute to the lack of a statistically significant association between living in one's own house and self-reported happiness.

These findings are in line with previous research. A positive association between happiness and home ownership has been reported in studies conducted in China (Hu, 2011), Japan (Tiefenbach & Kohlbacher, 2014), and Switzerland (Zimmermann & Wanzenried, 2019).

4.9 Subnational Macroeconomic Measures

The inclusion of the macroeconomic indicators at the subnational level (rather than the national level) into the multilevel mixed-level ordered logistic specification provides an enabling environment (which can have either positive or negative consequences) on respondents' self-reported level of happiness and life satisfaction. The extent to which the macroeconomic measures differ across subnational within a country opens up the possibility of controlling for these factors in determining happiness and life satisfaction. Better local economic conditions (such as domestic GRDP per capita) and more conducive living conditions (such as a low level of poverty, less inequality, better access to basic infrastructure, and a lower crime rate) probably increase the likelihood of happiness or satisfaction with one's life.

We systematically incorporate each contextual variable by introducing one subnational macroeconomic indicator at a time. The estimation results are shown in Table 4, where, for brevity, only the estimates for the subnational macroeconomic indicators are presented, and the estimates for other independent variables (individual traits and household characteristics) are omitted.

For Indonesia, the higher the GRDP per capita at the district level, the higher the likelihood of being happy (the estimate was statistically significant at the 15% level). This indicated that the respondents living in districts having high GRDP per capita (i.e., better overall district macroeconomic conditions) are more likely to report a favorable level of happiness. The estimation results also revealed that there was no association between happiness and subnational HDI, poverty incidence, or the Gini coefficient of per capita consumption.

In Thailand, the gross provincial product (GPP) per capita and the human achievement index (HAI) are inversely related to self-evaluated happiness and life satisfaction. Conversely, the Gini coefficient of expenditures per capita is positively linked to higher SWB evaluations. These three specific findings are counterintuitive, given that individuals residing in provinces with more conducive macroeconomic conditions tend to report lower SWB measures. In contrast, those in provinces with higher income inequality report higher SWB. One plausible interpretation is that in provinces with elevated GPP and HAI, individuals are more likely to engage in upward social comparisons, measuring themselves against those with higher economic well-being. Such comparisons can result in feelings of relative deprivation and contribute to lower self-reported happiness. Conversely, in regions characterized by higher income inequality, individuals may engage in fewer upward social comparisons, opting to evaluate themselves compared to those with lower economic status. This tendency can lead to higher SWB reports.

In Japan and South Korea, none of the subnational macroeconomic indicators had a statistically significant impact on happiness or life satisfaction. However, there is an exception in South Korea, where the HDI was found to have a modestly negative influence on happiness levels. The outcomes observed in Japan and South Korea, where subnational macroeconomic indicators displayed no substantial effect

Table 4 Multilevel mixed-effects ordered logit estimates: contextual covariates

	Happiness												Life satisfaction											
	Indonesia			Thailand			Japan			South Korea			Indonesia			Thailand			Japan			South Korea		
	[1]			[2]			[3]			[4]			[5]			[6]			[7]			[8]		
GRDP per capita[a]	0.167	(0.108)	+	–0.391	(0.124)	***	–0.001	(0.008)		–0.168	(0.171)		0.067	(0.116)		–0.461	(0.123)	***	–0.002	(0.008)		–0.004	(0.189)	
Human development index[b]	0.001	(0.013)		–4.449	(1.781)	**	1.958	(1.866)		–2.387	(1.371)	*	0.004	(0.022)		–5.621	(1.741)	***	1.649	(1.979)		–1.705	(1.711)	
Level of poverty	–0.024	(0.032)		0.020	(0.012)	*	–			–			–0.024	(0.032)		0.031	(0.011)	***	–			–		
Gini of expenditures per capita	–0.475	(2.131)		–			–			–			–0.475	(2.131)		–			–			–		

Note ***, **, *, + significant at the 1, 5, 10, and 15% levels

[a] Gross Province Product (GPP) per capita for Thailand; Gross National Income (GNI) per capita for Japan

[b] Human Achievement Index (HAI) for Thailand

on happiness or life satisfaction, may be explained by the relatively uniform distribution of economic well-being in both countries. In subnational with limited income disparity, access to resources, and living standards, these macroeconomic indicators may have a less pronounced impact on overall levels of happiness and life satisfaction.

International evidence on the effect of subnational contextual macroeconomic measures on happiness and life satisfaction is limited. In the case of GRDP per capita, a study in Spain by Cuñado and Gracia (2012) found no statistically significant relationship between GRDP per capita at the Spanish regional level and happiness. Moreover, Sujarwoto and Tampubolon (2015), who examined the determinants of happiness in Indonesia using the contextual variable at the district level, found a negative association between GRDP per capita and the reported level of happiness. Concerning HDI, a study conducted by Furwanti et al. (2021) used cross-sectional data from 34 Indonesian provinces and a path analysis model to examine the impact of provincial income inequality and happiness. The study found that provincial income inequality significantly and negatively affects Indonesian happiness.

In the context of income inequality, Alesina et al. (2004) employed state-level income inequality data within the United States. Their research revealed that the well-being of individuals with lower incomes is not significantly impacted by income inequality. However, it did have a notable effect on the well-being of wealthier individuals. The authors contended that their findings align with the prevailing perception that Americans live in a socially mobile society. In such a society, individual efforts can lead to upward or downward shifts on the income scale, thus influencing their overall happiness. Furthermore, Oshio and Kobayashi (2009) examined income inequality within Japanese prefectures. Their research substantiated that individuals residing in prefectures with substantial income inequality generally expressed lower happiness. The authors suggested that a plausible explanation for this trend is that individuals may hold a specific ideal concept of income distribution, and any deviation from it, particularly in the form of increased inequality or higher poverty rates, tends to diminish overall happiness.

4.10 Study Limitation

This study is based on a single cross-sectional data point. While valuable insights can be gained from this data, it does not allow for comparing the factors influencing happiness and life satisfaction across countries over time, which would be of significant interest and carry substantial policy implications. It is imperative to explore possibilities for conducting similar surveys, even if they do not necessarily involve panel data, to facilitate longitudinal analyses.

The analysis and conclusions are contingent, among other factors, on sample size. Sample size strongly influences regression significance, with larger samples yielding more reliable estimates and increased statistical power for effect detection and noise differentiation. The number of observations in this analysis varies significantly: 1004 for Thailand, 1232 (for happiness model) or 1246 (for life satisfaction model) for

Indonesia, 2000 for South Korea, and 11,804 for Japan. This variability naturally impacts the accuracy of estimates for each country in this study. This distinction becomes evident when examining the Japan case, where almost all covariates produce statistically significant point estimates, while the opposite holds for the Indonesia and Thailand cases. Therefore, increasing the number of observations for Indonesia and Thailand could enhance the analytical results.

The extent of subnational representation varies markedly among countries. In Japan, respondents are chosen from all 47 prefectures, while South Korea encompasses all seven metropolitan areas and nine provinces. In contrast, Indonesia includes only 17 out of 514 districts or seven out of 33 provinces, and Thailand covers respondents from 11 out of 77 provinces. As a result, surveys in Japan and South Korea represent the entire country, whereas Indonesia and Thailand cover less than one-fourth of their respective provinces. Enhancing representation in Indonesia and Thailand has the potential to enhance analytical outcomes.

5 Conclusion and Future Research Agenda

This research investigated the factors influencing two aspects of subjective well-being (SWB), namely perceived happiness and life satisfaction, across four Asian countries: Indonesia, Thailand, Japan, and South Korea. In addition to accounting for typical individual characteristics and household attributes, the study also attempted to account for subnational macroeconomic variables, such as Gross Regional Domestic Product (GRDP) per capita, Human Development Index (HDI), poverty rate, and indicators of income inequality (measured by the Gini coefficient of per capita expenditures). The research relied on data from multi-country surveys, specifically the Survey of Well-being in Southeast Asia (SoWSA), conducted in Asia from 2015 to 2018. To analyze the data, we employed a multilevel mixed-effects ordered logistic methodology for analysis.

The analysis findings indicate that various factors are associated with a higher likelihood of experiencing happiness and life satisfaction, regardless of the observed variations among different countries concerning these results. These factors include being female (as opposed to being male), having a higher level of education, having a higher household income, and being a homeowner. Conversely, the likelihood of happiness and life satisfaction tends to decrease with age (up to a certain point), being divorced or unmarried (in contrast to being married), having temporary or no employment (as opposed to permanent employment), and living in households with a larger number of family members.

Applying a multilevel model, where individuals are considered nested within their respective subnational when reporting self-perceived happiness and life satisfaction, indicates that regional disparities, cultural diversity, and differential access to resources have a more substantial impact in Indonesia and Thailand. Conversely, in the case of Japan and South Korea, the effects of subnational variations appear to be less pronounced, possibly due to a higher level of social and cultural homogeneity, fairer resource distribution, or effective policies that mitigate regional disparities in these countries. These insights offer valuable insight into how regional factors shape individuals' self-reported happiness in each studied nation.

By incorporating the subnational macroeconomic indicators, this study revealed limited evidence concerning their influence on Indonesia. Only GRDP per capita was marginally associated with the SWB measures. In Thailand, GRDP per capita, the Human Achievement Index (HAI), and the poverty rate were significant factors affecting happiness and life satisfaction. However, their effects had unexpected directional patterns. Similarly, in South Korea, the HDI was found to have a marginal negative impact on self-reported SWB. Moreover, in the case of Japan, none of the subnational macroeconomic indicators seemed to impact the levels of happiness or life satisfaction.

Further investigation into the determinants of happiness and life satisfaction, along with the influence of subnational macroeconomic conditions, should be directed toward shaping policy recommendations. Future research initiatives stand to gain from incorporating more precise and contemporary macroeconomic, as well as sociocultural, indicators. They can also benefit from advanced estimation methodologies and the utilization of panel datasets to gain deeper insights into the intricate relationship between SWB and subnational economic and social dynamics.

Competing Interests The author declares no competing interests.

Ethical Approval This article does not contain any study with human participants performed by the author.

Informed Consent This article does not contain any study with human participants performed by the author.

Appendix

See Table 5.

Table 5 Descriptive statistics

	Indonesia	Thailand	Japan	South Korea
Happiness (after recoding)				
1	0.107	0.135	0.190	0.137
2	0.087	0.100	0.168	0.248
3	0.219	0.182	0.128	0.187
4	0.295	0.277	0.178	0.191
5	0.144	0.128	0.196	0.153
6	0.148	0.178	0.140	0.085
Life satisfaction (after recoding)				
1	0.069	0.144	0.171	0.168
2	0.056	0.100	0.249	0.100
3	0.177	0.186	0.126	0.156
4	0.302	0.258	0.172	0.174
5	0.207	0.156	0.171	0.207
6	0.190	0.155	0.111	0.197
Man [base]	0.501	0.468	0.500	0.509
Woman	0.499	0.532	0.500	0.491
Age (year)	38.9	46.1	45.6	43.1
Education: group 1 [base]	0.206	0.423	0.350	0.201
Education: group 2	0.140	0.103	0.122	0.142
Education: group 3	0.448	0.178	0.449	0.547
Education: group 4	0.205	0.296	0.078	0.111
Marital status: married [base]	0.713	0.629	0.620	0.632
Marital status: divorced	0.067	0.128	0.060	0.058
Marital status: unmarried	0.221	0.242	0.320	0.311
Employment: permanent [base]	0.125	0.186	0.406	0.483
Employment: non-permanent	0.502	0.642	0.290	0.282
Employment: no	0.373	0.171	0.305	0.235
Household size (person)	5.2	3.9	2.8	3.1
Household income: low [base]	0.275	0.431	0.227	0.232
Household income: lower-middle	0.431	0.242	0.271	0.267
Household income: upper-middle	0.204	0.187	0.227	0.264
Household income: high	0.089	0.139	0.276	0.238
Do not live in own house [base]	0.453	0.314	0.310	0.386
Live in own house	0.547	0.686	0.690	0.614
Observations	1248	1005	11,804	2000

Note All figures are in proportion unless otherwise indicated

References

Alesina, A., Di Tella, R., & MacCulloch, R. (2004). Inequality and happiness: Are Europeans and Americans different? *Journal of Public Economics, 88*(9–10), 2009–2042. https://doi.org/10.1016/j.jpubeco.2003.07.006

Amirzai, F. R., & Sönmez, A. (2022). Socio-economic determinants of happiness: The case of Afghanistan. *Sosyo Ekonomi, 30*(52), 183–198. https://doi.org/10.17233/sosyoekonomi.2022.02.10

Bartram, D. (2021). Age and life satisfaction: Getting control variables under control. *Sociology, 55*(2), 421–437. https://doi.org/10.1177/0038038520926871

Blanchflower, D., & Graham, C. (2020). *The mid-life dip in well-being: Economists (who find it) versus psychologists (who don't)!* National Bureau of Economic Research. https://doi.org/10.3386/w26888

Blanchflower, D. G. (2021). Is happiness U-shaped everywhere? Age and subjective well-being in 145 countries. *Journal of Population Economics, 34*(2), 575–624. https://doi.org/10.1007/s00148-020-00797-z

Blanchflower, D. G., & Oswald, A. J. (2011). International happiness: A new view on the measure of performance. *The Academy of Management Perspectives, 25*(1), 6–22. http://www.jstor.org/stable/23045031

Boo, M. C., Yen, S. H., & Lim, H. E. (2016). A note on happiness and life satisfaction in Malaysia. *Malaysian Journal of Economic Studies, 53*(2), 261–277.

Chen, W.-C. (2012). How education enhances happiness: Comparison of mediating factors in four East Asian countries. *Social Indicators Research, 106*(1), 117–131. https://doi.org/10.1007/s11205-011-9798-5

Clark, A. E. (2017). Happiness, income and poverty. *International Review of Economics, 64*(2), 145–158. https://doi.org/10.1007/s12232-017-0274-7

Cuñado, J., & de Gracia, F. P. (2012). Environment and happiness: New evidence for Spain. *Social Indicators Research, 112*(3), 549–567. https://doi.org/10.1007/s11205-012-0038-4

Di Tella, R., MacCulloch, R. J., & Oswald, A. J. (2003). The macroeconomics of happiness. *The Review of Economics and Statistics, 85*(4), 809–827. http://www.jstor.org/stable/3211807

Diener, E., Scollon, C. N., & Lucas, R. E. (2009). The evolving concept of subjective well-being: The multifaceted nature of happiness. In *Assessing well-being* (pp. 67–100). Springer Netherlands.

Dolan, P., Peasgood, T., & White, M. (2008). Do we really know what makes us happy? A review of the economic literature on the factors associated with subjective well-being. *Journal of Economic Psychology, 29*(1), 94–122. https://doi.org/10.1016/j.joep.2007.09.001

Easterlin, R. A. (1995). Will raising the incomes of all increase the happiness of all? *Journal of Economic Behavior & Organization, 27*(1), 35–47. https://doi.org/10.1016/0167-2681(95)00003-b

Easterlin, R. A. (2004). The economics of happiness. *Daedalus, 133*(2), 26–32.

Ferrer-i-Carbonell, A. (2013). Happiness economics. *SERIEs: Journal of the Spanish Economic Association, 4*(1), 35–60. https://doi.org/10.1007/s13209-012-0086-7

Frey, B. S. (2018). *Economics of happiness*. Springer International Publishing. https://doi.org/10.1007/978-3-319-75807-7

Furwanti, R., Lestari, D. M., Muflikha, M., & Wibowo, M. G. (2021). Determinant of macroeconomics: Does income inequality influence happiness? Evidence from Indonesia. *JEJAK, 14*(1), 146–156. https://doi.org/10.15294/jejak.v14i1.28278

Helliwell, J., Layard, R., & Sachs, J. (Eds.). (2015). *World happiness report 2015*. Sustainable Development Solutions Network.

Helliwell, J., Layard, R., & Sachs, J. (Eds.). (2019). *World happiness report 2019*. Sustainable Development Solutions Network.

Hu, F. (2011). Homeownership and subjective well-being in urban China: Does owning a house make you happier? *Social Indicators Research, 110*(3), 951–971. https://doi.org/10.1007/s11205-011-9967-6

Kahneman, D., & Deaton, A. (2010). High income improves evaluation of life but not emotional well-being. *Proceedings of the National Academy of Sciences, 107*(38), 16489–16493. https://doi.org/10.1073/pnas.1011492107

Katsaiti, M. S. (2012). Obesity and happiness. *Applied Economics, 44*(31), 4101–4114. https://doi.org/10.1080/00036846.2011.587779

Landyanto, E. A., Ling, J., Puspitasari, M., & Irnanti, S. E. (2011). Wealth and happiness: Empirical evidence from Indonesia. *Chulalongkorn Journal of Economics, 23*, 1–17.

Lee, S. J. (2022). Determinants of happiness. In *Community quality-of-life and well-being* (pp. 105–142). Springer International Publishing. https://doi.org/10.1007/978-3-030-89643-0

Mehmetoglu, M., & Jakobsen, T. G. (2017). *Applied statistics using Stata: A guide for the social sciences*. Sage Publications Asia-Pacific Pte Ltd.

Muresan, G. M., Ciumas, C., & Achim, M. V. (2020). Can money buy happiness? Evidence for European countries. *Applied Research in Quality of Life, 15*. https://doi.org/10.1007/s11482-019-09714-3

Ngoo, Y. T., Tey, N. P., & Tan, E. C. (2015). Determinants of life satisfaction in Asia. *Social Indicators Research, 124*(1), 141–156. https://doi.org/10.1007/s11205-014-0772-x

Oshio, T., & Kobayashi, M. (2009). *Regional income inequality and happiness: Evidence from Japan* (PIE/CIS Discussion Paper 460). Center for Intergenerational Studies, Institute of Economic Research, Hitotsubashi University.

Oshio, T., Nozaki, K., & Kobayashi, M. (2011). Relative income and happiness in Asia: Evidence from nationwide surveys in China, Japan, and Korea. *Social Indicators Research, 104*(3), 351–367. https://doi.org/10.1007/s11205-010-9754-9

Rabe-Hesketh, S., & Skrondal, A. (2022). *Multilevel and longitudinal modeling using Stata* (4th ed.). Stata Press.

Rahayu, T. P. (2016). The determinants of happiness in Indonesia. *Mediterranean Journal of Social Sciences, 7*(2), 393–404.

Royo, M., & Velazco, J. (2006). *Exploring the relationship between happiness, objective and subjective wellbeing: Evidence from rural Thailand* (Wellbeing in Developing Countries Working Paper 16). Economic and Social Research Council.

Scoppa, V., & Ponzo, M. (2008). An empirical study of happiness in Italy. *The B.E. Journal of Economic Analysis & Policy, 8*(1). https://doi.org/10.2202/1935-1682.1965

Senasu, K., & Singhapakdi, A. (2017). Determinants of happiness in Thailand: The moderating role of religiousness. *Journal of Human Behavior in the Social Environment, 27*(4), 270–290. https://doi.org/10.1080/10911359.2017.1279580

Senasu, K., & Singhapakdi, A. (2018). Quality-of-life determinants of happiness in Thailand: The moderating roles of mental and moral capacities. *Applied Research in Quality of Life, 13*(1), 59–87. https://doi.org/10.1007/s11482-017-9506-y

Shams, K. (2014). Determinants of subjective well-being and poverty in rural Pakistan: A micro-level study. *Social Indicators Research, 119*(3), 1755–1773. https://doi.org/10.1007/s11205-013-0571-9

Sommet, N., & Morselli, D. (2017). Keep calm and learn multilevel logistic modeling: A simplified three-step procedure using Stata, R, Mplus, and SPSS. *International Review of Social Psychology, 30*(1), 203–218. https://doi.org/10.5334/irsp.90

Sönmez, A., & Sönmez, Ö. A. (2018). Life satisfaction and happiness with regard to human capital and religiosity in Turkey. *Bingöl Üniversitesi Sosyal Bilimler Enstitüsü Dergisi, 8*(16), 217–234. https://doi.org/10.29029/busbed.422920

Stutzer, A., & Frey, B. S. (2006). Does marriage make people happy, or do happy people get married? *The Journal of Socio-Economics, 35*(2), 326–347. https://doi.org/10.1016/j.socec.2005.11.043

Stutzer, A., & Frey, B. S. (2012). *Recent developments in the economics of happiness: A selective overview* (Discussion Paper 7078). Institute for the Study of Labor (IZA).

Sujarwoto, S., & Tampubolon, G. (2015). Decentralisation and citizen happiness: A multilevel analysis of self-rated happiness in Indonesia. *Journal of Happiness Studies, 16*, 455–475. https://doi.org/10.1007/s10902-014-9518-3

Tiefenbach, T., & Kohlbacher, F. (2013). *Happiness from the viewpoint of economics: Findings from recent survey data in Japan* (German Institute for Japanese Studies (DIJ) Working Paper 13/1).

Tiefenbach, T., & Kohlbacher, F. (2014). Happiness in Japan in times of upheaval: Empirical evidence from the national survey on lifestyle preferences. *Journal of Happiness Studies, 16*(2), 333–366. https://doi.org/10.1007/s10902-014-9512-9

Toshkov, D. (2022). The relationship between age and happiness varies by income. *Journal of Happiness Studies, 23*(3), 1169–1188. https://doi.org/10.1007/s10902-021-00445-7

Ura, K., Alkire, S., Zangmo, T., & Wangdi, K. (2012). *A short guide to gross national happiness index*. The Centre for Bhutan Studies.

Veenhoven, R. (2012). Does happiness differ across cultures? In H. Selin & G. Davey (Eds.), *Happiness across cultures: Views of happiness and quality of life in non-western cultures* (pp. 451–472). Springer Netherlands. https://doi.org/10.1007/978-94-007-2700-7_30

Ye, D., Ng, Y.-K., & Lian, Y. (2015). Culture and happiness. *Social Indicators Research, 123*(2), 519–547. https://doi.org/10.1007/s11205-014-0747-y

Yiengprugsawan, V., Somboonsook, B., Seubsman, S.-A., & Sleigh, A. C. (2012). Happiness, mental health, and socio-demographic associations among a national cohort of Thai adults. *Journal of Happiness Studies, 13*(6), 1019–1029. https://doi.org/10.1007/s10902-011-9304-4

Zhu, Z., Ma, W., Leng, C., & Nie, P. (2021). The relationship between happiness and consumption expenditure: Evidence from rural China. *Applied Research in Quality of Life, 16*(4), 1587–1611. https://doi.org/10.1007/s11482-020-09836-z

Zimmermann, Y. S., & Wanzenried, G. (2019). Are homeowners happier than tenants? Empirical evidence for Switzerland. In G. Brule & C. Suter (Eds.), *Wealth(s) and subjective well-being* (pp. 305–321). Springer International Publishing. https://doi.org/10.1007/978-3-030-05535-6_14

Indera Ratna Irawati Pattinasarany is an Associate Professor of Sociology at Universitas Indonesia. Her current research focuses on social stratification and mobility, subjective well-being, inequality, and sociology of education.

Comparative Analysis of Income and Happiness in Japan and Korea

Hiroo Harada and Eiji Sumi

Abstract International studies suggest that in contrast to relative income hypothesis, reference income has a positive effect on individual happiness. Higher reference income not only triggers a feeling of envy ("comparison effect") but also serves as a signal of bright future prospects ("information effect"). Moreover, the relative importance of the comparison effect and information effect depends on the degree of mobility in society and one's life stage. Japanese and Korean societies and labor markets are relatively immobile compared to those in Western countries. Thus, using a nationally representative individual-level data set from Japanese and Korean citizens, this study examined how reference income affected individual life satisfaction (LS) in both early life and later life in Japan and Korea. We found a significant negative association between LS and average income of the demographic reference group in the later life sample and no association between these factors in the early life sample in both countries. Our findings suggest that the relative importance of these effects depends on the degree of mobility in one's life stage in both Japan and Korea.

Keywords Relative income hypothesis · Life satisfaction · Reference group · Information effect · Comparison effect · Japan and Korea

H. Harada
Senshu University, Kawasaki, Japan
e-mail: h2@isc.senshu-u.ac.jp

E. Sumi (✉)
College of Economics, Nihon University, Tokyo, Japan
e-mail: sumi.eiji@nihon-u.ac.jp

J. Yee et al. (eds.), *Social Well-Being, Development, and Multiple Modernities in Asia*,
https://doi.org/10.1007/978-981-97-3866-3_13

1 Introduction[1]

The relative income hypothesis proposes that individual happiness depends both on one's own income and income relative to the reference group.[2] Established and developed by Duesenberry (1949) and Friedman (1957), this hypothesis is the foundation of the consumption function in economics. In line with the relative income hypothesis, individual happiness is positively affected by one's own income and negatively affected by reference income. Higher reference income triggers a feeling of envy or jealousy, and thus has a negative effect on individual happiness. This negative effect is referred to as the comparison effect. Alternatively, reference income could be positively associated with happiness, as individuals could observe the increase in income of reference groups and interpret this as a signal that their own position will improve soon (c.f., Fitzroy et al., 2014; Senik, 2004, 2008). Senik (2004)[3]terms this positive effect as the "information effect."

Which factors affect the relative importance of comparison and information effects? Senik (2008) argues that the relative importance of these effects depends on an individual's degree of societal mobility. Fitzroy et al. (2014) find that comparison effects are more prominent in individuals' later lives, while information effects dominate in one's early life in Germany and the UK. However, to the best of our knowledge, few studies have examined the relative importance of these effects on individual happiness in Asian countries. Harada and Sumi (2018) are the first to find that reference income has no effect on happiness for young individuals, but comparison effects are more prominent for older people in Japan.

Japan and Korea, which are developed in northeastern Asia, have a long archaeological and hereditary relationship divided by the Tsushima Channel. The mutual communication and interchange of the people in both countries has been historically strong, so that some tendencies would exist in their characters under different climates. Both Japanese and Korean are raised in a Confucian culture, so they are well-mannered and generally conservative. In recent times, their societies and labor markets are relatively immobile compared to those in Western countries. Thus, even young individuals in these countries have fewer opportunities to advance and change

---

[1] This study is extended research of Harada and Sumi (2018).

[2] The reference group is the set of relevant others to which individuals compare themselves; it is defined based on geographic location and demographic characteristics such as age, gender, and education.

[3] This relation between income and happiness has been the main subject of empirical studies (c.f., Frey and Stutzer 2002). However, no studies have reached a consensus on how reference income affects individual happiness. Prior international studies on the association between individual happiness and reference income have mixed results: Senik (2004), Shields et al. (2009), and Mangyo and Park (2011) find no association between happiness and reference income in Russia, Australia, and China, respectively, whereas Luttmer (2005), Helliwell and Huang (2005), and Brown et al. (2015) find a positive association between happiness and reference income in the United States, Canada, and the UK, respectively. Additional studies, such as Blanchflower and Oswald (2004) in the United States and Clark et al. (2009) in Denmark, argue that there is a negative association between happiness and reference income.

their careers, and individuals are more likely to see peer success as envy as they age. In short, the comparison effect has a greater impact on individuals' happiness in their later lives than in their early lives.

Thus, in this study, to clarify whether an individual's degree of societal mobility affects the relative importance of comparison and information effects, we empirically examined the association between reference income and happiness, based on nationwide survey data of Japanese and Korean citizens. We also explored similarities and differences in the associations between reference income and happiness in both countries.

The remainder of this paper is organized as follows. In Sect. 2, we describe the relative income hypothesis. Section 3 explains the model and data. Section 4 discusses the results of the ordered logit estimation and marginal effects, and Sect. 5 summarizes our conclusions.

2 Relative Income Hypothesis

2.1 Relative Importance of Comparison and Information Effects

Reference income may affect individual happiness in two ways (c.f., Fitzroy et al., 2014; Harada & Sumi, 2018; Senik, 2004, 2008). First, higher reference income triggers a feeling of envy or jealousy, and thus has a negative effect on individual happiness. The other is that a higher reference income serves as a signal of future prospects and thus has a positive effect on individual happiness. The former is referred to as the comparison effect, and the latter is referred to as the information effect.

To formalize the role of reference income, we introduce a utility function, which provides a theoretical framework in economics and presume that utility can serve as a proxy for happiness in this study. Suppose that individual utility depends on one's own income Y, expected income E, and reference income RI. We assume that an individual's expected income depends on the reference group's observed income: $E = E(RI)$. In short, it is presumed that as an individual observes a change in the income of people with similar characteristics, the individual expects this as a signal that their own income will change in the same way under uncertainty. Next, an individual's utility function can be expressed as[4]:

$$U = V(Y, E(RI), RI) \tag{1}$$

Clearly, the marginal utility of Y is positive ($\partial V/\partial Y > 0$), as is the marginal utility of expected income E ($\partial V/\partial E > 0$). However, the marginal utility of reference income RI is ambiguous. The partial derivative of the utility with respect to RI is

[4] See Hirschman and Rothschild (1973) and Senik (2008) for more information.

$$\frac{\partial U}{\partial RI} = \left[\left(\frac{\partial V}{\partial E}\right)\left(\frac{\partial E}{\partial RI}\right)\right] + \frac{\partial V}{\partial RI} \tag{2}$$

The first term of Eq. 2, which represents the information effect of reference income on individual utility, is positive. As noted above, the first part of this term, $\partial V/\partial E$, is the marginal utility of expected income E and positive; the second part of this term, $\partial E/\partial RI$, represents the effect of reference income on expected income (i.e., the information effect) and is also positive. The information effect means that a higher reference income serves as a signal of an individual's higher own expected income ($\partial E/\partial RI > 0$). The second term, $\partial V/\partial RI$, represents the direct effect of *RI* on individual utility (i.e., comparison effect); this sign depends on how an individual feels about their reference group. If individual feelings are dominated by envy, then this term will be negative.

Hence, the effect of an increase in reference income is unknown in advance and depends on the relative importance of the information and comparison effects. This suggests the need for an empirical examination of this term using regression analysis.[5]

2.2 Hypotheses

A question about the relative importance of the comparison and information effects is how to define the reference group. Previous studies defined reference groups based on individual characteristics ("people like you"). In this study, we adopted demographic reference groups based on age (20 s, 30 s, 40 s, 50 s, 60 s) and gender.

Another question is which factors affect the relative importance of comparison and information effects. Senik (2008) argues that the relative importance of these effects depends on an individual's degree of societal mobility.[6] Fitzroy et al. (2014) find positive effects of reference income on happiness for those under 45 and negative effects for those over 45 in Germany and the UK. Harada and Sumi (2018) find that reference income has no effect on happiness for those under 40 and negative effects for those over 40 in Japan. These studies indicate that comparison effects are more prominent in individuals' later lives, while information effects dominate in one's early life. This is because young individuals are more mobile and likely to interpret the reference group's success as a signal that their position will soon improve. In other

[5] If the coefficient of RI in our regression model is negative, then the comparison effect has more impact than the information effect. Inversely, if the coefficient of RI is positive, then the information effect dominates over the comparison effect. If the coefficient of RI is statistically insignificant, then the information and comparison effects offset each other. If the coefficient of RI is statistically insignificant, it is possible that both effects are too small to show up as statistically significant.

[6] Senik (2008) examined how subjective well-being depends on both individual and reference income and found that information effects dominate in transitioning European countries and the United States, both of which have high social mobility, while comparison effects are dominant in stable European countries with a low social mobility (such as the UK, Germany, the Netherlands, etc.).

words, younger people see reference income not in comparison to their own income, but rather as an information indicator of their own future prospects. Thus, in this study, to examine whether the effect of reference income on individual happiness is affected by one's mobility, we divided the entire sample into two sub-samples based on age: "early life" and "later life." Based on Harada and Sumi (2018), we adopted two types of age categories for each life stage: ages 20–34 or 20–39 as the "early life" and ages 35–69 or 40–69 as the "later life."

Because both Japanese and Korean societies and labor markets are relatively immobile, individuals aged 40 or over have few opportunities to advance and change their careers. In other words, when individuals are younger, advancing and changing their careers is easier. If a higher reference income serves as a signal of bright future prospects, then its impact should be greater for individuals in their early lives. In short, the information effect has a greater impact on individuals in their early lives than in their later lives.

Therefore, we used the following three hypotheses to test how reference income affects individual utility:

Hypothesis 1: There is a positive association between happiness and reference income for individuals in early life, because the information effect is likely to dominate the comparison effect in early life.

Hypothesis 2: There is a negative association between happiness and reference income for individuals in later life, because the comparison effect is likely to dominate the information effect in later life.

We used individual data from the Social Well-Being Survey in Asia from 2015 to 2017, V2.0 (International Consortium for Social Well-Being Studies, 2020) in Japan and Korea. This is an online survey of respondents aged 20–69 years. Participants were selected in proportion to the national distribution with regard to age, gender, city size, and region. Populations were sampled proportionately by gender, age, city scale, and region, and were considered representative of Japan and Korea as a whole. There were 10403 and 2000 valid responses in Japan and Korea, respectively.

3 Methods

3.1 Model

The empirical analysis uses a subjective measure of life satisfaction (LS) as a proxy for individual happiness.[7] To analyze the relative income hypothesis, based on Harada and Sumi (2018), we estimated individual LS functions using an ordered

[7] Responses to the standard life satisfaction question, "How satisfied are you currently with overall life?" are used to measure happiness (c.f., Ferrer-i-Carbonell 2005; Goerke and Pannenberg 2015).

logit regression[8]:

$$LS_i^* = \alpha + \sum_{q=1}^{l} \beta_q X_i^q + \delta Y_i + \pi RI_i + u_i$$

$$LS_i = \begin{cases} 0 \text{ if } -\infty < LS^* \leq k_1 \\ 1 \text{ if } \ k_1 < LS^* \leq k_2 \\ 2 \text{ if } \ k_2 < LS^* \leq k_3 \\ \vdots \\ 10 \text{ if } k_{10} < LS^* < \infty \end{cases} \quad (3)$$

where LS^* is a latent unobserved variable. LS is recorded on an 11-point Likert scale (10 = very satisfied, 0 = very unsatisfied) and has 10 thresholds over the latent variables. X is an individual-level variable, Y is an individual's own income (equivalized income), RI is reference income, u is the error term,[9] and α, β, δ, π, and the 10 threshold values k are the parameters to be estimated. Moreover, i represents an individual.

3.2 Data

Dependent Variable: Life satisfaction. We assessed subjective overall LS based on answers to the following question: "How satisfied are you currently with life overall?" In the survey, this variable was scored on an 11-point scale, from 0 (very unsatisfied) to 10 (very satisfied). As shown in Table 1, the distributions of overall LS in the Japanese and Korean samples are quite similar. The median and mode values of overall LS in Japanese and Korean samples were the same: 6 and 7.

Independent Variables. The independent variables were individual attributes, municipality size, individual income, and reference income. Individual attributes included age, gender, marital status, housing status, educational attainment, and occupational status. Our data included male and female Japanese and Korean residents aged between 20 and 69 years.

Among all respondents, 48.6% of the Japanese sample and 49.1% of the Korean sample were female. The mean age in Japanese and Korean sample were 45.1 and 43.1 years old. Marital status was categorized into married, unmarried, and divorced (including widowed). Overall, nearly 65% of the respondents were married, and nearly 70% were homeowners in both samples. Occupational status was categorized into regular employees (company executives, permanent employees, and

[8] An ordered logit/probit estimation was also used by Blanchflower and Oswald (2004), Helliwell and Huang (2005), and Shields et al. (2009).

[9] In the ordered logit model, u is logistically distributed with $F(z) = e^z/(1 + e^z)$.

Table 1 Distribution of life satisfaction (Unit: %, % point)

LS	Japan	Korea	Difference
0	3.33	0.90	2.43
1	1.86	2.10	– 0.24
2	4.20	5.30	– 1.10
3	7.35	8.45	– 1.10
4	7.28	9.95	– 2.67
5	16.69	15.60	1.09
6	12.69	17.35	– 4.66
7	17.75	20.65	– 2.90
8	17.56	13.10	4.46
9	6.49	5.20	1.29
10	4.81	1.40	3.41
Mode	7	7	
Median	6	6	

civil servants: 42.3% of respondents in the Japanese sample and 48.3% in the Korean sample), non-regular employees (part-time workers, temporary staff, contract workers, and fixed-term staff: 19.5% of respondents in Japanese sample and 11.0% in Korean sample), self-employed and family employees (9.0% of respondents in Japanese sample and 17.3% in Korean sample), unemployed (2.4% of respondents in Japanese sample and 5.8% in Korean sample), and economically inactive (the retired, homemakers, and students: 26.8% of respondents in the Japanese sample and 17.7% in the Korean sample). Educational attainment was categorized into upper secondary and below (24.9% of respondents in the Japanese sample and 20.1% in the Korean sample), short-cycle tertiary (21.6% of respondents in Japanese sample and 14.2% in Korean sample), and bachelors or above (53.5% of respondents in the Japanese sample and 65.8% in the Korean sample).

Municipality size was controlled using residential area variables (towns and villages, small cities [population < 200,000], medium-sized cities [population 200,000–700,000], and 20 major cities [population > 700,000] in Japanese samples; towns and villages, small and medium-sized cities (population < 200,000), and metropolitan cities (population > 200,000) in the Korean sample).

Household income in the Japanese sample was categorized into 25 income segments ranging from less than 500,000 yen a year to 20,000,000 yen or more per year. Household income in the Korean sample was categorized into 22 income segments ranging from 0 won a month to 10,000,000 won or more per month.[10] For an individual's own income, we adopted an equivalized income calculated by dividing household income by the square root of household size. The average income

[10] In Korean sample, annual income was calculated by multiplying the monthly base income by 12 months per year.

of the demographic reference groups was determined as the mean annual income of each age and gender group in 2015.[11]

Table 2 presents the descriptive statistics for the LS, individual-level variables, and income variables.

4 Results

4.1 Estimation Results

We performed an ordered logit regression with the overall LS as the dependent variable.[12] All models included all individual and regional variables, allowing us to isolate the association between LS and income after controlling for all variables, as shown in Eq. 3. In addition, to examine the relative importance of the comparison and information effects at different stages in life (Hypotheses 1 and 2), we divided the entire sample into two sub-samples: "early life" and "later life." We then defined Model 1 as including the entire sample, Model 2 as including the "early life" sample, and Model 3 as including the "later life" sample. The empirical results from the Japanese and Korean samples are shown in Tables 3 and 4, respectively.

Individual Attributes

In the Japanese sample, these results regarding individual attributes were generally as expected; overall, LS was affected by certain individual attributes. For example, LS and age showed a U-shaped association. The LS of individuals aged 45–50 years was low. Women reported a higher LS than men. Unmarried and divorced individuals reported lower satisfaction than married individuals. Homeowners reported higher satisfaction than renters. Individuals with junior college or vocational school degrees and undergraduate or postgraduate degrees reported higher satisfaction than other groups. Non-regular employees and unemployed individuals reported lower satisfaction than regular employees.

Unlike the Japanese results, individual attributes did not provide the expected results in the Korean sample. For example, LS and age were not found to be associated. Women in later life reported a lower LS than men. LS and educational attainment were not associated with LS.

Municipality Size

We found no associations between municipality size and LS in both Japanese and Korean samples.

---

[11] Data on annual personal income by gender and age obtained from Japanese National Tax Agency in Japan and Korean Ministry of employment and labor in Korea.

[12] The null hypothesis of the log likelihood ratio chi-square (LR χ^2) test that all predictor variables do not contribute to the model was rejected in all models.

Table 2 Descriptive statistics

Variables		Japan				Korea			
		Mean	S.D.	Min	Max	Mean	S.D.	Min	Max
Life Satisfaction		5.922	2.383	0	10	5.701	2.085	0	10
Age		45.137	13.576	20	69	43.052	12.365	20	69
Gender	[Male]	0.514	0.500	0	1	0.509	0.500	0	1
	Female	0.486	0.500	0	1	0.491	0.500	0	1
Marital status	[Married]	0.647	0.478	0	1	0.632	0.482	0	1
	Divorced	0.062	0.242	0	1	0.058	0.233	0	1
	Unmarried	0.291	0.454	0	1	0.311	0.463	0	1
Home ownership	[Renter]	0.286	0.452	0	1	0.306	0.461	0	1
	Owner	0.714	0.452	0	1	0.695	0.461	0	1
Occupational status	[Regular]	0.423	0.494	0	1	0.483	0.500	0	1
	Non-regular	0.195	0.396	0	1	0.110	0.312	0	1
	Self employed	0.090	0.286	0	1	0.173	0.378	0	1
	Unemployed	0.024	0.153	0	1	0.058	0.234	0	1
	Economically inactive	0.268	0.443	0	1	0.177	0.382	0	1
Educational attainment	[Upper secondary or below]	0.249	0.433	0	1	0.201	0.401	0	1
	Short-cycle tertiary	0.216	0.411	0	1	0.142	0.349	0	1
	Bachelors or above	0.535	0.499	0	1	0.658	0.475	0	1
Municipality size	[Town and Village]	0.082	0.275	0	1	0.028	0.165	0	1
	Small cities	0.373	0.484	0	1	0.063	0.243	0	1
	Medium-sized cities	0.251	0.434	0	1	0.358	0.480	0	1
	Large-sized cities	0.294	0.456	0	1	0.551	0.498	0	1
Own income		4.068	2.871	0.088	32.600	38.646	29.360	0.000	169.706
Reference income	Age and Gender	3.967	1.450	2.090	6.620	45.310	12.133	32.440	65.260

Note Unit of income: Millions of local currencies per a year. Reference is shown in brackets

Income Variable

We found positive associations between own income and LS in both Japanese and Korean samples, indicating that higher own income increases LS.

Table 3 Ordered logit regression estimation results: Japan

Variables		Model1		Model2				Model3			
		Entire		Age 20–34		Age 20–39		Age 35–69		Age 40–69	
		Coef.	[Z-value]	Coef.	[Z-value]	Coef.	[Z-value]	Coef.	[Z-value]	Coef.	[Z-value]
Individual attributes											
Age	Age	– 0.1176	[– 8.740][a]	– 0.6568	[– 5.129][a]	– 0.4098	[– 6.291][a]	– 0.1084	[– 3.439][a]	– 0.1106	[– 2.447][b]
	Age(squared)	0.0013	[8.710][a]	0.0104	[4.492][a]	0.0059	[5.688][a]	0.0011	[3.604][a]	0.0011	[2.626][a]
Gender [Male]	Female	0.2796	[3.582][a]	0.4458	[3.346][a]	0.4202	[3.660][a]	0.0056	[0.044]	– 0.1456	[– 0.950]
Marital Status	Divorced	– 0.6364	[– 8.518][a]	– 1.5589	[– 4.699][a]	– 1.0372	[– 5.874][a]	– 0.5571	[– 7.196][a]	– 0.5001	[– 6.021][a]
[Married]	Unmarried	– 1.0693	[– 23.136][a]	– 1.3238	[– 15.589][a]	– 1.2726	[– 19.176][a]	– 0.9388	[– 16.611][a]	– 0.8309	[– 12.322][a]
Home Ownership [Renter]	Owner	0.3011	[7.370][a]	0.1637	[2.349][b]	0.1809	[3.236][a]	0.3964	[7.760][a]	0.4734	[7.757][a]
Educational Attainment	Short– cycle tertiary	0.1738	[3.335][a]	0.2373	[2.119][b]	0.2902	[3.258][a]	0.1718	[2.905][a]	0.1237	[1.915][c]
[High School]	Bachelors or above	0.3093	[6.993][a]	0.3605	[4.013][a]	0.4054	[5.506][a]	0.3048	[5.902][a]	0.2454	[4.332][a]
Occupational Status	Non– regular	– 0.2974	[– 5.670][a]	– 0.4520	[– 4.499][a]	– 0.4389	[– 5.440][a]	– 0.2468	[– 3.935][a]	– 0.2141	[– 3.010][a]
[Regular]	Self employed	– 0.1521	[– 2.304][b]	– 0.2245	[– 1.291]	– 0.1365	[– 1.059]	– 0.1416	[– 1.948][c]	– 0.1583	[– 2.002][b]

(continued)

Table 3 (continued)

Variables		Model1		Model2				Model3			
		Entire		Age 20–34		Age 20–39		Age 35–69		Age 40–69	
		Coef.	[Z-value]	Coef.	[Z-value]	Coef.	[Z-value]	Coef.	[Z-value]	Coef.	[Z-value]
	Unemployed	– 1.0923	[– 9.298][a]	– 1.0513	[– 5.086][a]	– 1.0880	[– 6.534][a]	– 1.1218	[– 7.863][a]	– 1.1071	[– 6.703][a]
	Economically inactive	0.0757	[1.436]	– 0.0169	[– 0.174]	0.0191	[0.235]	0.0869	[1.341]	0.0912	[1.265]
Municipality size											
[Town and Village]	Small cities	0.0713	[1.071]	0.1151	[0.827]	0.1461	[1.302]	0.0465	[0.613]	0.0226	[0.272]
	Medium–sized cities	0.0018	[0.026]	– 0.1043	[– 0.724]	– 0.0261	[– 0.224]	0.0290	[0.363]	0.0168	[0.192]
	20 Major cities	0.0010	[0.014]	0.0422	[0.298]	0.1015	[0.883]	– 0.0310	[– 0.391]	– 0.0789	[– 0.911]
Income											
Own Income		0.1151	[16.821][a]	0.0946	[6.923][a]	0.1119	[9.677][a]	0.1245	[15.527][a]	0.1218	[14.057][a]
Reference Income	Age and gender	– 0.0747	[– 2.570][b]	0.0219	[0.225]	– 0.0354	[– 0.526]	– 0.1600	[– 3.782][a]	– 0.1899	[– 3.895][a]
K1		– 5.8053	[– 22.923][a]	– 13.4542	[– 7.208][a]	– 10.1860	[– 9.922][a]	– 6.0671	[– 9.319][a]	– 6.3391	[– 5.872][a]
K2		– 5.3257	[– 21.222][a]	– 12.9955	[– 6.967][a]	– 9.7051	[– 9.468][a]	– 5.5775	[– 8.584][a]	– 5.8590	[– 5.432][a]

(continued)

Table 3 (continued)

Variables		Model1		Model2				Model3			
		Entire		Age 20–34		Age 20–39		Age 35–69		Age 40–69	
		Coef.	[Z-value]	Coef.	[Z-value]	Coef.	[Z-value]	Coef.	[Z-value]	Coef.	[Z-value]
K3		– 4.6519	[– 18.697][a]	– 12.3607	[– 6.632][a]	– 9.0471	[– 8.840][a]	– 4.8854	[– 7.532][a]	– 5.1690	[– 4.795][a]
K4		– 3.9358	[– 15.918][a]	– 11.5999	[– 6.231][a]	– 8.3204	[– 8.143][a]	– 4.1841	[– 6.459][a]	– 4.4563	[– 4.136][a]
K5		– 3.4394	[– 13.954][a]	– 11.0831	[– 5.957][a]	– 7.7956	[– 7.637][a]	– 3.6934	[– 5.706][a]	– 3.9781	[– 3.694][a]
K6		– 2.5712	[– 10.476][a]	– 10.2066	[– 5.492][a]	– 6.8684	[– 6.739][a]	– 2.8235	[– 4.365][a]	– 3.1456	[– 2.922][a]
K7		– 1.9922	[– 8.131][a]	– 9.5961	[– 5.166][a]	– 6.2510	[– 6.138][a]	– 2.2517	[– 3.483][a]	– 2.5862	[– 2.403][b]
K8		– 1.1398	[– 4.656][a]	– 8.7677	[– 4.723][a]	– 5.3806	[– 5.288][a]	– 1.3868	[– 2.145][b]	– 1.7376	[– 1.615]
K9		0.1013	[0.413]	– 7.6796	[– 4.137][a]	– 4.2408	[– 4.167][a]	– 0.0933	[– 0.144]	– 0.4343	[– 0.404]
K10		1.0580	[4.272][a]	– 6.8676	[– 3.698][a]	– 3.4299	[– 3.366][a]	0.9192	[1.419]	0.6202	[0.576]
N		10,403		2667		4160		7736		6243	
LR Chi2		1716.8	a	505.5	a	825.4	a	1,241.8	a	916.5	a

Note [a] $p < 0.01$, [c] $p < 0.10$, [b] $p < 0.05$. The variable in brackets is reference

Table 4 Ordered logit regression estimation results: Korea

Variables		Model1		Model2				Model3			
		Entire		Age 20–34		Age 20–39		Age 35–69		Age 40–69	
		Coef.	[Z-value]	Coef.	[Z-value]	Coef.	[Z-value]	Coef.	[Z-value]	Coef.	[Z-value]
Individual attributes											
Age	Age	– 0.0564	[– 1.725][a]	– 0.3114	[– 0.921]	– 0.1753	[– 1.115]	– 0.0559	[– 0.778]	– 0.0522	[– 0.534]
	Age(squared)	0.0006	[1.618]	0.0048	[0.751]	0.0023	[0.893]	0.0005	[0.685]	0.0003	[0.325]
Gender [Male]	Female	– 0.0924	[– 0.705]	– 0.0067	[– 0.040]	0.0199	[0.139]	– 0.5385	[– 2.200][b]	– 1.2275	[– 2.733][c]
Marital status	Divorced	– 0.7028	[– 3.859][c]	– 2.1517	[– 4.016][c]	– 1.4667	[– 3.592][c]	– 0.4666	[– 2.424][b]	– 0.4399	[– 2.152][b]
[Married]	Unmarried	– 0.7475	[– 6.586][c]	– 0.9336	[– 4.561][c]	– 0.8464	[– 5.211][c]	– 0.6339	[– 4.498][c]	– 0.5895	[– 3.544][c]
Home ownership [Renter]	Owner	0.3468	[3.962][c]	0.1961	[1.274]	0.2129	[1.639]	0.4272	[3.966][c]	0.4962	[4.125][c]
Educational attainment	Junior college	0.1142	[0.811]	0.0190	[0.066]	– 0.0330	[– 0.140]	0.1462	[0.889]	0.2338	[1.293]
[High School]	University	0.2582	[2.392][b]	0.0358	[0.148]	0.1682	[0.852]	0.3182	[2.585][c]	0.2867	[2.179][b]
Occupational Status	Non regular	– 0.4181	[– 3.061][c]	– 0.3456	[– 1.373]	– 0.3026	[– 1.383]	– 0.4249	[– 2.594][c]	– 0.4914	[– 2.781][c]
[Regular]	Unemployed	– 0.3105	[– 2.736][c]	– 0.2175	[– 0.719]	– 0.5026	[– 2.131][b]	– 0.3151	[– 2.541][b]	– 0.2517	[– 1.916][a]
	Retired	– 1.0851	[– 6.143][c]	– 0.7863	[– 3.109][c]	– 0.9458	[– 4.041][c]	– 1.4060	[– 5.410][c]	– 1.3293	[– 4.704][c]
	Self employed	– 0.1875	[– 1.539]	– 0.4592	[– 1.924][a]	– 0.3413	[– 1.631]	– 0.0574	[– 0.380]	– 0.0654	[– 0.407]
Municipality size											
[Town and Village]	Small cities	– 0.1015	[– 0.357]	– 0.3851	[– 0.638]	– 0.1378	[– 0.257]	0.0122	[0.037]	– 0.1258	[– 0.366]

(continued)

Table 4 (continued)

Variables		Model1		Model2				Model3			
		Entire		Age 20–34		Age 20–39		Age 35–69		Age 40–69	
		Coef.	[Z-value]	Coef.	[Z-value]	Coef.	[Z-value]	Coef.	[Z-value]	Coef.	[Z-value]
	Medium-sized cities	− 0.1106	[− 0.451]	0.0004	[0.001]	0.1307	[0.268]	− 0.1620	[− 0.592]	− 0.3106	[− 1.084]
	Metropolitan city	− 0.1455	[− 0.600]	− 0.0062	[− 0.011]	− 0.0129	[− 0.027]	− 0.1800	[− 0.667]	− 0.2337	[− 0.830]
Income											
Own Income		0.0107	[7.353][c]	0.0049	[1.853][a]	0.0088	[3.654][c]	0.0131	[7.472][c]	0.0122	[6.513][c]
Reference income	Age and gender	− 0.0158	[− 2.528][b]	− 0.0097	[− 0.415]	0.0014	[0.081]	− 0.0325	[− 3.231][c]	− 0.0579	[− 3.380][c]
K1		− 6.6965	[− 9.896][c]	− 11.0525	[− 2.244][b]	− 8.3698	[− 3.453][c]	− 7.6520	[− 4.835][c]	− 9.5950	[− 3.697][c]
K2		− 5.4553	[− 8.436][c]	− 9.7766	[− 1.992][b]	− 7.1321	[− 2.972][c]	− 6.4137	[− 4.095][c]	− 8.3460	[− 3.230][c]
K3		− 4.3520	[− 6.827][c]	− 8.6676	[− 1.769][a]	− 5.9910	[− 2.503][b]	− 5.2965	[− 3.393][c]	− 7.2487	[− 2.810][c]
K4		− 3.5070	[− 5.530][c]	− 7.6631	[− 1.565]	− 5.0128	[− 2.097][b]	− 4.5002	[− 2.885][c]	− 6.4771	[− 2.512][b]
K5		− 2.8672	[− 4.533][c]	− 6.8852	[− 1.406]	− 4.3213	[− 1.810][a]	− 3.9137	[− 2.510][b]	− 5.8670	[− 2.276][b]
K6		− 2.1057	[− 3.336][c]	− 6.1253	[− 1.252]	− 3.5763	[− 1.499]	− 3.1416	[− 2.017][b]	− 5.0831	[− 1.973][b]
K7		− 1.3428	[− 2.130][b]	− 5.3986	[− 1.103]	− 2.7852	[− 1.168]	− 2.3518	[− 1.511]	− 4.3255	[− 1.680][a]
K8		− 0.2596	[− 0.412]	− 4.3226	[− 0.883]	− 1.6867	[− 0.707]	− 1.2518	[− 0.805]	− 3.2387	[− 1.259]
K9		1.0350	[1.633]	− 2.9056	[− 0.594]	− 0.2965	[− 0.124]	0.0143	[0.009]	− 1.9871	[− 0.772]
K10		2.6661	[4.066][c]	− 1.7556	[− 0.358]	0.9063	[0.378]	1.8513	[1.178]	− 0.0459	[− 0.018]

(continued)

Table 4 (continued)

Variables	Model1		Model2				Model3			
	Entire		Age 20–34		Age 20–39		Age 35–69		Age 40–69	
	Coef.	[Z-value]	Coef.	[Z-value]	Coef.	[Z-value]	Coef.	[Z-value]	Coef.	[Z-value]
N	2000		573		794		1427		1206	
LR Chi2	247.3		57.0		91.7		219.6		179.8	

Note [a] $p < 0.10$, [b] $p < 0.05$, [c] $p < 0.01$. The variable in brackets is reference

Comparison Effect Versus Information Effect

The empirical results from the demographic reference group in both Japanese and Korean samples showed a negative association between LS and average income among individuals of the same age and gender at the 1% significance level (Model 1 in Tables 3 and 4), and the comparison effect dominated the information effect.

The empirical results for the 35–69 and 40–69 age groups in both Japanese and Korean samples showed negative associations between LS and average income among individuals of the same age and gender group at the 1% significance level (Model 3 in Tables 3 and 4). However, empirical results for the 20–34 and 20–39 age groups in both Japanese and Korean samples showed no association between LS and average income among individuals in the same age and gender group (Model 2 in Tables 3 and 4). These results suggest that the information effect has a greater impact on individuals in their early life than in their later life; the information effect through ambition cancels out the comparison effect in early life. However, there is another possibility that the effect of reference income is insignificant because both effects are originally very small and insignificant, not because of cancelation.

4.2 Evaluation of Marginal Effects: Own Income vs. Reference Income

In the previous section, our empirical results indicated that higher own income increases LS, while higher demographic reference income decreases LS in later life. To examine how increases in both individuals' own income and reference income affect one's LS in later life, based on Harada and Sumi (2018), we compared the marginal effects of own income with reference income, obtained from ordered logit estimation results. A marginal effect measures the change in the probability of $LS = m$ for a change in the independent variable x_l. According to Long and Freese (2014), discrete change is the change in the probability of $LS = m$ for change in x_l from the start value to the end value, holding all other variables constant. For example, a discrete change is the change in the probability of $LS = m$ for a change in any amount (such as 1 million yen) of income, holding all other variables constant. Therefore, we used discrete changes in our analysis.

The average discrete change (ADC) is the mean of the discrete change calculated at the observed values for all observations in the sample.

$$\text{ADC} = \frac{1}{N}\sum_{i=1}^{N}\frac{\Delta \Pr\left(LS_i = m|X = x_i\right)}{\Delta x_l} \tag{4}$$

Here, $m = 0, \ldots, 10$. ADC implies, on average, that a discrete change in x_l increases the probability of $LS = m$ by z percentage points.

Tables 5 and 6 show how increases in both one's own and reference income affect the predicted probability based on the estimation results from Japanese and Korean samples. Because the median value of LS was 6, we adopted $LS = 7$ as the threshold for relatively higher satisfaction.

For the Japanese entire sample (Model 1), a 2.5-million-yen increase (about \$20,000 [1USD = 120 JPY]) in own income increased the probability of choosing 7 and over by 6.5 percentage points ($\Delta Pr(LS \geq 7)/\Delta Y$). However, a 2.5-million-yen increase in reference income decreased the probability of choosing 7 and over by 4.2 percentage points ($\Delta Pr(LS \geq 7)/\Delta RI$). In the entire Korean sample (Model 1), a 25 million won increase (about \$20,000 [1USD = 0.0008 KRW]) in their own income increased the probability of choosing 7 and over by 6.0 percentage points ($\Delta Pr(LS \geq 7)/\Delta Y$). A 25 million won increase in reference income decreased the probability of choosing 7 and over by 8.4 percentage points (ΔPr(LS $\geq$ 7)/ΔRI).

Among Japanese people between the ages of 35 and 69 (Model 3), a 2.5-million-yen increase in own income increased the probability of choosing 7 and over ($LS \geq 7$) by 6.9 percentage points. Contrarily, a 2.5-million-yen increase in reference

Table 5 Average discrete change (ADC) of increased income: Japan (Unit: %, % point)

Sample	LS	0	1	2	3	4	5	6	7	8	9	10	LS≥7
Entire	Pr(LS)	3.3	1.9	4.2	7.4	7.2	16.7	12.8	17.8	17.5	6.5	4.8	46.6
Entire	⊿Pr/⊿Y	– 0.8	– 0.4	– 0.9	– 1.3	– 1.1	– 1.6	– 0.4	0.8	2.6	1.6	1.5	6.5
	⊿Pr/⊿RI	0.6	0.3	0.6	0.9	0.7	0.9	0.1	– 0.8	– 1.7	– 0.9	– 0.8	– 4.2
Age 35–69	⊿Pr/⊿Y	– 0.8	– 0.4	– 0.9	– 1.3	– 1.1	– 1.8	– 0.6	0.7	2.9	1.8	1.5	6.9
	⊿Pr/⊿RI	1.4	0.7	1.4	1.9	1.5	1.8	0.1	– 1.7	– 3.8	– 1.9	– 1.4	– 8.8
Age 40–69	⊿Pr/⊿Y	– 0.8	– 0.4	– 0.9	– 1.3	– 1.1	– 1.8	– 0.6	0.6	2.9	1.9	1.5	6.9
	⊿Pr/⊿RI	1.7	0.8	1.7	2.4	1.7	2.1	0.1	– 2.0	– 4.6	– 2.3	– 1.7	– 10.6
Entire	Difference	0.2	0.1	0.3	0.4	0.4	0.7	0.3	0.0	0.9	0.7	0.7	2.3
Age 35–69	Difference	– 0.6	– 0.3	– 0.5	– 0.6	– 0.4	0.0	0.5	– 1.0	– 0.9	– 0.1	0.1	– 1.9
Age 40–69	Difference	– 0.9	– 0.4	– 0.8	– 1.1	– 0.6	– 0.3	0.5	– 1.4	– 1.7	– 0.4	– 0.2	– 3.7

Note LS: Life Satisfaction, Y: Own Income, RI: Reference income
Pr(LS): Predicted Probability of Choosing LS = m, Unit: %
ΔPr/ΔY: Marginal effect of predicted probability for 2.5-million-yen increase in own income, Unit: % point
ΔPr/ΔRI: Marginal effect of predicted probability for 2.5-million-yen increase in reference income, Unit: % point
Difference: |ΔPr/ΔY|-|ΔPr/ΔRI|, Unit: point

Table 6 Average discrete change (ADC) of increased income: Korean (Unit: %, % point)

Sample	LS	0	1	2	3	4	5	6	7	8	9	10	LS≥7
Entire	Pr(LS)	0.9	2.1	5.3	8.5	10.0	15.6	17.3	20.5	13.1	5.2	1.4	40.2
Entire	⊿Pr/⊿Y	– 0.2	– 0.5	– 1.1	– 1.5	– 1.3	– 1.3	– 0.2	1.7	2.5	1.4	0.4	6.0
	⊿Pr/⊿RI	0.4	0.9	2.0	2.4	1.9	1.3	– 0.6	– 3.1	– 3.2	– 1.6	– 0.5	– 8.4
Age 35–69	⊿Pr/⊿Y	– 0.3	– 0.6	– 1.3	– 1.6	– 1.5	– 1.6	– 0.4	1.9	2.9	1.9	0.5	7.2
	⊿Pr/⊿RI	1.2	2.4	4.7	4.7	3.2	1.9	– 2.0	– 6.4	– 5.9	– 3.1	– 0.7	– 16.1
Age 40–69	⊿Pr/⊿Y	– 0.3	– 0.6	– 1.3	– 1.5	– 1.4	– 1.5	– 0.3	1.8	2.7	1.9	0.4	6.8
	⊿Pr/⊿RI	3.0	5.7	9.7	7.9	4.4	0.4	– 5.3	– 11.2	– 9.0	– 4.6	– 0.9	– 25.7
Entire	Difference	– 0.2	– 0.4	– 0.9	– 0.9	– 0.6	0.0	– 0.4	– 1.4	– 0.7	– 0.2	– 0.1	– 2.4
Age 35–69	Difference	– 0.9	– 1.8	– 3.4	– 3.1	– 1.7	– 0.3	– 1.6	– 4.5	– 3.0	– 1.2	– 0.2	– 8.9
Age 40–69	Difference	– 2.7	– 5.1	– 8.4	– 6.4	– 3.0	1.1	– 5.0	– 9.4	– 6.3	– 2.7	– 0.5	– 18.9

Note LS: Life Satisfaction, Y: Own Income, RI: Reference income
Pr(LS): Predicted Probability of Choosing LS = m, Unit: %.
ΔPr/ΔY: Marginal effect of predicted probability for 2.5-million-yen increase in own income, Unit: % point.
ΔPr/ΔRI: Marginal effect of predicted probability for 2.5-million-yen increase in reference income, Unit: % point.
Difference: |ΔPr/ΔY|-|ΔPr/ΔRI|, Unit: point.

income decreased the probability of choosing 7 and over ($LS \geq 7$) by 8.8 percentage points. Among those between the ages of 40 and 69 (Model 3), a 2.5-million-yen increase in own income increased the probability of choosing 7 and over ($LS \geq 7$) by 6.9 percentage points. Contrarily, a 2.5-million-yen increase in reference income decreased the probability of choosing 7 and over ($LS \geq 7$) by 10.6 percentage points.

Among Koreans between the ages of 35 and 69 (Model 3), a 25 million won increase in own income increased the probability of choosing 7 and over ($LS \geq 7$) by 7.2 points. In contrast, a 25 million won increase in reference income decreased the probability of choosing 7 and over ($LS \geq 7$) by 16.1% points. Among those between the ages of 40 and 69 (Model 3), a 25 million won increase in own income increased the probability of choosing 7 and over ($LS \geq 7$) by 6.8 percentage points. However, a 25 million won increase in reference income decreased the probability of choosing 7 and over ($LS \geq 7$) by 25.7 percentage points.

In Tables 5 and 6, "difference" represents the difference (i.e., ($|\Delta Pr/\Delta Y|-|\Delta Pr/\Delta RI|$) between absolute value of marginal effect of the predicted probability for increase in an individual's own income ($|\Delta Pr/\Delta Y|$) and marginal effect of the predicted probability for increase in reference income (|ΔPr/ΔRI|). When "difference" is positive, then the marginal effect of increase in own income is larger than the marginal effect of increase in reference income (i.e., $|\Delta Pr/\Delta Y| > |\Delta Pr/\Delta RI|$). Inversely, when "difference" is negative, then the marginal effect of increase in reference income is larger than the marginal effect of increase in own income (i.e., $|\Delta Pr/\Delta Y| < |\Delta Pr/\Delta RI|$). The "difference" in the entire sample was positive. Contrarily, the "difference" of the later life sub-sample was negative (for example, the probability of choosing high *LS* ($Pr(LS \geq 7)$) was –1.9 point in age 35–69 and –3.7 point in age 40–69 sub-samples in the Japanese sample; although the probability of choosing high *LS* ($Pr(LS \geq 7)$) was – 8.9 point in age 35–69, that the probability of this was – 18.9 point in age 40–69 sub-samples in the Korean sample), which means that the marginal effect of an increase in reference income is larger than the marginal effect of an increase in own income as one ages.

In addition, the marginal effect of an increase in Korean people's own income in later life is almost the same as that of Japanese people in later life (concretely, the probability of choosing a high *LS* ($Pr(LS \geq 7)$) of Korean was larger than that of Japanese by 0.3 point at the age of 35–69: the probability of choosing a high *LS* ($Pr(LS \geq 7)$) of Korean was smaller than that of Japanese by 0.1 point at the age of 40–69). Furthermore, the marginal effect of an increase in the reference income of Korean people in later life is considerably larger than that of Japanese people in later life (concretely, the probability of choosing a high *LS* ($Pr(LS \geq 7)$) of Koreans was larger than that of Japanese people by 7.3 point at the age of 35–69: the probability of choosing high LS ($Pr(LS \geq 7)$) of Korean was larger than that of Japanese by 15.1 point at the age of 40–69).[13]

5 Conclusions

While the relative income hypothesis proposes that higher reference income triggers a feeling of envy and thus has a negative effect on individual happiness, empirical studies have not yet reached a consensus on how reference income affects individual happiness. Thus, in this study, we distinguished the information effect from the comparison effect and examined the factors that affect the relative importance of comparison and information effects using Japanese and Korean nationwide survey data from 2015.

Our main findings are as follows. First, our empirical findings from the "later life" sample (ages 35–69 or 40–69) show a negative association between LS and average income of the demographic reference group. Our empirical results from the "early life" sample (ages 20–34 or 20–39) show no association between LS and average income of the demographic reference group in both countries. These results indicate that the information effect cancels out the comparison effect in one's early life, while the comparison effect dominates the information effect in one's later life.

[13] Further research is needed to fully understand this finding.

In short, these results indicate that individuals in later life envy the increased income of their demographic reference group, while young individuals are more mobile and more likely to be ambitious when faced with increased income of their demographic reference group. Consequently, our results partially support Hypothesis 1 and fully support Hypothesis 2.[14]

Second, we found that among those in the "later life" sample, the marginal effect of an increase in reference income tends to be larger than the marginal effect of an increase in individual income in both countries. Thus, they may be more likely to feel jealous in the economic success of their peers.

Third, the marginal effect of an increase in the reference income of Korean people in later life is larger than that of Japanese people in later life.

Both Japanese and Korean labor markets are characterized by a low risk of unemployment and a short duration of joblessness spells. According to the OECD (2018), the traditional Japanese employment system, characterized by lifetime employment and strong seniority-based wage profiles, is a possible cause of high wage inequality between regular workers and non-regular workers. Korean earnings quality is substantially below the OECD average because of the relatively low average wages and high wage inequality. This is associated with a high share of workers employed by very small firms. In addition, the low enrollment rate in employment insurance among self-employed and non-regular workers in small firms contributes to low benefit coverage in Korea. Thus, growing inequality in the labor market in both countries may cause a feeling of strong jealousy at the economic success of their peers in later life. However, further research is needed to provide a more detailed explanation of this larger comparison effect in later life.

Our contribution to the study of happiness is that we verified the relative importance of comparison and information effects depending on the degree of mobility in life stages in East Asian developed countries such as Japan and Korea. This is consistent with the results of previous international studies, such as Senik (2008) and Fitzloy et al. (2014). In addition, our results imply that the estimations of reference income across all age samples make the mistake of interpreting the relative importance of comparison and information effects, as pointed out by Fitzloy et al. (2014).

Acknowledgements This work was supported by the MEXT-Supported Program for the Strategic Research Foundation at Private Universities of Japan, 2014–2018 (S1491003).

[14] To assume that the insignificant effect means the cancelation of comparison effect by information effect, we need to rigorously show that information and comparison effect have independently positive and negative effects on LS. Further research is needed to examine these effect.

References

Blanchflower, D. G., & Oswald, A. J. (2004). Well-being over time in Britain and the USA. *Journal of Public Economics, 88*, 1359–1386.

Brown, S., Gray, D., & Roberts, J. (2015). The relative income hypothesis: A comparison of methods. *Economic Letters, 130*, 47–50.

Clark, A. E., Westergård-Nielsen, N., & Kristensen, N. (2009). Economic satisfaction and income rank in small neighborhoods. *Journal of European Economic Association, 7*(2–3), 519–527.

Duesenberry, J. S. (1949). *Income, saving and the theory of consumer behavior*. Harvard University Press.

Ferrer-i-Carbonell, A. (2005). Income and well-being: An empirical analysis of the comparison income effect. *Journal of Public Economics, 89*, 997–1019.

FitzRoy, F., Nolan, M., Steinhardt, M., & Ulph, D. (2014). Testing the tunnel effect: Comparison, age and happiness in UK and German panels. *IZA Journal of European Labor Studies, 3*, 1–30.

Frey, B. S., & Stutzer, A. (2002). What can economists learn from happiness research? *Journal of Economic Literature, 40*(2), 402–435.

Friedman, M. (1957). *A theory of the consumption function*. Princeton University Press.

Goerke, L., & Pannenberg, M. (2015). Direct evidence for income comparisons and subjective well-being across reference groups. *Economics Letters, 137*, 95–101.

Harada, H., & Sumi, E. (2018). Happiness and relative income hypothesis in contemporary Japan: Study of lifestyle and values. *The Senshu Social Well-Being Review, 5*, 63–74.

Helliwell, J, F. & Huang, H. (2005). *How's the job? Well-being and social capital in the workplace*. NBER Working Paper No. 11759.

Hirschman, A. O., & Rothschild, M. (1973). The changing tolerance for income inequality in the course of economic development with a mathematical appendix. *The Quarterly Journal of Economics, 87*(4), 544–566.

International Consortium for Social Well-Being Studies. (2020). Social well-being sur-vey in Asia, 2015–2017. (Indonesia) Universitas Indonesia, (Japan) Senshu University, (South Korea) Seoul National University, (The Philippines) Ateneo de Manila University, (Thailand) Chulalongkorn University, (Taiwan) Academia Sinica, (Vietnam) Vietnam Academy of Social Sciences[Producers]. Ko-rea Social Science Data Archive (KOSSDA) [Distributors], 2020–06–25, A1-CUM-0022, V2.0, http://hdl.handle.net/20.500.12236/23941

Long, J. S., & Freese, J. (2014). *Regression models for categorical dependent variables using stata* (3rd ed.). Stata Press.

Luttmer, E. F. (2005). Neighbours as negatives: Relative earnings and well-being. *Quarterly Journal of Economics, 120*(3), 963–1002.

Mangyo, E., & Park, A. (2011). Relative deprivation and health: Which reference groups matter? *Journal of Human Resources, 46*(3), 459–481.

OECD. (2018). *Employment outlook 2018*.

Senik, C. (2004). When information dominates comparison: Learning from Russian subjective panel data. *Journal of Public Economics, 88*(9), 2099–2123.

Senik, C. (2008). Ambition and Jealousy: Income interactions in the 'Old' Europe versus the 'New' Europe and the United States. *Economica, 75*(299), 495–513.

Shields, M. A., Price, S. W., & Wooden, M. (2009). Life satisfaction and the economic and social characteristics of neighbourhoods. *Journal of Population Economics, 22*, 421–443.

Hiroo Harada is Professor Emeritus of Economics at Senshu University. His research interests are in the fields of public finance, taxation, regional economy, public choice, and social capital/well-being.

Eiji Sumi is Professor of Economics at Nihon University. His research interests and publications are in the fields of public choice, local public finance, and subjective wellbeing.

Trust in Strangers and Well-Being: A Comparison in Asian Societies

Keitaro Yazaki

Abstract In recent years, social sciences have focused on the positive effects of generalized trust on individuals and society. Although trust in most people and trust in strangers are directed toward a wide range of people, a pertinent question that arises in our mind is "are both types of trust theoretically and empirically equivalent?" This paper explains the theoretical differences between trust in most people and trust in strangers based on the sociology of strangers and examines the effect of both types of trust on individual well-being using data from the Social Well-being Survey in Asia (SoWSA). Paradoxically, in societies with more solid social ties and fewer strangers, the effect of strangers on well-being increases. In contrast, in a more urbanized society with weaker social ties surrounded by strangers, trust in strangers has no significant effect on well-being, and instead, social ties such as "trust in most people" have a positive effect on individual well-being. The Ordinary Least Squares regression results showed that trust in strangers had no significant effect on individual well-being in East Asia, whereas it had a positive effect in Southeast Asian societies. In contrast, trust in most people positively affected well-being in East Asia but had a negative effect in Southeast Asia.

Keywords Strangers · Generalized trust · Well-being

1 Introduction

Portes suggest that trust and social capital have negative effects on society. In some cases, they can create a closed and exclusive community such as a mafia or hate group and divide the society (Portes, 1998, 2014).

Many researchers have reacted to this concern by insisting that generalized trust, as trust in a wider range of people, overcomes the exclusivity of a closed group. In contrast to the narrow closed trust, such as that fostered among family

K. Yazaki (✉)
Department of Fine Arts, Tainan University of Technology, Tainan City, Taiwan
e-mail: kei.yzk.15@gmail.com

J. Yee et al. (eds.), *Social Well-Being, Development, and Multiple Modernities in Asia*,
https://doi.org/10.1007/978-981-97-3866-3_14

members or kinship, wider trust forms mutual relationships without any exclusivity (Fukuyama, 2001). Putnam emphasizes the role of bridging social capital, which enables establishment of links between closed communities or groups across borders (Putnam, 2000). Generalized social trust helps in creation and development of a civil society, enhances democratic stability (Putnam et al., 1993), reduces economic inequality (Rose, 2011), and promotes individual well-being (Helliwell, 2003). Thus, generalized trust functions as a cure for the whole society.

However, does not trust in a wide range of people also include exclusivity? Looking back at the history of nationalism, we are often confronted with the ambiguity of the concept of "the people." Much of the early nationalism, especially in the nineteenth century, demanded the political and social inclusion of most people, as opposed to the dictatorship of a few, such as kings and aristocrats, which is the basis of today's concept of a welfare state that calls for inclusion of all people. However, nationalism has often been associated with racism or exclusionism. According to Pelinka (2012), "the people," as articulated by Abraham Lincoln, demanded inclusive relationships with a wider range of others, but the concept did not include African-American people or women. During the period of German reunification, the concept of people (*Volk*) promoted social inclusion, but later transformed into a slogan, leading to nationalism and populism (Pelinka, 2012). During Monday demonstrations in 1989, many people advocated the slogan "We are the people" (Wir sind das Volk) against the dictatorship of the Socialist Unity Party of Germany and for a democratic and more inclusive society. Nevertheless, right-wing groups such as Pegita used the exact phrase, "We are the people," for anti-immigration propaganda in 2014. Inclusive trust can overlook the existence of minorities, and extremists often justify the exclusion of minorities for the sake of "people." The concept of people is highly ambiguous, and who are the "people" strongly depends on the context, time, and the society.

This type of ambiguity has been highlighted in the recent social surveys. People who trust well-known people are likely to trust most people (Sturgis & Smith, 2010), and the determinants of a wider range of trust include not only trust in unknown others, but also well-known others. The tendency to trust most people, and not only well-known people, has been observed more in East Asian societies than in Western societies (Delhey et al., 2011).

To avoid the ambiguity of the concept of "people," which can include both wide and narrow trust, Naef and Schupp (2009) suggest using the idea of trust in strangers instead of trust in most people. This study assumes that trust in strangers is sufficient for determining trust within a wider radius of trust. However, the concept of "stranger" must not be handled simply as an improved measure of trust among most people. Trust in most people and trust in strangers should be distinguished as being qualitatively different, and their effects should be compared simultaneously at the same level. In the following section, we explain the characteristics of the concept of "stranger" as compared to "most people" considering a theoretical perspective of the sociology of strangers.

1.1 Stranger as Untrusted

Sociological theories have traditionally focused on strangers because of the assumption that modernization was caused by accepting strangers (Simmel, 1908; Sombart, 1991; Tönnies, 2005). Strangers try to minimize the extent to which they deal with local people to avoid getting close to them. Rapid trade that requires no intimate association leads to the rationalization of the society. Social norms and lifestyles, which are naively believed, are also fluidized by strangers who do not fit into the local culture (Simmel, 1908).

Modern society cannot exist without a symbiosis with strangers. However, Simmel (1908) did not assume the opportunistic expectation of mutual understanding between natives and strangers, describing strangers as a paradoxical combination of "nearness" and "farness." On the one hand, due to modernization the number of strangers increases; on the other hand, the gaps between them are not bridged. Thus, despite the observable increase in number of strangers in the society, the possibility of existence of sympathy between them does not increase. Thus, from Simmel's perspective, we can hypothesize that a society physically close to strangers is mentally or socially distanced from them.

Schütz (1994) contrasts between strangeness and trust from a phenomenological perspective. According to him, "thinking as usual," which is fostered naturally by the circumstances in which one is brought up, provides "trustworthy recipes" that encompass acceptable values and behaviors in social life. For strangers, however, the self-evident worldview shared by the members of the host society is totally unnatural and doubtful because it provides them the impression that its prescriptions are inconsistent and incongruent. Moreover, strangers' worldview inherited from their home society becomes questionable because it does not conform to the host society. Consequently, strangers tend to distance themselves from establishing a trusting relationship rather than judging the world as trustworthy.

Rumford ascertains that routinized interactions with strangers in the age of globalization make the world more complex and incomprehensible rather than uniting it as one (Rumford, 2013). Recent studies on strangers demand a more abstract perspective than Simmel and Schütz, who emphasized that all people are likely to be considered as potential strangers along with the increase in modernization (Bauman, 1998; Hahn, 1994; Marrota, 2010; Nassehi, 1995; Stichweh, 2007). A characteristic of strangers is that they have no reference group. Today, not only newcomers, whom Simmel and Schütz regarded as strangers, but also most of the other people have lost their reference groups. Individualization, in which people are separated from any group or community (Beck & Beck-Gernsheim, 1994) promotes the generalization of strangers. Immigrants are still regarded as strangers in most societies, but it is not rare that neighbors, even if they have the same ethnicity and lifestyle as the natives or the majority, can also be regarded as a stranger, especially in urban cities. What do we really know about residents who live in the same apartment and have the same ethnicity? If we restrict ourselves to formal greetings only and do not talk to residents about their backgrounds, occupations, hobbies, and political opinions, what is the difference between natives and immigrants? The difference between native and immigrant is nowadays quite slight. Both are objectively the same strangers, but they differ in that natives rarely label themselves as strangers.

Thus, the definition of strangers should be defined abstractly as *constructed* when non-understanding occurs, or when this non-understanding is structured as distrust in some communication process (Hellmann, 1998: 434). Therefore, we cannot specify a priori as to who strangers are: a stranger does not have an objective character but is a relational concept (Hahn, 1994). This constructed character of strangers is exactly the same as the concept of ethnicity, which is constructed abstractly in relation to other groups (Banton, 2008: 1275–6). The context in each situation determines the stranger. A neighbor can be a stranger in an urban city, but in a certain political context, can be considered as a sibling. We can define strangers as untrustworthy at an abstract level, as distrust in communication may make us consider someone as a stranger.

1.2 Trust in the Untrusted

If we regard strangers as untrustworthy, how can trust in strangers be explained? It seems paradoxical to trust someone who is untrustworthy. Using the term "civil inattention," Goffman showed us that such contradictory behaviors play out in everyday life. While people in urban cities must detach themselves from others, they must also make use of gestures or pay attention through eye contact (Goffman, 1963: 84). Baumann said, when we face strangers, we are undecided whether to view them as friends or enemies (Bauman, 1998: 25). Trust in strangers functions in this gray zone, preventing hasty judgment as to whether a stranger is trustworthy. We trust and distrust strangers at the same time, trust them as neighbors but distrust them as citizens, or stop doubting them temporally and trust them successively (Hellmann, 1998: 439). Minimal sympathy and indifference with unknown others (Stichweh, 2010) constitute the core of trusting strangers. Many city people are exposed to so many strangers that it takes some time to get comfortable around them, and they imply a minimum level of trust with gestures or greetings.

Considering the paradoxical and ambivalent trust directed toward strangers, we must distinguish it from the trust defined by social capital and generalized trust studies.

The social capital theory stems from Smith's concept of sympathy. Based on the notion of sympathy as a basic human need, the theory of social capital links a person's consumption to that of others, without calculating the return (Robison et al., 2002). In addition to it being adopted for people with whom a person is well acquainted with, such as family, relatives, friends, and neighbors, this concept has been extended to a wider range of people, such as strangers, beyond one's interpersonal networks and unknown people (Stolle, 2002).

In contrast to Smith's theory, the concept of a stranger assumes that sympathy between random people is practically impossible. Simmel (1903) criticized Smith's concept of sympathy, claiming that it was only possible for small communities, such as the *polis* in ancient Greece, in which people are fairly homogeneous and their interests are relatively simple and undifferentiated. Modern society is characterized by urbanization, social differentiation, and diversity, rendering sympathy increasingly impossible.

We do not argue whether sympathy between a wider range of people is possible; instead we argue that the difference between trust in most people and trust in strangers should be considered. If we can reduce the trust in most people to *sympathy*, then trust in strangers can be characterized as *tolerance* (Yazaki, 2018). Thinking as usual, as Schütz explained, is nourished in childhood by the parents, which helps in consolidation of trust and sympathy. This facilitates a wider radius of trust if the worldview, as extended to the culture or nation, becomes a common sense. On the contrary, trust in strangers suspends such mutual trust and displays only temporary tolerance toward others, accompanied by indifference. This form of trust rarely offers an opportunity to sympathize, but rather provides an opportunity to interact with people, regardless of their worldview.

From this theoretical background, we build up the following two hypotheses.

1.3 Hypotheses

The first hypothesis examines the qualitative difference between trust in most people and trust in strangers, and its relationship with trust in family members (see Fig. 1). Trusting most people is positively correlated with trusting family, since these forms of trust are based on sympathy under "thinking as usual." Trust in most people is also positively correlated with trust in strangers, since both are oriented toward a wider radius of people. With respect to these points, trust in family and strangers do not have anything in common, and the elementary worldview constructed by family can be broken through the existence of strangers. Therefore, it was assumed that trust in family and trust in strangers were negatively correlated. This analysis aims to provide an empirical constellation of trust that we have described theoretically. Each type of trust can function as a cause and a result.

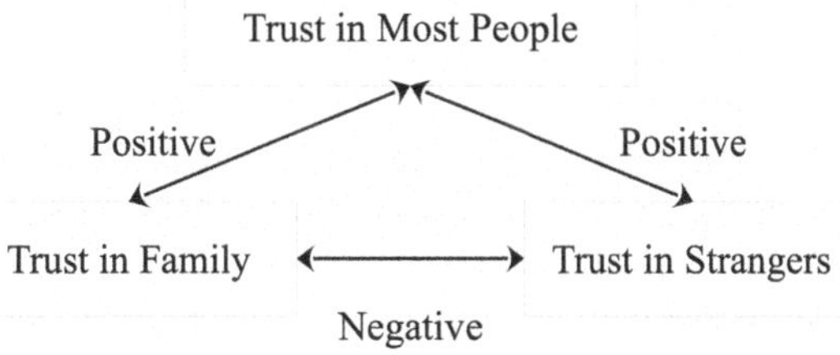

Fig. 1 Relation between the three forms of trust

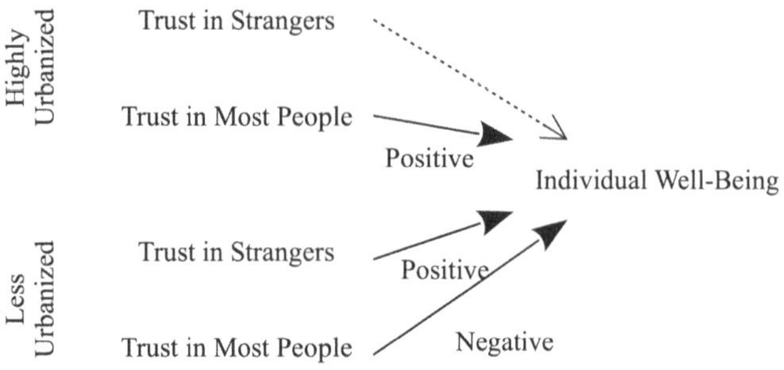

Fig. 2 Effects of generalized forms of trust on well-being

The second hypothesis examines the effect of both kinds of trust on individuals' well-being considering Simmel's proposition that explains strangers as the paradoxical combination of "nearness" and "farness." Thus, we can conclude that a society physically close to strangers is mentally distanced from them. We assumed that this theoretical proposition could operate as the relationship between the types of trust and the well-being of individuals (see Fig. 2).

In a more urbanized society, where everyone is a stranger, the trust for strangers does not affect individuals' well-being, because people distance themselves from strangers. On the contrary, in a society where the degree of urbanization is relatively low and strangers are rare, people can accept them mentally. As Stichweh (2010) points out, people in traditional societies do not necessarily regard strangers as enemies. In a society where there was little contact with the outside world, the presence of merchants was precious, so if their stay was temporary, the host of the house could welcome them as guests. In contemporary less urbanized societies, people can be benefitted when they are receptive to tourists, merchants, and executives from global corporations looking to invest, even if they do not trust strangers.

This framework of assuming the effects of trust in strangers can also be applied to trust in most people in highly urbanized societies where sympathy is fundamentally difficult because there are strangers everywhere, and hence gaining sympathy is preferred but is scarce, and isolated people long for community. In this type of society, trust in most people has a positive effect on the well-being. On the contrary, in less urbanized societies, where living with the same kind of people is preferred, having sympathy for others is not only mundane but also ubiquitous because it is difficult to live alone, and cooperation with various people is essential for survival. However, at the same time, social networks can demand many services or even self-sacrifice from the community, which works exactly like social pressure. In this form of society, trust has a negative effect on well-being. Strong peer pressure in a community may make strangers more attractive. Interacting with the strangers is an oasis to escape from the day-to-day pressure, when people can forget about the community's norms and become individuals. Thus, strangers can bring not only material profits but also mental benefits.

Table 1 Survey data study description

	JP	KR	TW	ID	PH	TH	VN
Date	2015	2015	2017	2017	2016	2016	2015
Age	20–70	20–69	20–69	20–82	18–80	17–90	18–74
N	2300 (11,786)	2000	2303	1248	1065	995	1094

2 Data and Methods

This study compared the differences in the effects of the two types of generalized trust, trust in most people and trust in strangers, using data from *the Social Well-Being Survey in Asia* (*SoWSA*). This survey offers data from seven Asian countries, namely Japan (JP), South Korea (KR), Taiwan (TW), Indonesia (ID), Philippines (PH), Thailand (TH), and Vietnam (VN). Only the sample size of the Japanese was extremely large; hence, it was resampled and reduced to 2300[1] (see Table 1).

As this survey measured various forms of trust on the same five-point scale, it was found to be suitable for comparing trust in strangers and trust in most people. Both forms of trust were measured through the following statement: "To what degree do you feel you can trust or not trust strangers" "The possible answers and scores ranged from "Can trust a lot" (5), "Can trust" (4), "Can trust somewhat" (3), "Can hardly trust" (2), and "Cannot trust at all" (1).

In order to test the first hypothesis, we examined the partial correlation between trust in strangers, trust in most people, and trust in family. Trust in neighbors and trust in government staff were included as control variables. As trusting relationship with the neighbors can result due to sympathy, like trust in family and trust in most people, the relationship between them can be established, but its range with respect to both forms of trust should be distinguished. Trust in government staff should be regarded as an indicator of trust in an abstract system related to bureaucracy and managed by anonymous people (Giddens, 1990; Luhmann, 1973). Although compliance with an abstract system can be enforced to a large extent, it can also be correlated with trust in strangers and trust in most people, yet it considers trust in an abstract system to be impersonal. In this study, the social attributes were not considered as control variables because their purpose was to aggregate the various forms of trust at an abstract level. For the same reason, we did not examine the characteristics of each of the societies of the seven countries by integrating the survey data obtained from each of them into one.

The third and the last hypothesis, which involved Ordinary Least Squares regression (OLS), examined the effects of trust in strangers and in most people on individual well-being. As a dependent variable of general life satisfaction (Helliwell et al., 2016: 13–4), we used the Cantril ladder on an 11-point scale with the following statement:

[1] The after-sampling of the Japan survey was conducted, using the set.seed (453,058) function in R.

> Please imagine a ladder with steps numbered from 0 at the bottom to 10 at the top. Suppose we say that the top of the ladder represents the best possible life for you, and the bottom of the ladder represents the worst possible life for you. On which step of the ladder would you say you personally feel you stand at this time, assuming that the higher the step, the better you feel about your life, and the lower the step, the worse you feel about it? Which step comes closest to the way you feel?

This item measured general well-being and helped in assessing one's life as a whole from a more reflective perspective than happiness. Abstract well-being is highly associated with generalized trust, which measures more abstract relationships with others.

In order to test the second hypothesis, the control variables, like forms of trust including trust in family, trust in neighbors, and trust in government staff were entered, along with social attributes including gender, education, household income, marital status, age, and employment status. The score on household income was converted to a decile score (i.e., the 10th-quartile of each of the seven societies.[2]

During conduction of the 2nd analysis, the population was divided into East Asian and Southeast Asian societies (See Tables 2 and 3). The second hypothesis assumes that the effect of the two types of trust on well-being varies with the degree of urbanization or modernization. This analysis regarded Japan, Korea, and Taiwan as more urbanized societies, whereas Indonesia, the Philippines, Vietnam, and Thailand as being less urbanized. Kobayashi and Aldar (2018) analyzed the SoWSA data and revealed that the East Asia and Southeast Asia also differed on mechanisms associated with well-being, so we should not merge these seven countries into one population. After analyzing each of the seven countries separately (Yazaki, 2018), we combined them into Eastern and Southeast Asian countries.

First, the dependent variable of the second hypothesis, the mean value of the individual well-being on the Cantril Ladder was found to be higher for Southeast Asian (6.96) than for East Asian (5.54) countries. While trust in most people did not differ significantly between the two groups (East Asia: 2.87; Southeast Asia: 2.79), trust in strangers tended to be higher in East Asia (2.11) than in Southeast Asia (1.79). A key sociodemographic feature of these data is the percentage of self-employed people, including farmers. Self-employed people in Southeast Asia comprise 39.76%, which is higher than that in East Asia (12.10%). This suggests that Southeast Asia still has a relatively low level of urbanization.

[2] Household income in Indonesia could be split only into the 3-quartiles, because the variance is extremely low as a result of the inadequate setting of the response category. However, to keep comparability with the income of other societies divided into decline, it was converted based on the median values when divided into tenths: 0–29% as the 2nd, 30–69% as the 5th, 70–89% as the 8th, and 90–100% as the 10th.

Table 2 Descriptive statics of East Asia ($N = 6603$)

Label	NA (%)	Mean (or %)	S.D	Median	Range
Cantril ladder (well-being)	0	5.54	1.97	6	0–10
Trust in strangers	0	2.11	0.81	2	1–5
Trust in most people	0	2.87	0.72	3	1–5
Trust in family	0	3.73	0.86	4	1–5
Trust in neighbors	0	2.83	0.76	3	1–5
Trust in government staff	0	2.6	0.83	3	1–5
Regular worker (Ref)	0	52.70%			
Temporary		12.16%			
Self-employed		12.10%			
Un-employed		4.39%			
Non-employed		18.64%			
Age	0	42.62	12.75	42	20–69
Female (Ref)	0	49.69%			
Married (Ref)	0	57.73%			
University Graduates (%)	0.18	60.61%			
Household Income (deciles)	3.57	5.69	2.84	6	1–10
JP (ref)	0	34.83%			
KR		30.29%			
TW		34.88%			

3 Results

Our first hypothesis concerns the constellation among trust in most people, trust in strangers, and trust in family. The results of Spearman's partial correlation (see Table 4) show that trust in most people was positively correlated with trust in family ($r_s = 0.10$) and trust in strangers ($r_s = 0.37$), whereas there was a negative correlation between trust in strangers and trust in family ($r_s = 0.20$). This supported our hypothesis that trust in most people as well as trust in family is fostered by sympathy, and trust in a wider range of people enhances both (i.e., trust in most people and trust in strangers). Contrarily, trust in strangers hinders creation of sympathy, can lessen the significance of "thinking as usual" that is cultivated through sympathy within the household.

The second hypothesis pertains to the relationship between trust and well-being: In a more urbanized and stranger-surrounded society, people exhibit "civic indifference" toward them and do not get well-being from strangers. Furthermore, people feel lonely because of their weakened social ties. In this situation, trust in most people enhances mental stability. In less urbanized societies, trust in various people and mutual help are essential for survival. However, such trust can lead to peer pressure to involve people in the community and can lower individuals' well-being. At times,

Table 3 Descriptive statics of Southeast Asia ($N = 4402$)

Label	NA (%)	Mean (or %)	S.D	Median	Range
Cantril ladder (well-being)	0.14	6.96	1.66	7	0–10
Trust in strangers	0.93	1.74	0.87	2	1–5
Trust in most people	0.41	2.79	0.98	3	1–5
Trust in family	0.25	4.3	0.74	4	1–5
Trust in neighbors	0.16	3.36	0.88	3	1–5
Trust in government staff	3.34	3.04	0.94	3	1–5
Regular worker (Ref)		14.59%			
Temporary		20.30%			
Self-employed		39.76%			
Un-employed		4.51%			
Non-employed		20.83%			
Age	0	41.36	13.53	41	20–69
Female (Ref)	0	51.02%			
Married (Ref)	0.05	69.86%			
University Graduates (%)	3.25	5.54	2.77	5	
Household Income (deciles)	0.41	18.11%			1–10
JP (ref)	0	28.35%			
KR		24.19%			
TW		22.60%			

Table 4 Partial correlation between the forms of trust ($N = 11{,}125$)

Trust in …	Most people		Family		Strangers		Neighbors		Government Staff	
Most People	1.00									
Family	0.10	***	1.00							
Strangers	0.37	***	-0.2	***	1.00					
Neighbors	0.22	***	0.34	***	0.13	***	1.00			
Government Staff	0.10	***	0.15	***	0.14	***	0.23	***	1.00	

*p < 0.05, **p < 0.01, ***p < 0.001

the presence of strangers is rare, and trusting them provides material and mental benefits beyond the strong social ties. Tables 5 and 6 illustrate the effects of the various forms of trust on individual well-being measured by the Cantril ladder as generalized individual well-being by using the OLS regression.

In East Asia (see Table 5), Model 1 focuses on the effects of trust variables, while controlling for country variables. This proves that trust in most people enhances individual well-being, while trust in strangers has no significant effect. Model 2,

Table 5 Regression of the dependent variable of the Cantril ladder (East Asian Model)

Predictors	Model 1		Model 2		Model 3	
	Est	*Beta*	*Est*	*Beta*	*Est*	*Beta*
(Intercept)	1.79[a] (0.13)	0.04 (0.02)	0.91[a] (0.15)	− 0.21 (0.03)	1.18[a] (0.21)	− 0.23 (0.03)
Trust in strangers	0.03 (0.04)	0.01 (0.01)	0.05 (0.03)	0.02 (0.01)	0.01 (0.06)	0.00 (0.02)
Trust in most people	0.41[a] (0.04)	0.15 (0.02)	0.36[a] (0.04)	0.13 (0.02)	0.17[b] (0.07)	0.06 (0.03)
Trust in family	0.40[a] (0.03)	0.17 (0.01)	0.37[a] (0.03)	0.16 (0.01)	0.45[a] (0.04)	0.19 (0.02)
Trust in neighbors	0.23[a] (0.04)	0.09 (0.02)	0.17[a] (0.04)	0.07 (0.02)	0.18[a] (0.04)	0.07 (0.02)
Trust in government staff	0.19[a] (0.03)	0.08 (0.01)	0.19[a] (0.03)	0.08 (0.01)	0.19[a] (0.03)	0.08 (0.01)
Job: Temporary (ref: Regular workers)			− 0.22[c] (0.07)	− 0.11 (0.04)	− 0.22[c] (0.07)	− 0.11 (0.04)
Job: Self− employed			− 0.05 (0.07)	− 0.03 (0.04)	− 0.05 (0.07)	− 0.02 (0.04)
Job: Un− employed			− 0.80[a] (0.11)	− 0.41 (0.06)	− 0.79[a] (0.11)	− 0.40 (0.06)
Job: Non− employed			0.05 (0.06)	0.02 (0.03)	0.06 (0.06)	0.03 (0.03)
Sex: Female (dummy)			0.33[a] (0.05)	0.17 (0.02)	0.32[a] (0.05)	0.16 (0.02)
Marital Status: Married(dummy)			0.47[a] (0.05)	0.24 (0.03)	0.46[a] (0.05)	0.23 (0.03)
Age			0.00 0.00	0.01 (0.01)	0.00 0.00	0.01 (0.01)
Household income (deciles)			0.12[a] (0.01)	0.17 (0.01)	0.11[a] (0.01)	0.17 (0.01)
University graduates (dummy)			0.15[c] (0.05)	0.08 (0.02)	0.16[a] (0.05)	0.08 (0.02)
KR (ref: JP)	0.00 (0.06)	0.00 (0.03)	0.01 (0.06)	0.01 (0.03)	− 0.64[b] (0.28)	0.03 (0.03)
TW	− 0.22[a] (0.06)	− 0.11 (0.03)	− 0.14[b] (0.06)	− 0.07 (0.03)	− 0.41 (0.28)	− 0.07 (0.03)
Trust in strangers × KR					0.06 (0.08)	0.02 (0.03)
Trust in strangers × TW					0.09 (0.08)	0.04 (0.03)
Trust in most people × KR					0.34[a] (0.10)	0.12 (0.04)

(continued)

Table 5 (continued)

Predictors	Model 1		Model 2		Model 3	
	Est	*Beta*	*Est*	*Beta*	*Est*	*Beta*
Trust in most people × TW					0.27[c] (0.09)	0.10 (0.03)
Trust in family × KR					− 0.10 (0.07)	− 0.04 (0.03)
Trust in family × TW					− 0.19[c] (0.07)	− 0.08 (0.03)
Observations	6355		6355		6355	
R^2/R^2 adjusted	0.138/0.137		0.213/0.211		0.217/0.214	
AIC	25,690.091		25,123.285		25,106.198	
VIF	< 1.5		< 1.5		< 6.0	

[a] $p < 0.001$, [b] $p < 0.05$, [c] $p < 0.01$, † < 0.1

in which both trust variables and social attributes were entered, showed the same effects as Model 1 did. In Model 3, which examined the interaction effect between each society, trust in most people in South Korea and Taiwan had a positive impact on well-being, whereas the effect of trust in strangers was not significant in any of the three societies. These models suggest that the trust in strangers is ineffective in establishing individual well-being in East Asia, whereas trust in most people can establish it.

Table 6 shows the results of Southeast Asian societies. Similarly, Models 1 and 2 demonstrate that trust in strangers has a positive effect on well-being, while trust in most people has a negative impact. In Model 3, we confirmed that, in Thailand and Vietnam, trust in strangers positively influenced well-being, even though the effect in the case of Thailand was found to be unstable ($p < 0.1$). As for trust in most people, the result for Vietnam suggested a negative effect on well-being, even though the p-value was less than 0.1. However, if we consider the results of Models 1 and 2, trust in most people is likely to lower individual well-being, thus functioning as a social pressure requiring conformity.

4 Discussion

This study was based on the premise that trust in most people and trust in strangers have different characteristics. Trust in most people is based on sympathy and has a positive correlation with trust in the family (see Table 5), which cultivates thinking as usual. Trust in strangers hinders the possibility of creation of sympathy, creating momentary attitudes and behaviors of tolerance, and demands refraining from "thinking as usual," which depicts a negative correlation with trust in the family

Table 6 Regression of the dependent variable of the Cantril ladder (Southeast Asian Model)

	Model 1		Model 2		Model 3	
Predictors	Est	Beta	Est	Beta	Est	Beta
(Intercept)	5.27[a] (0.18)	−0.01 (0.03)	4.99[a] (0.22)	− 0.10 (0.06)	4.00[a] (0.42)	− 0.10 (0.06)
Trust in strangers	0.10[b] (0.03)	0.05 (0.02)	0.08[c] (0.03)	0.04 (0.02)	− 0.04 (0.06)	− 0.02 (0.03)
Trust in most people	− 0.07[c] (0.03)	− 0.04 (0.02)	− 0.08[b] (0.03)	− 0.05 (0.02)	− 0.04 (0.06)	− 0.02 (0.04)
Trust in family	0.28[a] (0.04)	0.12 (0.02)	0.26[a] (0.04)	0.11 (0.02)	0.51[a] (0.09)	0.23 (0.04)
Trust in neighbors	0.03 (0.03)	0.02 (0.02)	0.07[c] (0.03)	0.04 (0.02)	0.06[d] (0.03)	0.03 (0.02)
Trust in government staff	0.13[a] (0.03)	0.08 (0.02)	0.14[a] (0.03)	0.08 (0.02)	0.15[a] (0.03)	0.08 (0.02)
Job: Temporary (ref: Regular workers)			− 0.25[b] (0.09)	− 0.15 (0.05)	− 0.25[b] (0.09)	− 0.15 (0.05)
Job: Self-employed			− 0.04 (0.08)	− 0.02 (0.05)	− 0.03 (0.08)	− 0.02 (0.05)
Job: Un-employed			− 0.37[b] (0.14)	− 0.22 (0.09)	− 0.36[c] (0.14)	− 0.22 (0.09)
Job: Non-employed			− 0.15 (0.09)	− 0.09 (0.06)	− 0.14 (0.09)	− 0.08 (0.06)
Sex: Female (dummy)			0.21[a] (0.05)	0.13 (0.03)	0.21[a] (0.05)	0.13 (0.03)
Marital status: Married(dummy)			0.16[b] (0.06)	0.10 (0.04)	0.16[b] (0.06)	0.10 (0.04)
Age			− 0.01[b] (0.00)	− 0.05 (0.02)	− 0.01[b] (0.00)	− 0.05 (0.02)
Household income (deciles)			0.07[a] (0.01)	0.12 (0.02)	0.07[a] (0.01)	0.12 (0.02)
University graduates (dummy)			0.24[b] (0.08)	0.14 (0.04)	0.25[a] (0.08)	0.15 (0.04)
PH (ref: ID)	− 0.23[b] (0.07)	− 0.14 (0.04)	− 0.20[b] (0.07)	− 0.12 (0.04)	0.78 (0.48)	− 0.15 (0.05)
TH	0.38[a] (0.08)	0.23 (0.05)	0.35[a] (0.08)	0.21 (0.05)	1.31[c] (0.52)	0.22 (0.05)
VN	− 0.02 (0.08)	− 0.01 (0.05)	− 0.09 (0.08)	− 0.05 (0.05)	1.51[b] (0.55)	− 0.05 (0.05)
Trust in strangers × PH					0.11 (0.08)	0.06 (0.04)
Trust in strangers × TH					0.17 † (0.10)	0.09 (0.05)

(continued)

Table 6 (continued)

	Model 1		Model 2		Model 3	
Predictors	Est	Beta	Est	Beta	Est	Beta
Trust in strangers × VN					0.20[c] (0.09)	0.11 (0.05)
Trust in most people × PH					0.07 (0.09)	0.04 (0.05)
Trust in most people × TH					− 0.07 (0.08)	− 0.04 (0.05)
Trust in most people × VN					− 0.15 † (0.09)	− 0.09 (0.05)
Trust in family × PH					− 0.33[b] (0.11)	− 0.15 (0.05)
Trust in family × TH					− 0.24[c] (0.11)	− 0.11 (0.05)
Trust in family × VN					− 0.36[b] (0.12)	− 0.16 (0.05)
Observations	4009		4009		4009	
R^2/R^2 adjusted	0.048/0.046		0.084/0.080		0.089/0.083	
AIC	15,316.606		15,181.835		15,177.393	
VIF	< 1.5		< 1.5		< 7.0	

[a] $p < 0.001$, [b] $p < 0.01$, [c] $p < 0.05$, [d] < 0.1

(see Table 4). Both types of trust are directed toward numerous people and can be called generalized trust; however, their characteristics are different.

These two qualities also differ with respect to their effects on individual well-being. In urbanized societies, where strangers are ubiquitous, trust no longer has a specific effect on well-being. However, in urban societies where social ties have weakened and hence the desire for various social ties has increased, trust in most people is likely to enhance individual well-being. This hypothesis is consistent with the data from East Asian societies, where trust laid on most of the people enhances well-being (Table 5). In contrast, in less urbanized societies, social ties are essential for survival but can also act as a source of peer pressure on the individual. Therefore, trust in most people is likely to reduce individuals' well-being (see Table 6), while at the same time yield enormous benefits in their daily life. Nevertheless, in societies where social ties are strong, strangers are extremely rare and hence are likely to appear attractive. The presence of strangers, such as tourists and individuals working in foreign companies, stand out and the material benefits of interacting with them are more pronounced. Alternatively, strangers may provide an oasis for peer pressure. In any case, trusting strangers was found to have a positive effect on the personal well-being in Southeast Asian societies (see Table 1.6).

In both cases, as suggested by our hypothesis, people try to mentally distance themselves from those who are physically close to them. In this sense, it is understandable that the effect of trust in family and that of neighbors on well-being seems to be higher in East Asia than in Southeast Asia. Although we cannot say for sure, considering the standard errors of the coefficients (see Tables 5 and 6), the results imply that the positive effect of emotional ties, such as family and neighbors, on well-being is higher in societies having weak social ties. On the contrary, in societies with strong social ties, this kind of trust may not contribute much to well-being. This trend has also been observed among East Asian societies. The effect of trust in most people on well-being in Japan is lower than in Taiwan and Korea (see Model 4 in Table 5). The results reflect that Japan is a homogeneous society, and peer pressure among most people is high in everyday life. The history of Japan also seems to prove that trust on the majority of people can quickly turn into peer pressure, which can be harmful not only to foreigners but also to the citizens. Apparently, people in Japan are aware of the violent nature of the concept of "most people."

This study argues that different social conditions have differential effects on trust. In recent years, the concept of social capital has become popular in social sciences, and many researchers have demonstrated its positive effects on the society and the individuals. However, this study raises the possibility that, even if social capital is bridging and open, its effects may vary from society to society. In urban societies, where social ties are generally weak, social capital is adequate for individual well-being. By contrast, in a less urbanized society having strong social ties and social capital can also lower individuals' well-being, even though it may offer solutions to many social problems.

In this context, this study emphasizes on the relationship between inclusion and exclusion. Any principle of social inclusion necessarily involves exclusivity; hence, inclusion and exclusion must be observed simultaneously. Luhmann (1995) uses the concept of "observer" to explain this relationship. We cannot see everything simultaneously; therefore, we always make something invisible while looking at something. If one looks forward, one cannot see backward, but if one looks backward, one cannot see forward. According to Luhmann, the nature of the observer depends on the inclusion principle: any principle of inclusion can be exclusive in some way or the other. Hence, the concerns expressed by Portes (1998) and Sen (2006) about the exclusivity of social capital cannot be dismissed, and it cannot simply be concluded that a broader range of trust avoids exclusivity. To ensure simultaneity of inclusion and exclusion, it is necessary to focus on "trust in strangers." Although Luhmann's way of considering inclusion through the concept of the "observer" is quite abstract, it fits well with the concept of the "stranger" because a stranger is a person who remains *invisible* (Luhmann, 1995). When we analyze ways of bridging social capital, we need to consider and investigate regarding the invisible people who fall through the cracks.

However, this study does not claim that trust in most people is imperfect and trust in strangers can be accurately measured. We must focus on the qualitative differences between those two variables. Trust in strangers has the potential to reduce the trust one has in the family members. The "thinking as usual" or sympathy cultivated within the family is a fundamental principle of trust in others and a basic human need. Trust in strangers, such as trust in most people, has a socially facilitative value but should never be pursued without considering when this kind of trust can be effective for individuals and societies.

For facilitating social well-being and achieving social diversity, the policies must distinguish between East Asian and Southeast Asian societies. The positive effect that trust in most people has on well-being in East Asian societies suggests that trust functions on a large scale to maintain diversity without any peer pressure. As a result, these societies are diverse. However, the fact that trust in strangers does not affect the well-being in East Asia suggests that people are already more interested in restoring social ties rather than in diversity. In this sense, these societies are not diverse. Therefore, it is necessary to consider policies that ensure that trust in strangers enhances individual well-being.

In Southeast Asian societies, trust in strangers enhances individual well-being. There is a high level of concern for those outside the community, and people are subjectively motivated to accept strangers. Thus, these societies are said to be diverse. However, trust in most people negatively impacts individuals' well-being. This may be attributed to the wide range of ties operant in peer pressure and exclusiveness. Hence, social diversity cannot be ensured. Therefore, further research should be conducted to explore the specific conditions under which trust can oppress individuals to a large extent.

In a society that lacks social integration, its promotion can enhance individual well-being, whereas in a society with strong social integration, creating relationships that hamper social integration can enhance individual well-being. From these perspectives, we should seek more flexible solutions depending on the context of each society.

5 Conclusions

We made a qualitative distinction between trust in most people and trust in strangers, based on the sociology of strangers that was initiated by Simmel, who explained strangers as mental distancing from physically close others. Trust in most people is based on more widespread trust that stems from the sympathy that one has for the family members, whereas trust in strangers depends upon the tolerance that temporarily suspends trustworthiness and sympathy. Trust in most people can result into warm relationships and enhancement of well-being, but it can also create peer pressure. Particularly in societies where social bonds are essential for survival and one cannot avoid such bonds, trust in most people can be oppressive to individuals. While on the contrary, trust in strangers does not impact well-being because it is a cold trust that is not based on sympathy. However, in societies where social ties are strong and strangers are scarce, trusting a stranger offers a way of escaping peer pressure and acting freely as an individual. Alternatively, trust in strangers facilitates dealing with outsiders such as tourists and provides material benefits that cannot be obtained from majority of members of the group. In such cases, it enhances an individual's well-being.

From this perspective, we first distinguished the following qualities of trust: Trust in most people correlates positively with trust in family members because it is based on sympathy and correlates with trust in strangers because it is broadly directed. In contrast, trust in strangers correlates positively with trust in most people because of its wide range but negatively with trust in the family because of the lack of sympathy. We analyzed the SoWSA data by employing partial correlations, and the results supported the hypothesis.

After identifying the qualitative difference between trust in most people and trust in strangers, we analyzed the different effects of trust on the Cantril ladder for individual well-being. We divided the SoWSA data into two groups: East Asia (Japan, South Korea, and Taiwan) and Southeast Asia (Indonesia, the Philippines, Thailand, and Vietnam), and assumed that East Asia is a more urbanized society, with weakened ties and surrounded by strangers, while Southeast Asia that is still undergoing urbanization, is characterized by strong social ties, but relatively few strangers. In East Asia, trust in strangers does not affect the well-being, whereas trust in most people positively affects the well-being of individuals. In Southeast Asia, trust in strangers affects well-being, whereas trust in most people has a negative effect on well-being. The results of OLS supported this hypothesis.

This study had certain limitations. It could not determine the relatively stable effect of both forms of trust in the model that examined the interaction effect between societies as compared to the models that integrate societies. The various causal mechanisms that differ from society to society could not be considered. In addition, whether the stability of the effect in the integrated models adequately reflected the characteristics of East Asia and Southeast Asia or was simply a result of the large sample size could not be examined. This survey was limited to seven Asian societies; hence, it could not be determined whether these results are valid only for Asian societies or can be generalized to other regions. The relationship between trusting strangers and individual well-being is perhaps more positive and significant in Western societies. However, considering the slogan "Überfremdung (over-foreignization)" that blames increasing "Fremde (strangers)" is being yelled in Germany, the difference between West and East Asia may not be so large.

References

Banton, M. (2008). The sociology of ethnic relations. *Ethnic and Racial Studies, 31*(7), 1267–1285.

Bauman, Z. (1998). Moderne und Ambivalenz. In U. Bielefeld (Ed.), *Das Eigene und das Fremde: neuer Rassismus in der Alten Welt?* (pp. 23–49). Hamburger Edition.

Beck, U. (1996). How neighbors become Jews: The political construction of the stranger in an age of reflexive modernity. *Constellations, 2*(3), 378–396.

Beck, U., & Beck-Gernsheim, E. (1994). Individualisierung in modernen Gesellschaften: Perspektiven und Kontroversen einer subjektorientierten Soziologie. In U. Beck & E. Beck-Gernsheim

(Eds.), *Riskante Freiheiten: Individualisierung in modernen Gesellschaften* (pp. 10–39). Suhrkamp Verlag.
Delhey, J., Newton, K., & Welzel, C. (2011). How general is trust in "most people"? Solving the radius of trust problem. *American Sociological Review, 76*(5), 786–807.
Fukuyama, F. (2001). Social capital, civil society and development. *Third World Quarterly, 22*(1), 7–20.
Giddens, A. (1990). *The consequences of modernity*. Polity Press.
Goffman, E. (1963). *Behavior in public places: Notes on the social organization of gatherings*. The Free Press.
Hahn, A. (1994). Die soziale Konstruktion des Fremden. In W. M. Sprondel (Ed.), *Die Objektivität der Ordnungen und ihre kommunikative Konstruktion: Für Thomas Luckmann*. Suhrkamp Verlag.
Helliwell, J. F. (2003). How's life? Combining individual and national variables to explain subjective well-being. *Economic Modelling, 20*(2), 331–360. https://doi.org/10.1016/s0264-9993(02)00057-3
Helliwell, J. F., Haifang, H., & Shun, W. (2016). The distribution of world happiness. In J. Helliwell, R. Layard & J. Sachs (Eds.), *World happiness report* (pp. 8–49). Sustainable Development Solutions Network.
Hellmann, K.-U. (1998). Fremdheit als soziale Konstruktion: Eine Studie zur Systemtheorie des Fremden. In H. Münkler (Ed.), *Die Herausforderung durch das Fremde* (pp. 401–459). Akademie Verlag.
International Consortium for Social Well-Being Studies. (2015–2017). Social Well-Being Survey in Asia, 2015–2017. (Indonesia) Universitas Indonesia, (Japan) Senshu University, (South Korea) Seoul National University, (The Philippines) Ateneo de Manila University, (Thailand) Chulalongkorn University, (Taiwan) Academia Sinica, (Vietnam) Vietnam Academy of Social Sciences[Producers]. Korea Social Science Data Archive (KOSSDA) [Distributors], 2020-06-25, A1-CUM-0022, V2.0, http://hdl.handle.net/20.500.12236/23941
Kobayashi, J., & Aldar, D. (2018). Inequality of well-being in Asia: A comparative analysis of happiness in eight countries. *The Senshu Social Well-Being Review, 5*, 75–82.
Luhmann, N. ([1968] 1973). *Vertrauen, ein Mechanismus der Reduktion sozialer Komplexität*. Ferdinand Enke Verlag.
Luhmann, N. (1995). Inklusion und Exklusion. In *Soziologische Aufklärung 6: Die Soziologie und der Mensch* (pp. 237–264). Westdeutscher Verlag.
Marotta, V. (2010). The Cosmopolitan Stranger. In H. Stan & W. Vandekerckhove (Eds.), *Questioning cosmopolitanism* (pp. 105–120). Springer.
Marotta, V. (2012). Georg Simmel, the stranger and the sociology of knowledge. *Journal of Intercultural Studies, 33*(6), 675–689.
Naef, M., & Schupp, J. (2009). Measuring trust: Experiments and surveys in contrast and combination. *SOEPpaper*, 167. https://doi.org/10.2139/ssrn.1367375
Nassehi, A. (1995). Der Fremde als Vertrauter. Soziologische Beobachtungen zur Konstruktion von Identitäten und Differenzen. *Kölner Zeitschrift für Soziologie und Sozialpsychologie, 47*(3), 443–463.
Pelinka, A. (2012). Populismus: zur Karriere eines Begriffes. In S. P. U. Institut (Ed.), *Populismus. Herausforderung oder Gefahr für die Demokratie?* (pp. 9–20). New Academic Press.
Portes, A. (1998). Social capital: Its origins and applications in modern sociology. *Annual Review of Sociology, 24*(1), 1–24.
Portes, A. (2014). Downsides of social capital. *Proceedings of the National Academy of Sciences, 111*(52), 18407–18408.
Putnam, R. D. (2000). *Bowling alone: The collapse and revival of American community*. Simon and Schuster.
Putnam, R. D., Leonardi, R., & Nanetti, R. Y. (1993). *Making democracy work: Civic institutions in modern Italy*. Princeton University Press.

Robison, L. J., Schmid, A. A., & Siles, M. E. (2002). Is social capital really capital? *Review of Social Economy, 60*(1), 1–21.
Rose, D. C. (2011). *The moral foundation of economic behavior*. Oxford University Press.
Rumford, C. (2013). *The globalization of strangeness*. Palgrave Macmillan.
Schütz, A. (2002 [1944]). Der Fremde. Ein sozialpsychologischer Versuch. In G. Wagner, & P. U. Merz-Benz (Eds.), *Der Fremde als sozialer Typus* (pp. 73–92). UVK Verlagsgesellschaft.
Sen, A. (2006). *Identity and violence: The illusion of destiny*. Penguin Books.
Simmel, G. (1903). Die Lehre Kants von Pflicht und Glück. *Das Freie Wort: Frankfurter Halbmonatsschrift Für Fortschritt Auf Allen Gebieten Des Geistigen Lebens, 3*(14), 548–553.
Simmel, G. (1908). *Soziologie: Untersuchungen über die Formen der Vergesellschaftung*. Duncker & Humblot.
Sombart, W. (1991 [1928]). *Der moderne Kapitalismus: Historisch-systematische Darstellung des gesamteuropäischen Wirtschaftslebens von seinen Anfängen bis zur Gegenwart*. DTV Deutscher Taschenbuch.
Stichweh, R. (2007). Fremdheit in der Weltgesellschaft: Indifferenz und Minimalsympathie. https://www.fiw.uni-bonn.de/demokratieforschung/personen/stichweh/pdfs/28_25stwfremdheitinderweltgesellschaft.pdf. Accessed May 30, 30, 2018.
Stichweh, R. (2010). *Der Fremde: Studien zu Soziologie und Sozialgeschichte*. Suhrkamp.
Stolle, D. (2002). Trusting strangers: The concept of generalized trust in perspective. *Österreichische Zeitschrift Für Politikwissenschaft, 31*(4), 397–412.
Sturgis, P., & Smith, P. (2010). Assessing the validity of generalized trust questions: What kind of trust are we measuring? *International Journal of Public Opinion Research, 22*(1), 74–92. https://doi.org/10.1093/ijpor/edq003
Tönnies, F. (2005). *Gemeinschaft und Gesellschaft: Grundbegriffe der reinen Soziologie*. Wissenschaftliche Buchgesellschaft.
Yazaki, K. (2018). Sympathy or tolerance? A comparison of the effects of trusting most people and trusting strangers in Asian societies. *The Senshu Social Well-Being Review, 5*, 21–36.
Yazaki, K. (2019). Social inclusion in systems theory: Art and science as blind spot observatioin. *Social Well-Being Kenkyu Ronsyu, 5*, 47–65.

Keitaro Yazaki is an Assistant Professor of Sociology at a Department of Fine Arts, Tainan University of Technology. His research focuses on social system theory, sociology of art, well-being. He is also a member of the Center for Social Well-being Studies at Senshu University.

War Experience, Fear of War, and Social Unrest

Kiyohisa Shibai

Abstract This study examines the correlation among people's war experiences, happiness, and social unrest in both ordinary and extraordinary situations. War can radically transform societies, and often has severe negative impacts, including the loss of social capital. Therefore, even in ordinary situations (i.e., the daily lives of citizens), the experience of war is expected to cause unhappiness and degradation of the values of social capital. The fear of war can result in social unrest because people lose trust in the government, which is the only organization that can prevent wars. Moreover, this fear of war causes the security dilemma, which can trigger social unrest in extraordinary situations involving a direct threat of war. However, research has yet to derive a complete understanding of how war experiences negatively impact people's lives in ordinary and extraordinary situations. This study uses survey data from numerous countries in the Asia–Pacific region containing a diverse range of cultures and war experiences to analyze the effects of war experience and fear of war on people's happiness, values of social capital, and distrust in the government.

Keywords War experience · Fear of war · Happiness · Social capital · Trust in government

1 Introduction

Preventing war outbreaks is one of the most important challenges for international and domestic societies. Wars involving the use of modern weaponry typically lead to higher casualties, destroy social industries, and have a severely negative impact on social capital. Even among populations with access to substantial social capital, including strong family ties, large number of friends, and strong local community, war can radically affect people's lives. Once a war breaks out, it would be impossible for

K. Shibai (✉)
Joint Support-Center for Data Science Research (ROIS-DS), The Institute of Statistical Mathematics, Tokyo, Japan
e-mail: kshibai@ism.ac.jp

J. Yee et al. (eds.), *Social Well-Being, Development, and Multiple Modernities in Asia*, https://doi.org/10.1007/978-981-97-3866-3_15

a single person to stop it. According to Putnam (2000, 2002, 2007), social solidarity and social capital can be inhibited by social change, such as immigration, in the short and medium terms. It is clear that war-related damage causes radical societal changes with severe causalities and loss of social capital. Therefore, war experiences and fear of war are expected to give rise to social unrest caused by the fear of losing social capital.

However, scant research has been conducted on war experiences and their impact on social capital. The experience of war is a multifaceted phenomenon that differs for each person, nation, state, and region. Memories of war vary substantially based on age, residential area, and nation, and have a substantial effect on the value and ethics of people experiencing them. In addition, the repercussions of the memories of war depend on an individual's life and national history. Therefore, comparative analyses of different national contexts through which citizens have derived various war experiences may be useful in understanding the effects of war on social unrest.

Based on the research questions described above, the current study focused on three main academic issues (hypotheses):

(1) The correlations between war experiences and happiness, as well as that of war experiences and fear of war,
(2) The correlations between war experiences and citizens' values of social capital, which can affect the mental health of a whole citizenry and is a potential cause of social unrest, and
(3) The correlations between fear of war and trust in the state, which brings about social unrest.

The first correlation is conducted to examine whether past war experiences influence people's happiness and fear of future wars. The first correlation is needed to analyze with the second and third issues because the analysis of the first serves as the basis of this study.

To examine the second correlation, this study analyzes whether what kind of past war experience affected citizens' values of social capital which was destroyed by wars in detail. If war experiences lead to negative effects on values of social capital, which positively affects people's daily lives, they indirectly influence the social order.

To examine the third issue, the current study analyzes whether citizens' fear of war affects their trust in the government. The objective of this study is to elucidate the direct effects of war experience on society and determine whether it leads to social unrest. Distrust in the government can destabilize the social order and exacerbate the fear of war, because it is impossible for citizens to prevent wars or safeguard themselves against it. If a government does not adequately respond to citizens' fear, their anxiety related to war may increase, thereby impacting social order, and this chain reaction may repeat in a cycle. This issue is examined by focusing on extraordinary situations wherein people were aware of direct war threats. The effect is likely to be stronger in democratic states, compared with nondemocratic states. Politicians in a democracy are likely to be concerned about public opinion and future election prospects to a greater extent than those in nondemocratic states, because they are more directly affected by the "audience cost" (Fearon, 1994; Tomz, 2007). Therefore, high audience cost is more likely to occur in a democratic state.

Distrust in government is related to insufficient social capital because damages caused by war can lead people to lose their lives and assets, thereby causing them to lose trust in the government. War and the fear of war can lead to citizens' disapproval of the government. War damage causes a decline in government support due to the adverse effects on nation's lives, such as economics, social welfare, infrastructure, social networks, and families and friends. In addition, war often leads to other problems, such as terrorism, genocide, and refugees. They significantly destroy victims' social capital. Citizens cannot protect themselves from such disasters. Only the government has the capability to protect the nation from such problems. Therefore, losing or fear of losing social capital is correlated to distrust in the government.

Citizens understand the underlying causes that lead to their loss of social capital and thus complain about the government causing them to incur such losses. Complaints about and distrust in the government can accumulate if a war continues over the course of several years or repeats multiple times. The accumulated burden of war, which continuously damages the nation's social capital, eventually becomes the burden and dissatisfaction of the citizens. Therefore, in this study, it is assumed that the degree of trust in the government reflects the nation's experiences of war and losing social capital, albeit in a partial one, and social unrest and distrust in government caused by war experiences are correlated to loss of social capital.

The third correlation is related to social unrest and the outbreak of war. In the past, policymakers have sometimes decided to engage in undesired wars due to changes in security and defense policies and deepening mutual distrust. This cause-and-effect relationship is known as the "security dilemma," which is a serious cause of war and fear of war being repeated several times. For example, if State A's armament policy for defense is considered aggressive by rival State B, State B may proceed with further armament for defense; then if State A also considers State B's policy to be aggressive, this continuation of mutual uncertainty can lead to war if mutual distrust peaks, despite each state selecting their policies for their own security, rather than to attack each other (Glaser, 1992, 1997, 2000; Herz, 1950; Jervis, 1976, 1978; Montgomery, 2006; Roe, 2005). Jervis (1978: 169) explained the security dilemma as follows: "many of the means by which a state tries to increase its security decrease the security of others." The security dilemma can lead to the development of nuclear weapons, as noted in the case of North Korea. The threat of war and security dilemma can disturb the social order, thereby causing citizens and governments to become unstable.

In this study, war is considered to constitute conflicts between states, as well as those within states. Interstate wars have decreased in recent years, and the biggest state powers have not directly engaged in war with each other since World War II. In contrast, particularly in the post-Cold War period, intrastate violence and ethnic conflicts have been responsible for large numbers of deaths internationally. Data from the Uppsala Conflict Data Program (UCDP) indicate that many casualties have been noted in Southeast Asian countries (Table 1), mostly in intrastate and ethnic conflicts, including anti-government insurgencies. Therefore, in this study, "war" is also used to refer to interstate wars and intrastate conflicts. Both types of war severely impact social unrest and induce the fear of violence among citizens.

The security dilemma can also emerge in intrastate conflicts because a key element of it comprises windows of opportunity and vulnerability (Van Evera, 1984). Posen (1993) argued that "Isolated ethnic groups—ethnic islands—can produce incentives for preventive war." Some theorists have argued that perceived offensive advantages make preventive war more attractive; if one side has an advantage that will not be present later, and if security can be achieved through offensive military action, leaders will be inclined to attack during this "window of opportunity." Posen (1993: 32–33) provided the following example: "If a surrounding population will ultimately be able to fend off relief attacks from the home territory of an island group's brethren, but is currently weak, then the brethren will be inclined to attack sooner rather than later." Various studies have examined intrastate conflicts involving security dilemmas (Arfi, 1998; Lake & Rothchild, 1996; Pischedda, 2018; Posen, 1993; Roe, 2005). Roe (2005: 4) provided the following description of the societal security dilemma: "With European security no longer concerned so much about security dilemmas between states, security dilemmas between societies thus seem to acquire some importance." Furthermore, Arfi (1998: 152) noted that "social identity endows social interactions with predictability around a set of expectations, a necessary ingredient to sustain social life. Changes in the social identities of ethnic groups destabilize established patterns of interethnic relations, decrease interethnic predictability, and create uncertainty about future relations."

Although the security dilemma is an overarching theory of armed conflict, its internal processes, such as how the fear of war affects citizens' lives and public opinion, and how such social unrest affects policy-making, have yet to be explained. This study investigates the detailed effects of security dilemmas on societies in real-world situations.

Figure 1 shows why the exchange of armaments for a country's own security can eventually lead to war. However, it is unclear how the fear of war affects societies and how governments deal with challenges to social order. Understanding the direct

Table 1 Number of deaths in 1989–2017 (UCDP)[a]

	Total number of deaths	State-based violence	Non-state violence	One-sided violence
Indonesia (ID)	8113	3627	2119	2367
Japan (JP)	0	0	0	0
South Korea (KR)	0	0	0	0
Philippines (PH)	19,003	17,477	220	1306
Thailand (TH)	4077	2168	6	1903
Taiwan (TW)	0	0	0	0
Vietnam (VN)	0	0	0	0

[a] UCDP Battle-Related Deaths Dataset ver. 18.1, UCDP One-sided Violence ver. 18.1, Dataset, and UCDP Non-State Conflict Dataset ver. 18.1

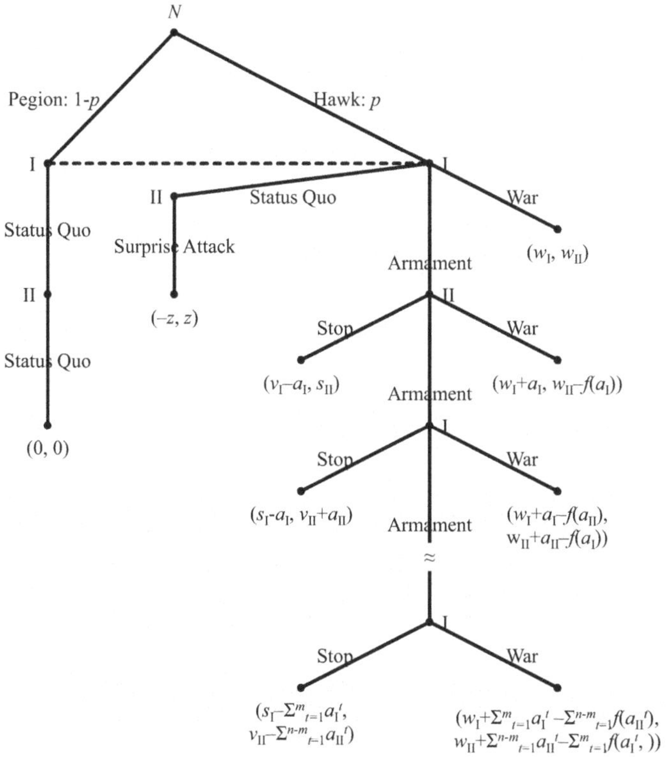

Fig. 1 Process of the security dilemma[1]

and indirect effects of war experience and fear of war on society can elucidate the processes underlying the security dilemma. In addition, clarifying these issues can reveal whether high social capital can prevent the deepening of the security dilemma, because multiple human networks, reciprocity, and revitalization of communities can weaken the fundamental basis of the dilemma. According to Butterfield (1951: 21), the fundamental basis of the dilemma is uncertainty among individuals: "For you know that you yourself mean him no harm, and that you want nothing from him save guarantees for your own safety; and it is never possible for you to realise or remember properly that since he cannot see the inside of your mind, he can never have the same assurance of your intentions that you have."

---

[1] w: profit by selecting War. s: profit by selecting Stop. a: cost for Armament. v: profit by the rival selecting Stop. $f(a)$: utility function of the effect on the rival's expected utility of War and Stop. m: the number of player I's selecting Armament in the period n. (SQ, SQ) becomes the Nash equilibrium if player II is the Pigeon type. In this game, it is an incomplete information that a player i can select Armament or not in a time t: this figure assumes I cannot Armament at last. A preference order of Hawk type is $z > v > s = w > 0$. Pigeon type's preference order is $z > v > 0 > w = s$. Player I's preference order is $v > 0 > w = s > -z$. Player I selects Armament at t because of $w_I < w_I + a_I$ and $s_I - f(a_I) < w_I + a_I$. Players selecting more Armament will get more loss if they choose Stop

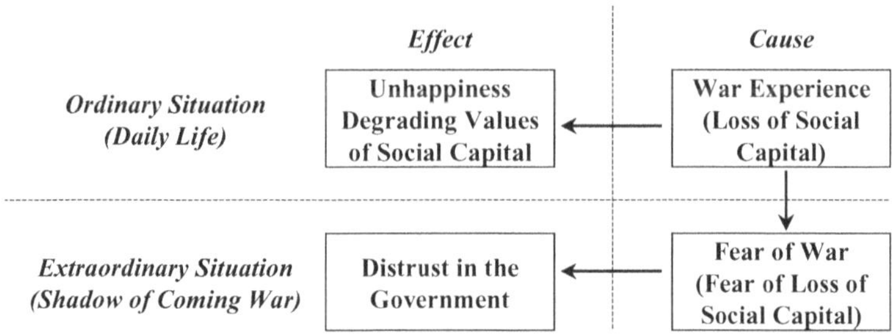

Fig. 2 Depiction of the research question

Therefore, the security dilemma leads to increased fear of war, which will, in turn, lead to loss of the nation's social capital, thereby causing people to lose confidence in their government.

The relationships among the three issues are explained in Fig. 2. Understanding past war experiences is the starting point of this study, because war experiences affect social capital and fear of war. The primary research question in this study is how the war experience affects daily life and the extraordinary situation in the presence of signs that the security dilemma or war is threatened. If both the extraordinary and ordinary situations become exacerbated by the war experience, it indicates that war experience is a serious cause of social unrest and declining social order.

To analyze these three topics, this study analyzed two cross-national comparative surveys: the Social Well-being Survey in Asia (SoWSA) version 2.0 and the Cross-National Comparative Survey on National Character in the 2000s and 2010s (hereinafter, the survey conducted in the 2000s is abbreviated as PRVS, and the other is abbreviated as APVS) (Yoshino, 2009, 2015). The SoWSA includes data regarding social capital, which enables the analysis of ordinary situations. The PRVS and APVS include data related to fear of war, thus enabling the analysis of extraordinary situations, although differences in the data used restricts the analysis to correlations between the two situations.

2 Data and Methods

East Asia (Northeast and Southeast Asia) comprises many countries with distinct cultures, political institutions, and economic development features. Residents of East Asia have a range of experiences of armed conflict and violence. Many wars have broken out in this region in the process of gaining independence from former colonies,

---

because the costs of choosing Armament and the expected loss produced by the rival's Armament cumulatively increase. They keep selecting Armament until one of both cannot select it. The final decision is War, unless the value of an expected war cost $\sum_{t=1}^{n-m} f\left(a_{\mathrm{II}}^{t}\right))$ is higher than $2 \cdot \sum_{t=1}^{m} a_{\mathrm{I}}^{t}$.

confrontations between democratic and communist governments, and ethnic and religious enmity. According to the UCDP, 19,003 people were killed in the Philippines during the post-Cold War era (1989–2017) due to state-based, non-state, and one-sided violence. In contrast, no person has been killed due to these three types of violence in Japan during this period. Interstate wars can completely destroy societies, and intrastate conflicts also disrupt social communities and depress social capital, which is closely related to "civic virtue" (Putnam, 2000: 19). People find it difficult to accept morality and virtue when their lives are in jeopardy. Based on the aforementioned issues, this study presents a hypothesis that the experience of armed conflict and violence will negatively impact people's daily lives.

Before analyzing the research hypotheses, basic information about the study samples was summarized. Table 2 shows the level of well-being in the populations of interest. A high proportion of the populations in Indonesia, the Philippines, Thailand, and Vietnam reported being happy or very happy: more than 40% respondents answered with scores ranging from 8 to 10. In contrast, Japanese, Korean, and Taiwanese respondents reported lower happiness levels, and more than 10% respondents in these populations reported scores between 0 and 3. The two groups are clearly distinguished by the region and level of economic development. Happier populations were located in developing countries in Southeast Asia, whereas the less happy populations were located in developed countries in Northeast Asia. These distributions are in accordance with an explanation based on social capital, wherein it is predicted that even wealthy people will not feel happy if the human networks and local communities wherein they live have fallen into decay.

Furthermore, these countries can be distinguished based on their public order. Table 1 shows the number of deaths caused by armed conflict between 1989 and 2017. The data shows that there have been no war casualties in Northeast Asia, whereas many people have been killed in armed conflicts in Southeast Asian countries during this period. These results indicate that the war experiences of nations in East Asia are diverse. However, even countries with few conflict-related deaths may experience security problems. Vietnam, Taiwan, and Japan have experienced serious territorial disputes with China, which may result in armed conflict in the future. Moreover, South Korea is in a state of war with North Korea. Such problems can impinge on

Table 2 Response rates of respondents' happiness (0–10 scores) (SoWSA)

	0–3 scores	4–7 scores	8–10 scores	*N*
ID	0.013	0.402	0.585	1249
JP	0.130	0.535	0.335	11,804
KR	0.137	0.625	0.238	2000
PH	0.041	0.515	0.444	1137
TH	0.012	0.410	0.577	1126
TW	0.108	0.625	0.267	2303
VN	0.024	0.374	0.602	1202

people's perspectives. Although no war deaths have been noted in Vietnam since the Cold War, many Vietnamese people have experienced prolonged armed conflict for independence and unity, including the Indochina War and the Vietnam War. These war experiences have been reported to exert an influence Vietnamese values (Shibai, 2015).

In the current analysis, I examined people's experience of war using data from the UCDP and Correlates of War (COW) datasets (Interstate war data version 4.0). Four types of wars were included in the UCDP: Side A, Side A2, Side B, and Side B2 (UCDP/PRIO armed conflict dataset version 18.1). Side A includes the country/countries on the offensive side in a conflict and the government side in internal conflicts. Thus, this database includes respondents who are part of the primary party in the conflict. Side A2 refers to a party that supports Side A in the conflict. Side B refers to the country/countries on the defensive side of a conflict. Internal conflict includes militarized opposition organizations, which are primary parties in the conflict. Side B2 refers to a party that supports Side B in the conflict.

I classified the war experience based on these four types and measured the number of war experiences within each person's living years. I classified war records before 1945 in the COW based on these four types and added the data along with that of the UCDP, because the UCDP does not include data before 1945 (Table 3). For example, the number of war experiences for Side A in Japan in 1940 was one because Japan attacked China. There were two Side A in Japan in 1941, because Japan attacked China and the United States. Therefore, the total number of war experiences in Side A in Japan from 1940 to 1941 was three. Consequently, the data for Japanese individuals aged 70 in 2015 (surveyed year) were as follows: two war experiences for Side A, because Japan attacked China and India in 1945; one war experience for Side A2, because Japan supported the United States in 2002; one war experience for Side B, because Japan was attacked by the United States in 1945; and no war experiences for Side B2.

People in the Philippines, Thailand, and Indonesia have many war experiences, because several ethnic conflicts and anti-government armed insurgencies have occurred in these countries. A high number of war experiences are noted for Side A because state forces engaged in conflict in these cases. Table 3 shows distinctions in the number of war experiences and includes many zero values.

The number of war experiences of a person is directly proportional to their age, but the numbers of each type are diverse. Distinctions among divergent war experience are important. Both Side A and B war experiences cause deterioration of the living environment, tax increases, and military casualties, but only Side B causes the destruction of society and civilian deaths. Therefore, the experience of Side B is expected to lead to greater fear of war and social unrest, compared with the experience of Side A.

To express the cumulative pain of prolonged war, the number of war experiences is measured in years. The reason is that when the war extends for a longer period, more damage occurs. For example, the Vietnam War (1965–75) counts as 10, and not 1, if a sample had lived experiences of the war. The measuring method used can

Table 3 Number of war experiences in each country (COW and UCDP)

	Age	Side A	Side A2	Side B	Side B2		Age	Side A	Side A2	Side B	Side B2
ID	70	47	5	4	0	TH	70	25	9	6	4
	60	45	5	0	0		60	24	9	6	0
	50	36	5	0	0		50	24	7	6	0
	40	31	5	0	0		40	21	0	6	0
	30	16	5	0	0		30	15	0	3	0
	20	10	5	0	0		20	15	0	1	0
	10	0	5	0	0		10	11	0	1	0
JP	70	2	1	1	0	TW	70	0	0	5	0
	60	0	1	0	0		60	0	0	1	0
	50	0	1	0	0		50	0	0	0	0
	40	0	1	0	0		40	0	0	0	0
	30	0	1	0	0		30	0	0	0	0
	20	0	1	0	0		20	0	0	0	0
	10	0	0	0	0		10	0	0	0	0
KR	70	0	19	5	0	VN	70	0	11	43	19
	60	0	19	0	0		60	0	11	34	19
	50	0	19	0	0		50	0	11	24	17
	40	0	10	0	0		40	0	11	13	3
	30	0	10	0	0		30	0	5	3	0
	20	0	10	0	0		20	0	0	0	0
	10	0	9	0	0		10	0	0	0	0
PH	70	104	5	0	4						
	60	95	5	0	0						
	50	95	5	0	0						
	40	82	1	0	0						
	30	62	1	0	0						
	20	44	1	0	0						
	10	26	0	0	0						

reflect the scale of each war and each person's experience in the data, albeit to a limited extent.

In the Asia–Pacific region, many political disputes and armed conflicts occurred in the 2000s and 2010s. The most serious conflicts included the India–Pakistan conflict, which involved rivalry based on nuclear powers; the North Korean nuclear development; the territorial disputes between China and Japan, Taiwan, and many Southeastern countries; and ethnic conflicts in multinational countries, such as Philippines and Indonesia. The PRVS and APVS data showed variance in fear of war in

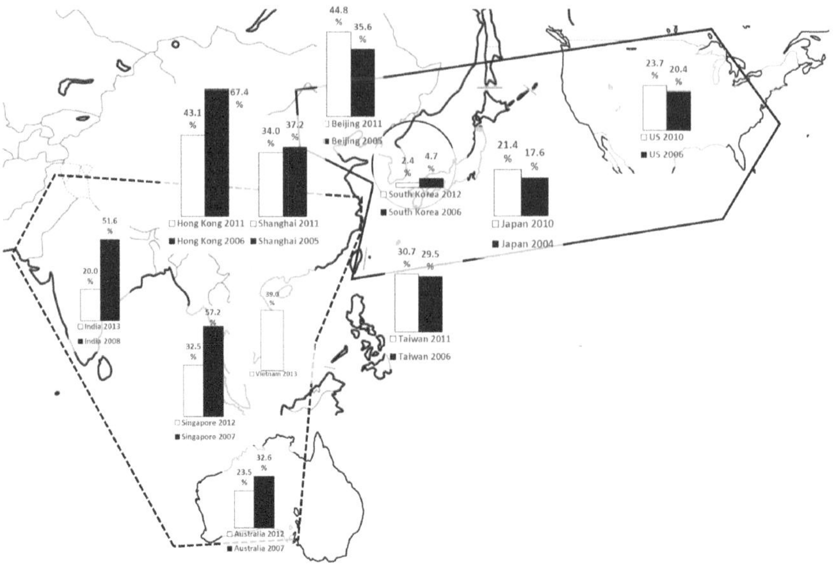

Fig. 3 Response rates of the fear of war in the 2000s and 2010s (PRVS and APVS)

the 2000s and 2010s (Fig. 3). Trends in fear of war can be distinguished based on location. In the northeast, fear of war increased slightly during the 2010s. In contrast, fear drastically decreased, compared to that of the 2000s, in the southwest, where many citizens had a strong fear of war in the 2000s. The most unique case was noted in South Korea, on the Korean peninsula, the center of armed conflicts in the Asia–Pacific region. People in South Korea did not report fear of war in the 2000s and 2010s in both relative or absolute terms. The data indicated that people in South Korea did not fear war more than they did 20 years ago, because the response rate for fear of war did not change from the 2000s to 2010s, despite North Korea developing nuclear weapons and the confrontation between North Korea and the United States deteriorating further. The diversity of values regarding war experiences is academically interesting and supports the need for analyzing the relationship between the war experience and social capital.

3 Results

To ascertain the psychological effects of the war experience, this study analyzed the relationships between the war experience and social capital, fear of war and social capital, and fear of war and trust in the state. Shibai (2018) reported several findings regarding the fear of war: education level and income were negatively correlated with fear of war; people's fear of war was correlated with dissatisfaction in their own lives and/or families; and those who supported the state tended to worry about war more than others.

The war experience, particularly memories of one's homeland being attacked, tends to influence citizens, regardless of the number of war experiences. For example, Americans have particularly strong memories of the 9/11 terrorist attack (Svendsen & Campbell, 2010). The coefficients in the current analysis indicate two possibilities regarding the effects of war experiences: the experience of offensive wars may decrease fear of war, and more importantly, defensive wars may increase fear of war. These results partially correspond to conventional understanding of the effects of memories of war-related damage to one's homeland and resistance to self-determination, which can lead to increased fear of invasion because experiencing war-related casualties plays a key role in the development of national memories, national identities, and nationalism (Grant, 2005; Harrison, 2003; Hutchinson, 2007; Schori-Eyal et al., 2015; Smith, 1981, 2009; Svendsen & Campbell, 2010). It is clear that wars often impact nations' values, although previous research has focused exclusively on historically important or "great" wars. Grant (2005: 521) explained the American national identity and the effect of the war experience as a myth: "It was in the context of Memorial Day rituals and against the backdrop of the Civil War cemeteries that America constructed its own version of what Mosse termed the 'Myth of the War Experience', a myth 'designed to mask war and to legitimize the war experience', reshaping it into 'a sacred experience which provided the nation with a new depth of religious feeling, putting at its disposal ever-present saints and martyrs, places of worship, and a heritage to emulate'."

According to the COW data, the number of battle deaths on the defensive side after World War II was notably higher than that of the offensive side (the average number of battle deaths on the offensive side was 21,395.84, and the average number on the defensive side was 29,731.93). In addition, the number of battle deaths for countries on the offensive side in the post-Cold War period was zero for some countries. However, the indirect effects of war are likely to affect citizens' values.

The following analysis is divided into three steps. The first step is to focus on the correlations between war experience and happiness, and between war experience and fear of war. The second step analyzes the correlation between war experience and values of social capital to determine whether the war experience influences citizens' values in daily life. The third step explores the effect of the fear of war to assess whether past experience of war affects the likelihood of fear of future wars.

Correlations between war experience and happiness. Wars destroy social infrastructures, and damage the human networks that social capital is based on. Happiness is also decreased due to war in the long term. By examining the correlations between war experience and happiness, this section focuses on the basic variables of the samples, thus clarifying the distribution of happiness.

Table 4 shows simple correlations among happiness and war experience, damage experience against war, and current life with the multivariate analysis and the SoWSA data: "How happy are you currently?" (happy); "When did your household experience the following things latest?—War or armed conflict" (past_exp); "Which of the following large disasters or damages apply in the following questions?—War" (damage); "Which of the following large disasters or damages apply in the following questions?"—War (res_area); and "How satisfied are you currently with the following?—Current life overall" (current_life).

There were no clear patterns in common among the nations. Past_exp is significant at the 5% level in Indonesia, Japan, and Taiwan. Damage is significant at the 5% level only in South Korea and Thailand. Res_area is significant in South Korea, Philippines, Taiwan, and Vietnam. There is no country in which all past_exp, damage, and res_area is significant at the 5% level. However, the results indicate that war in residential areas impacts many countries.

Few interactions are noted among past_exp, damage, and res_area at the 5% level. The effects of war experiences is expected to not be strong among East Asian people, contrary to the clear effect of current_life. The most significant variables and interactions are noted in Japan, but these results should be verified carefully because almost all Japanese samples (11,291/11,786) answered "never experienced" in past_exp.

It is important to note that correlations exist between the war experience and social capital variables. The interaction between past_exp and current_life is significant in Japan and Vietnam, and the interaction among past_exp, res_area, and current_life is significant in the Philippines and Vietnam. These results indicate that war experience has little effect on social capital. Only Japan has many interactions, but these results

Table 4 *P*-value of analysis of variance between happiness scores and war experience (SoWSA)

	ID	JP	KR	PH	TH	TW	VN
Dependent variable: happiness score (0–10 scores)							
Past_exp	*	***				*	
Damage			*		*		
Res_area			**	***		**	*
Current_life	***	***	***	***	***	***	***
Past_exp: damage							*
Past_exp: res_area				**			**
Damage: res_area		***					
Past_exp: current_life		***					**
Damage: current_life		*					
Res_area: current_life		*	*				
Past_exp: damage: res_area		*					
Past_exp: damage: current_life		**					
Past_exp: res_area: current_life				*			*
Damage: res_area: current_life		*					
Past_exp: damage: res_area: current_life							

Significance codes: 0***, 0.001**, 0.01*, 0.05

must be considered carefully because the reason for this outcome is believed to be the number of Japanese samples.

3.1 Correlations Between War Experience and Fear of War

This section examines the correlation between war experience and the fear of war by using data from the PRVS and APVS. The objective is to verify the effects of war experience in extraordinary situations wherein war was likely to break out, rather than in citizens' daily lives. This question is also closely related to the security dilemma theory. The fear of war can cause the security dilemma if it weakens citizens' trust in the state and instils social unrest. Governments must cope with the distrust of citizens, thereby making their inadequate policy and social unrest part of the internal process of the security dilemma. In the PRVS and APVS, the age of the samples was encoded as classified age data in intervals of 5 years; thus, the war experience data were also changed to mean values within these intervals.

The correlation between war experience and fear of war is confirmed to some extent with the combination data of PRVS and APVS. Countries that have a correlation between fear of war and Side A are China, Taiwan, and India. Countries that have a correlation between fear of war and Side B are China, South Korea, and India. There is no interaction between Sides A and A2. The interaction between Sides B and B2 is significant only in the Australian data. These results reveal that war experiences have an effect on fear of war, especially when a country is the primary player in the war. The derived results allow this study to address the next issue (Table 5).

Table 5 *P*-value of analysis of variance between war experience and fear of war (PRVS and APVS)

	JP	CN	TW	KR	AU	SG	IN	VN
Dependent variable: fear of war (4 very much > 3 somewhat > 2 slightly > 1 not at all)								
Side A		***	**				**	
Side A2				*		***	***	
Side B		***		***			***	
Side B2					**			
Side A: Side A2								
Side A: Side B							**	
Side A: Side B2								
Side A2: Side B		*						
Side A2: Side B2								
Side B: Side B2					**			

Significance codes: 0***, 0.001**, 0.01*, 0.05
There is no significant interaction among 3 or more variables

3.2 Correlations Between War Experience and Values of Social Capital

According to Putnam (2000), the presence of a high level of social capital has a positive impact on children's health and growth, safer and improved education, longer lifespan, happiness, democratic institutions, and economic institutions. Social capital has multiple effects, in terms of reciprocity, including public health, education, politics, and the economy. If the war experience has any effect on these factors, the war experience and values of social capital is expected to be negatively correlated. It is assumed to be more difficult for people to have positive thoughts if they have experienced a sudden loss or fear of loss of social capital in the past.

Table 4 indicates few interactions among the variables of war experience and social capital. Only Japanese people have interactions between war experience and social capital. There is only an interaction between past_exp and current_life in Korea, and interactions among past_exp, res_area, and current_life in the Philippines and Vietnam. Unfortunately, this interaction is rarely observed.

Therefore, this study conducted a principal components analysis (PCA) to derive detailed results on correlations among the variables—war experience, social capital, happiness, and attributes (gender, education, and the number of family)—because correlations are noted among each value of social capital and each war experience.

The PCA results are as shown in Fig. 4. Unfortunately, there are no key differences or patterns. The variables of war experience and attributions are plotted together, and the variables of social capital are plotted on the opposite side. The results show that the study hypothesis about war experience and variables of social capital being negatively correlated is not supported by the data, and war experience and social capital are independent of each other in all of the East Asian countries, which have unique cultural characteristics.

Indonesia, Philippines, and Thailand, wherein many conflict-related casualties have occurred, exhibit a common feature—the plot of Side A is isolated from the other plots. The plots of Side B are located at almost (0, 0). The plots of war experience in the other countries are also not close to social capital, but are near (0, 0). Overall, these results indicate that the war experience is largely independent of social capital and happiness, or that war experience has almost no effect. The factors affecting social capital are correlated with happiness in all the countries examined, but these factors of war experience are not related to social capital.

The previous analyses—the analysis of variance and PCA—did not support the hypothesis of correlations between war experience and the values of social capital. To determine any correlation between war experience and the values of social capital, an additional analysis is performed for the effects of war experience and social capital in ordinary situations.

To comprehensively clarify the correlations among war experience, happiness, and social capital, this section examines data regarding the war experience and citizens' satisfaction levels with relation to social capital: current life, family life, married

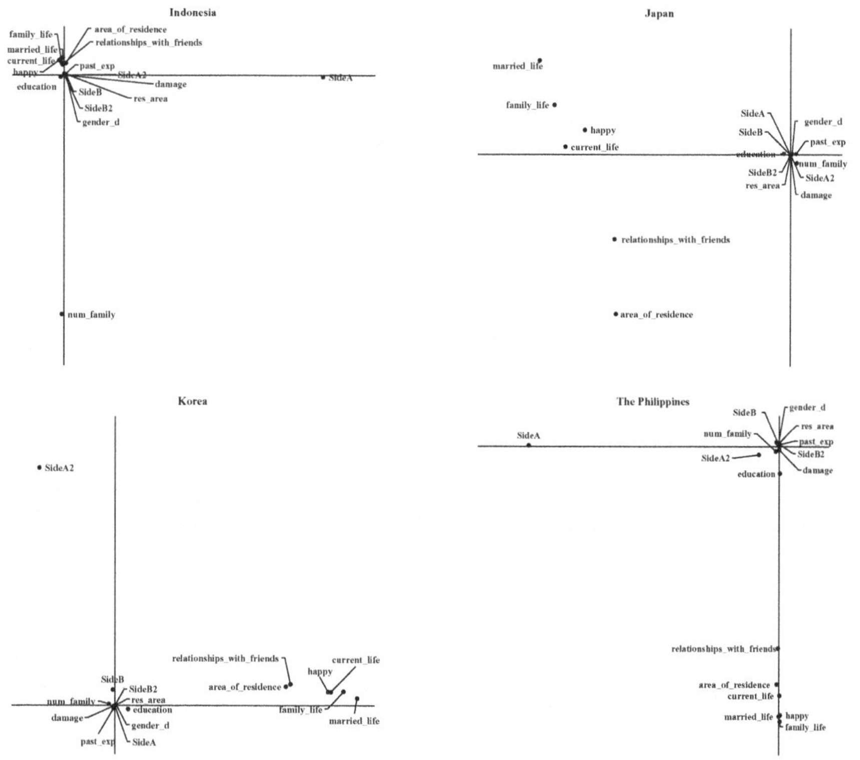

Fig. 4 PCA of happiness, war experience, and social capital (SoWSA)

life, relationships with friends, and area of residence. The number of a nation's war experiences is included as more detailed information on war experience.

Table 6 shows the results of regression analysis for each country with more detailed independent variables. In this analysis, almost all variables of war experience are not significant, and the significant variables are only Side A in Indonesia, res_area in Taiwan, and damage in Vietnam. The coefficient of Side A in Indonesia is negative, which supports the first hypothesis. However, the regression analysis also indicates no interaction effect between war experience and social capital because almost no significant effect is noted for detailed variables of war experience and the variables of values of social capital have a significant effect, regardless of war experience, which is typically consistent with the social capital theory.

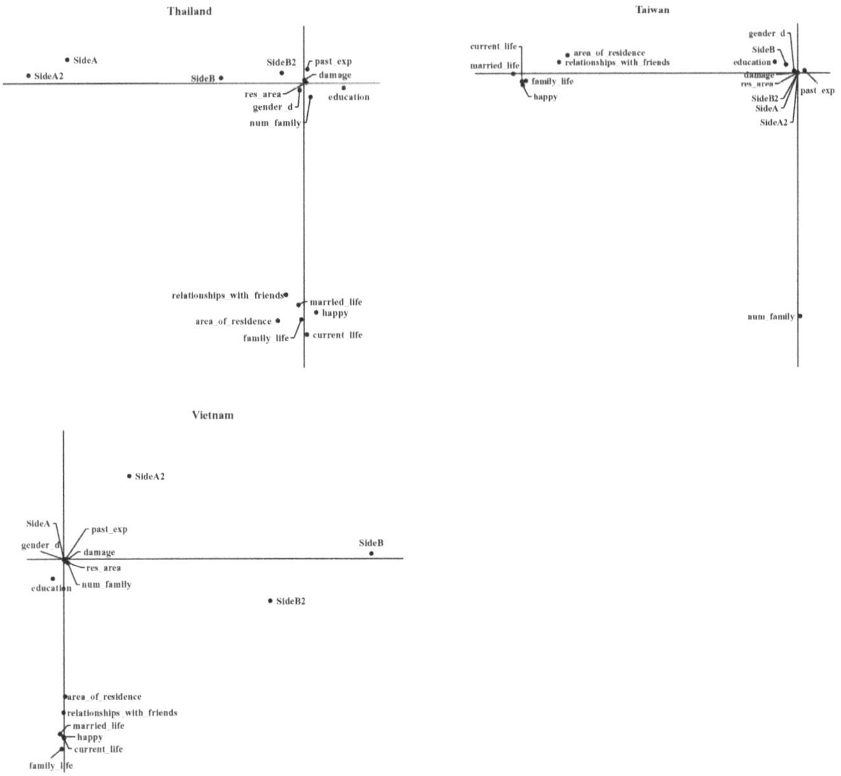

Fig. 4 (continued)

3.3 *Correlations Between Fear of War and Trust in the Government*

The correlation between fear of war and trust in the state is then analyzed. To derive detailed results regarding general trends in the effects of fear of war in extraordinary situations, regression analyses of data from each country is used in this section. Two survey topics of PRVS and APVS were useful for measuring citizens' trust in the state: the level of trust in the national government bureaucracy, and the level of trust in the national assembly (congress). These two factors are measured using a 4-point Likert scale: very confident (4), somewhat confident (3), not confident (2), and not confident at all (1). The relationship between fear of war and trust in the state indicates that governments lose citizens' trust when citizens' fear of war becomes exacerbated, because this situation indicates that the government has not utilized adequate countermeasures to address security problems.

The results of these analyses are presented in Tables 7 and 8. Table 7 shows the effects of war experience on fear of war. Although the amount of data for each war

Table 6 Effects of war experience on happiness (estimates and *p*-values) (SoWSA)

	ID		JP		KR		PH	
Dependent variable: happiness score (0–10 scores)								
Adjusted R^2	0.341		0.714		0.802		0.431	
Past_exp	0.092		0.051		0.044		0.039	
Damage	– 0.005		0.519		0.311		– 0.399	
Res_area	0.036		– 0.022		– 0.300		– 0.179	
Side A	– 0.011	**	n.a.		n.a.		– 0.002	
Side A2	n.a.		n.a.		0.000		– 0.025	
Side B	– 0.200		n.a.		0.020		n.a.	
Side B2	n.a.		n.a.		n.a.		– 0.028	
Current_life	0.275	***	0.503	***	0.728	***	0.415	***
Family_life	0.091	*	0.219	***	0.160	***	0.106	*
Married_life	0.210	***	0.074	***	0.030		0.241	***
Relationships_with_friends	0.102	**	0.043	***	0.006		0.118	***
Area_of_residence	0.068	*	0.016	*	0.014		– 0.009	
Number_of_family	– 0.005		0.022	*	0.034		0.027	
	TH		TW		VN			
Adjusted R^2	0.503		0.748		0.594			
Past_exp	– 0.030		0.042		0.092			
Damage	– 0.134		– 1.226		0.474	*		
Res_area	– 0.020		1.576	**	– 0.384			
Side A	– 0.005		n.a.		n.a.			
Side A2	– 0.020		n.a.		– 0.008			
Side B	– 0.061		0.030		– 0.004			
Side B2	0.020		n.a.		0.010			
Current_life	0.557	***	0.772	***	0.363	***		
Family_life	0.217	***	0.072	*	0.206	***		
Married_life	– 0.024		0.022		0.250	***		
Relationships_with_friends	0.069		0.081	**	0.040			
Area_of_residence	– 0.020		0.001		0.029			
Number_of_family	– 0.003		0.003		0.027			

Significance codes: 0***, 0.001**, 0.01*, 0.05

was insufficient, several general trends can be observed. First, the Side A conflict has a negative effect on fear of war. This effect is significant in the regression analyses of data from the United States, China, Australia, and India. These results are in accordance with the research hypothesis. In contrast, the results of Side B and Side A2 conflicts were complex. China and Korea's Side B war experience had a significant positive effect on fear of war, but other estimates were significantly negative for

Australia and India. Findings regarding the Side A2 conflict did not support the research hypothesis, because results for the United States, Korea, and Singapore show a negative effect on fear of war. The results for the Side B2 conflict in Australia support the research hypothesis, and reveal positive effects on fear of war. However, data were limited because the number of Side B2 conflicts was very low. Only the results for Side A conflicts show a significant general trend, whereas that of the other cases indicate that each nation shows unique characteristic effects of war. These differences may be caused by differences in culture, national memory, and national identity between countries.

Table 8 shows the existence of a slight effect of fear of war on citizens' trust in the state (bureaucracy and government). The results for Taiwan, Australia, and India in the analyses of congress support the research hypotheses because the values of coefficients show that fear of war negatively affects trust in the congress. In addition, Sides A and A2 of the US in the analyses of bureaucracy, and Side A2 of Singapore and Side B of India in the analyses of congress support the hypotheses.

A general trend is noted in the control variables regarding living conditions ("Over the next five years do you think your living conditions will change for better or worse?" 5 = "Much better," 4 = "Slightly better," 3 = "About the same," 2 = "Slightly

Table 7 Regression analysis of war experience and fear of war (estimates and *p*-values) (PRVS and APVS)

	JP		US		CN	
Dependent variable: fear of war (4 very much > 3 somewhat > 2 slightly > 1 not at all)						
Adjusted R^2	0.002		0.089		0.021	
Side A	0.011		– 0.073	***	– 0.026	***
Side A2	– 0.032		– 0.150	**	– 0.004	
Side B	– 0.551		0.004		0.074	***
Side B2	n.a.		– 0.004		n.a.	
	TW		KR		AU	
Adjusted R^2	0.007		0.040		0.006	
Side A	0.021	**	n.a.		– 0.065	**
Side A2	0.009		– 0.034	**	n.a.	
Side B	– 0.061		0.081	***	– 0.012	*
Side B2	n.a.		n.a.		0.077	**
	SG		IN		VN	
Adjusted R^2	0.061		0.019		0.003	
Side A	n.a.		– 0.012	***	n.a.	
Side A2	– 0.151	***	0.195	***	0.006	
Side B	n.a.		– 0.562	***	– 0.012	
Side B2	n.a.		n.a.		– 0.003	

Significance codes: 0***, 0.001**, 0.01*, 0.05

Table 8 Effects of fear of war on trust in the state (estimates and *p*-values) (PRVS and APVS)

	JP		US		CN	
Dependent variable: trust in the bureaucracy (4 very confident > 3 somewhat confident > 2 not confident > 1 not confident at all)						
Adjusted R^2	0.035		0.047		0.180	
War_fear	– 0.028		– 0.018		– 0.014	
Side A	0.008		– 0.036	***	0.020	***
Side A2	0.049		– 0.099	*	– 0.002	
Side B	– 0.230		0.000		– 0.017	
Side B2	n.a.		– 0.005		n.a.	
Living_condition	0.091	***	0.051	*	0.243	***
Number_of_family	0.012		0.026		0.005	
Education	0.039		– 0.058		– 0.089	***
Income	0.042		0.015		– 0.010	
	TW		KR		AU	
Adjusted R^2	0.044		0.029		0.032	
War_fear	– 0.002		– 0.004		0.003	
Side A	0.007		n.a.		n.a.	
Side A2	0.006		0.010		n.a.	
Side B	– 0.001		0.023	***	0.002	
Side B2	n.a.		n.a.		– 0.008	
Living_condition	0.146	***	0.091	***	0.101	***
Number_of_family	– 0.002		0.008		0.010	
Education	– 0.007		– 0.045		0.100	**
Income	0.039		– 0.062	**	0.048	
	SG		IN		VN	
Adjusted R^2	0.038		0.026		0.000	
War_fear	0.002		– 0.024		– 0.022	
Side A	n.a.		– 0.003		n.a.	
Side A2	– 0.033	***	0.078	**	0.001	
Side B	n.a.		– 0.346	**	– 0.011	
Side B2	n.a.		n.a.		0.002	
Living_condition	0.077	***	0.110	***	0.036	
Number_of_family	0.007		0.004		0.001	
Education	– 0.005		– 0.005		0.011	
Income	– 0.066	**	0.140	***	– 0.036	
Dependent variable: trust in the congress (4 very confident > 3 somewhat confident > 2 not confident > 1 not confident at all)						
	JP		US		CN	

(continued)

Table 8 (continued)

	JP		US		CN	
Adjusted R^2	0.017		0.076		0.111	
War_fear	– 0.036		– 0.021		0.024	**
Side A	0.015		0.046	***	0.018	***
Side A2	– 0.038		0.003		– 0.018	***
Side B	– 1.394	***	– 0.001		– 0.002	
Side B2	n.a.		0.023	*	n.a.	
Living_condition	– 0.011		0.009		0.149	***
Number_of_family	– 0.025		0.035	*	0.032	***
Education	– 0.014		0.007		– 0.019	
Income	0.094	**	0.050		– 0.063	***
	TW		KR		AU	
Adjusted R^2	0.052		0.229		0.080	
War_fear	– 0.038	*	– 0.004		– 0.071	***
Side A	– 0.029	***	n.a.		n.a.	
Side A2	0.026		0.010		n.a.	
Side B	0.056	*	0.023	***	0.012	**
Side B2	n.a.		n.a.		– 0.024	
Living_condition	0.071	***	0.091	***	– 0.059	**
Number_of_family	0.009		0.008		0.011	
Education	– 0.113	**	– 0.045		0.038	
Income	0.164	***	– 0.062	**	0.269	***
	SG		IN		VN	
Adjusted R^2	0.021		0.082		0.015	
War_fear	0.005		– 0.051	**	– 0.023	
Side A	n.a.		0.009	***	n.a.	
Side A2	– 0.032	***	– 0.169	***	0.001	
Side B	n.a.		0.449	***	– 0.014	*
Side B2	n.a.		n.a.		0.000	
Living_condition	0.039	***	– 0.068	***	0.058	**
Number_of_family	0.020	*	– 0.014		0.001	
Education	– 0.002		– 0.122	***	0.011	
Income	– 0.030		0.233	***	– 0.066	

Significance codes: 0***, 0.001**, 0.01*, 0.05

worse," and 1 = "Much worse"): they have a positive effect in many countries. This tendency indicates that more improvements in a person's living conditions will lead to increased trust in their states. This finding corresponds to a general consideration in which citizens support the government that improved their standard of living. In addition, richness should be a cause of the fear of war, because the damage values are expected to be higher if war destroyed higher quality of life. These findings indicate that the fear of war has a negative effect on trust in the state in some countries.

The results presented in the section indicate that fear of war is partially correlated with war experience and citizens' trust in the state.

4 Conclusion

This study analyzed the correlations between war experience and social unrest on two levels, in ordinary and extraordinary situations. The first hypothesis was partly supported (Tables 4, 5, 6, and 7), but support for the second hypothesis (Fig. 4, and Tables 4, 6) and the third hypothesis (Table 8) were notably weaker.

The effect of war experience on citizens remains unclear because many interactions between the variables were not significant. War has multiple negative effects on society, both in terms of physical and psychological factors. Conversely, social capital has multiple positive effects on society. Post-traumatic stress disorder among retired soldiers is a well-established health issue, but widely recognized war-related health issues have yet to be determined in connection with citizens. This study clarifies the relationship between the war experience and social unrest. Three primary issues were selected to analyze the research question. Unfortunately, the results did not reveal clear correlations between war experience and the variables of interest. Nonetheless, some interesting findings were revealed through statistical analyses.

The analyses of the first hypothesis partly supported the research hypothesis. The war experience of people on the aggressive side of a conflict (Side A) negatively affects the fear of war. In contrast, the effect of the war experience of people on the defensive side of a conflict (Side B) on fear of war is either positive or negative, depending on the country. This finding is particularly interesting because it indicates that the experiences of being invaded and the destruction of one's own society have a two-way effect, instead of a one-way effect. However, particularly through the analyses of SoWSA data, it is difficult to examine the effects of Sides A2 and B2 because almost no respondents reported experiences of both types of war (Table 3). Comparative analyses of countries in the Asia–Pacific region revealed that the Side A war experience negatively affects fear of war. An effect of the Side B war experience was found in the analyses of Australia and India.

The current analyses did not clearly support the second hypothesis that war experience and values of social capital are negatively correlated. If war experience has no effect on citizens' values of social capital, negative psychological impacts of war memories would not be expected, with the exception of rare cases wherein individuals experienced direct serious harm or the loss of loved ones.

In connection with the third hypothesis, this study analyzed the extraordinary situation and the results indicate that fear of war does not have a strong effect on citizens' trust in the state. This finding reveals that increasing citizens' fear of war does not directly lead to dissatisfaction with the state. In addition, the progression of the security dilemma and outbreak of war is unrelated with social unrest. In this case, even democratic states should be able to avoid war with relative ease. Politicians in democratic states are inevitably more concerned about public opinion and future election prospects than those in nondemocratic states, because they are more directly impacted by their audience. Ironically, this result does not align with the democratic war theory (Geis et al., 2006). In this study, the analyses of the United States, which is one of the main players of Side A and one of the most democratic states in the post-Cold War period, supported the hypothesis that the war experience and fear of war had negative effects.

Therefore, the correlation between the war experience and social unrest is not strongly supported by analyzing data from the SoWSA, PRVS, APVS, and UCDP. However, this conclusion is not definitive because key limitations are noted in the statistical analyses used, such as the insufficiency of the sample of people who experienced all four types of wars. Overall, few interstate wars have occurred since World War II, and many countries have not participated in any interstate wars, thus indicating that only older people possess this type of war experience. For example, only Japanese people aged 70 years or above have experienced Sides A and B conflicts, and Japanese people from younger age groups have no such experience. Therefore, there are many zero-value cells in data regarding war experience. This result indicates that it is difficult to conduct robust quantitative analyses. Moreover, it is difficult to increase the sample size because of the necessity of surveying large numbers of older people. Even in East Asia, where there are many diverse countries, the data were insufficient to analyze the effects of the war experience.

There are several other limitations related to the research sample. Quantifying the war experiences of Vietnamese people is a difficult task, because South Vietnam can be classified as Side A when fighting against North Vietnam and the communist insurgencies alongside the United States (which can be considered Side A2 in this war) between the 1950s and 1970s. Therefore, North Vietnam can be considered Side B in this conflict, although North Vietnam finally became Side A in the final phase of the war. However, in this study, the war experience of North Vietnam was considered as the national data for Vietnam, thus indicating that Vietnamese people were not considered to have experienced Side A conflict, although ex-South Vietnamese people currently live in a united Vietnam.

In conclusion, evidence for the correlations between war experience and social unrest in ordinary and extraordinary situations is weak, but cannot be excluded. Some effects of Side A war experiences are observed in countries with sufficient Side A data. Extensive data from other countries with multiple war experiences are required for future research aiming to address this research question in more detail. Overall, research regarding the correlations between war experience and social unrest is in the beginning stage; thus, further development of this research area is necessary.

Acknowledgements International Consortium for Social Well-Being Studies. Social Well-Being Survey in Asia, 2015–2017 [Dataset]. (Indonesia) Universitas Indonesia, (Japan) Senshu University, (South Korea) Seoul National University, (The Philippines) Ateneo de Manila University, (Thailand) Chulalongkorn University, (Taiwan) Academia Sinica, (Vietnam) Vietnam Academy of Social Sciences [Producers]. Korea Social Science Data Archive (KOSSDA) [Distributors], 2020-06-25, A1-CUM-0022, V2.0, http://hdl.handle.net/20.500.12236/23941.

References

Arfi, B. (1998). Ethnic fear: The social construction of insecurity. *Security Studies, 8*(1), 151–203.
Butterfield, H. (1951). *History and human relations*. Collins Clear-Type Press.
Fearon, J. D. (1994). Domestic political audiences and the escalation of international disputes. *American Political Science Review, 88*(3), 577–592.
Geis, A., Brock, L., & Müller, H. (Eds.). (2006). *Democratic wars: Looking at the dark side of democratic peace*. Palgrave Macmillan.
Glaser, C. L. (1992). Political consequences of military policy: Expanding and refining the spiral and deterrence models. *World Politics, 44*(4), 497–538.
Glaser, C. L. (1997). Security dilemma revisited. *World Politics, 50*(1), 171–201.
Glaser, C. L. (2000). The causes and consequences of arms races. *Annual Review of Political Science, 3*, 251–276.
Grant, S. (2005). Raising the dead: War, memory and American national identity. *Nations and Nationalism, 11*(4), 509–529.
Harrison, R. P. (2003). *The dominion of the dead*. The University of Chicago Press.
Herz, J. (1950). Idealist internationalism and the security dilemma. *World Politics, 2*(2), 157–180.
Hutchinson, J. (2007). Warfare, remembrance and national identity. In A. Leoussi & S. Grosby (Eds.), *Nationalism and ethnosymbolism* (pp. 42–54). Edinburgh University Press.
Jervis, R. (1976). *Perception and misperception in international politics*. Princeton University Press.
Jervis, R. (1978). Cooperation under the security dilemma. *World Politics, 30*(2), 167–214.
Lake, D. A., & Rothchild, D. (1996). Containing fear: The origins and management of ethnic conflict. *International Security, 21*(2), 41–75.
Montgomery, E. B. (2006). Breaking out of the security dilemma: Realism, reassurance, and problem of uncertainty. *International Security, 31*(2), 151–185.
Pischedda, C. (2018). Wars within wars: Why windows of opportunity and vulnerability cause inter-rebel fighting in internal conflicts. *International Security, 43*(1), 138–176.
Posen, B. R. (1993). Security dilemma and ethnic conflict. *Survival, 35*(1), 27–47.
Putnam, R. D. (2000). *Bowling alone: The collapse and revival of American community*. Simon & Schuster.
Putnam, R. D. (Ed.). (2002). *Democracies in flux: The evolution of social capital in contemporary society*. Oxford University Press.
Putnam, R. D. (2007). E pluribus unum: Diversity and community in the twenty-first century the 2006 Johan Skytte prize lecture. *Scandinavian Political Studies, 30*(2), 137–174.
Roe, P. (2005). *Ethnic violence and the societal security dilemma*. Routledge.
Schori-Eyal, N., Tagar, M. R., Saguy, T., & Halperin, E. (2015). The benefits of group-based pride: Pride can motivate guilt in intergroup conflicts among high glorifiers. *Journal of Experimental Social Psychology, 61*, 79–83.
Shibai, K. (2015). Vietnamese characteristics of social conscience and values: National character, differences between north and south, and gaps between the Vietnam War generation and the post-war generation. *Behaviormetrika, 42*(2), 167–189.
Shibai, K. (2018). Behind the shadow of coming war: An experimental test for antiwar sentiments. *The Senshu Social Well-Being Review, 5*, 3–19.

Smith, A. D. (1981). War and ethnicity: The role of warfare in the formation, self-images and cohesion of ethnic communities. *Ethnic and Racial Studies, 4*(4), 375–397.
Smith, A. D. (2009). *Ethno-symbolism and nationalism: A cultural approach.* Routledge.
Svendsen, E. S., & Campbell, L. K. (2010). Living memorials: Understanding the social meanings of community-based memorials to September 11, 2001. *Environment and Behavior, 42*(3), 318–334.
Tomz, M. (2007). Domestic audience costs in international relations: An experimental approach. *International Organization, 61*(4), 821–840.
Van Evera, S. (1984). The cult of the offensive and the origins of the first world war. *International Security, 9*(1), 58–107.
Yoshino, R. (2009). *The Asia-Pacific values survey summary report: Data analysis on peoples' sense of trust.* The Institute of Statistical Mathematics.
Yoshino, R. (2015). *The Asia-Pacific values survey summary report: Cultural Manifold Analysis (CULMAN) on people's sense of trust.* The Institute of Statistical Mathematics.

Kiyohisa Shibai is Project Assistant Professor at the Joint Support-Center for Data Science Research (ROIS-DS) and the Institute of Statistical Mathematics, the Research Organization of Information and Systems. His research theme is nuclear disarmament, conflict resolution, and international security.

Politics of Belonging and Citizenship: Relational Well-Being Based on Gender and Religious Identities in Indonesia and South Korea

Lugina Setyawati and Francisia S. S. E. Seda

Abstract Discussions regarding the relationship between citizenship and social well-being have primarily focused on the role of the state in providing welfare programs for citizens. In this context, citizens are regarded as political and legal categories, based on their membership in and belonging to the nation-state. Therefore, discourses on citizenship primarily consider its vertical dimension. However, citizens' cultural identities contribute to their social well-being; thus, the social relations between individuals and collectives from different groups must also be reviewed as the horizontal dimension of citizenship. This chapter focuses on the status and position of citizens based on their gender and religious identities, and how their status influences their relational well-being. Using an intersectional approach, this chapter adopts the politics of belonging and citizenship as the theoretical framework. The argument presented in this chapter is that the grand narrative concerning membership in the nation frames the status and position of citizens. This implies that the perception of well-being among people from minority groups is lower than that of those who are members of majority groups. In addition, the gender ideology of the state affects the subjective perception of well-being of men and women. A comparative analysis is conducted between Indonesia and South Korea to analyze the dataset derived from the Social Well-Being Survey in Asia in 2015–2017. The findings indicate that gender and religious identity are separate independent variables influencing relational well-being in both Indonesia and South Korea. However, the intersectional analysis results indicate that the combination of both identities is not necessarily indicative of low happiness and life satisfaction in minority groups, as indicated in the case of Indonesia. This study demonstrates that political and cultural contexts contribute to this relationship.

L. Setyawati (✉) · F. S. S. E. Seda
Department of Sociology, Universitas Indonesia, Depok, Indonesia
e-mail: lugina.setyawati09@ui.ac.id

F. S. S. E. Seda
e-mail: ery.seda09@ui.ac.id

J. Yee et al. (eds.), *Social Well-Being, Development, and Multiple Modernities in Asia*,
https://doi.org/10.1007/978-981-97-3866-3_16

Keywords Politics of belonging · Citizenship · Social well-being · Gender · Religious identity

1 Introduction

This chapter focuses on the correlation of gender and religion with social well-being. Citizenship is the primary framework wherein the gender and religious identities of individuals determines their membership in a nation-state. The concept of citizenship helps to frame an individual's status and position vis-à-vis the state and other members of the nation. According to the vertical dimension, citizenship grants the same rights and duties to members to access existing resources for their well-being and welfare. However, according to the horizontal dimension, citizenship marks an equal membership status for every citizen, despite their diverse identities. The intersectional approach is employed in this chapter to understand the intersection of gender and religious identity in influencing relational well-being. According to Yuval-Davis (2011), intersectionality is an effective strategy for analyzing social stratification because it allows us to examine the intersections of multifaceted social differences.

Most studies have considered citizenship as a political and legal membership category in the nation-state. Therefore, citizenship is defined based on the individual's "political rights and duties" with relation to the sovereignty of the state (Jónsdóttir, 2016; Vincent, 2002). In a welfare context, this discussion includes the rights of citizens in association with the roles of the state in terms of the quality of life and welfare of their citizens, which can be observed based on the implementation of policies related to those issues, as well as citizens' responsibility in fulfilling their obligations. Therefore, this concept is primarily linked to the vertical dimension of citizenship. However, the cultural aspect of citizenship found in the horizontal relation is rarely discussed, particularly with regard to the relationship with social well-being. However, cultural identity determines the status and position of individuals in their daily life in society. Cultural identity includes ethnic and religious identities. Cooper (2018) noted that "citizens exist in relation not just to a leader in abstract sense to a state, but to each other." This study focuses on how gender and religious identities serve as the basis for defining the state of "belonging" in a group. This affects the individual's subjective perception while positioning themselves in their community and will, in turn, contribute to their happiness and well-being.

The horizontal dimension of social exclusion is based on social cleavages, including gender, sexual orientation, religious groupings, ethnicity, racial groupings, political ideology, and other aspects related to primordial relations, rather than social stratification. Social stratification is related to the vertical dimension of social exclusion. The gender and religious groupings discussed in this chapter are related to the horizontal dimension of social exclusion. In sociological conceptual terminology, social stratification is closely related to the vertical dimension of social exclusion wherein social strata based on educational attainment, employment specifications, and personal income are the primary indicators. In the context of this chapter, the horizontal dimension, specifically social cleavages based on gender relations and religious groupings, are highlighted.

In South Korea, class identity and horizons are intertwined with gender, families, households, and transgenerational factors in the context of post-war history, wherein rapid structural changes have occurred and early mobility opportunities were presented (Abelmann, 1997). After gaining independence, South Korea adopted Western-oriented legal institutions. In addition, the cultural orientation of ordinary people is changing in accordance with universal values. Both these processes are perceived as indicators of the modernization process, which is not linear or straightforward. The modernization process is constantly reshaped by the model of gender equality led by local actors in the context of local, national, and global events (Nam, 2010). In the context of the processes of modernization and digitalization in South Korea, citizens continue to prioritize materialistic values more than post-materialistic values. Positive assessments of their standard of living and marriage are the most powerful influences on quality of life (Park, 2009).

To further explore the relationship between these factors, this chapter focuses on the cases of Indonesia and South Korea. On the one hand, both countries differ demographically; Indonesia is known for its ethnically and religiously diverse population, whereas South Korea is known to have a more homogenous population, in terms of ethnicity or religious diversity. On the other hand, both countries have similarities in that gender continues to strongly affect the relationship between men and women in society. Hence, our objective when presenting the case studies of the two countries is to demonstrate the variations and complexities of inter-relations among gender, religion, and relational well-being.

Religion, in particular, has gained attention in the discourse on relational well-being because in a society that continues to respect religious values and orientation as a guide for daily life, as well as in their social relations, religion is an important social capital among its adherents. This is particularly true for heterogeneous societies. This position also refers to Putnam's (2007) description of his study in the USA, wherein he noted that in the short term, ethnic diversity tends to reduce social solidarity and social capital. However, in the long term, this may have positive implications. He emphasized this argument to explain the increasing number of immigrants in various developed countries, including the USA. Regarding Putnam's argument, this chapter focuses on the inter-relations of social and cultural diversity with relational well-being.

In the Indonesian context, the religious identity of each citizen plays important role in their personal lives, community activities, and state administrative matters. Religion remains a key identity attached to each individual. The state regulates religious issues. The involvement of the state in religious affairs can be observed through the existence of the Ministry of Religious Affairs. In contrast, in South Korea, religious affiliation is considered an individual's personal and private matter, and the state is expected to not intervene. In this case, the religious life of citizens is not considered part of the state's domain. Accordingly, the state does not regulate nor organize the religious lives of its citizens. In fact, religion is no longer considered a

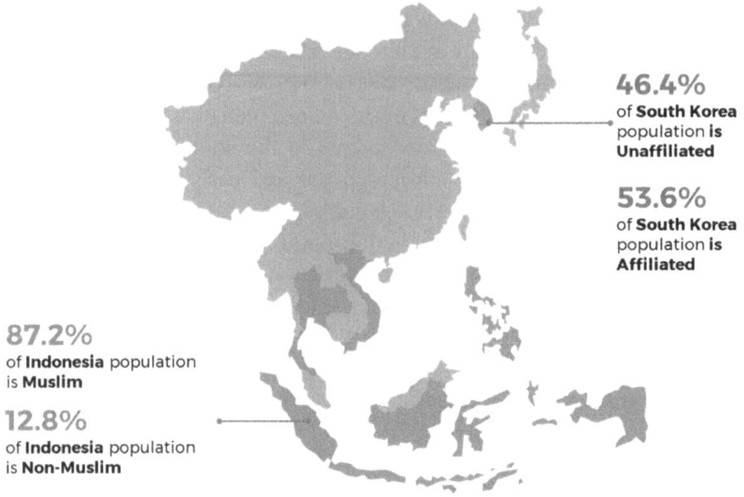

Fig. 1 Population by Religion in Indonesia and South Korea. (*Sources* https://www.pewresearch.org/religion/feature/religious-composition-by-country-2010-2050/)

primary identity, as indicated based on a significant proportion of the population not being affiliated with a particular religion. Nevertheless, understanding the difference between these two countries is crucial for clarifying the basis of this research that religious affiliation and activities play an important role in enhancing an individual's trust, participation, and interaction in their community (Fig. 1).

In terms of gender, the cases of Indonesia and South Korea are important because the division of labor based on gender remains effectively valid and applied on a daily basis in both countries. Despite the strong presence of the women's movement in both countries, several studies on gender roles in South Korea and Indonesia have shown that gender oppression and inequality continue to exist (Kim, 2009; You & Yoo, 2016). The World Economic Forum Report on the Gender Gap Index (GGI) confirmed that issues related to gender inequality remain prominent in both countries. Based on the 2018 report, South Korea ranked 115 with a GGI score of 0.657, whereas Indonesia ranked 85 with a score of 0.69. However, governments in both countries have made good will efforts aimed to address gender equality and justice through the formation of specific ministries to oversee matters related to gender. In South Korea, the relevant institution was called the Ministry of Gender Equality in 2001 and was later changed in 2005 to the Ministry of Gender Equality and Family. Similarly, in Indonesia, this institution was named the Ministry of Women's Role in the era of President Soeharto; however, after the reformation, the name has been changed several times and is now referred to as the Ministry of Women's Empowerment and Child Protection.

Based on analysis results derived from the 2015–2017 Social Well-Being Survey in Asia (SoWSA) dataset, the relationship of gender and religious identities with relational well-being in Indonesia and South Korea shows a similar trend, wherein men have a higher relational well-being score, compared to that of women, although the gap is not significant. Furthermore, the results of data processing indicate that religion contributes to relational well-being. However, the scores between the two countries are different, with Indonesia demonstrating a higher level of relational well-being.

This chapter argues that the politics of belonging applied to an individual's gender and religious identities affects their relational well-being because the status and position of the individual or group are cemented in their community. First, gender ideology continues to be active, marked by the tendency to associate women with their domestic roles. Women's status and position affects their happiness and life satisfaction. Consequently, women's relational well-being is lower than that of men. Second, in a society that values religious perspectives in their daily life and uses them as a basis for social relations, religious activities provide life satisfaction and happiness. With relation to this condition, in a diverse society, being part of a dominant or majority religious group is a form of social capital that contributes to the relational well-being of followers. As a result, the average relational well-being score among individuals of the dominant/majority group was better than that of the less dominant or minority groups.

This chapter is divided into three sections. The first section "Positioning Gender and Religious Identities in the Citizenship Discourse" provides a theoretical framework for understanding the issues and describes the method employed in this study. The second section is "Relational Well-Being in Indonesia and South Korea" and provides an overview of the association between gender identity and relational well-being, as well as the association between religious identity and relational well-being. The final section demonstrates the correlation of gender and religious identities with relational well-being. This section also describes the intersection of gender and religious identities.

1.1 Positioning Gender and Religious Identities in the Citizenship Discourse

This section discusses the key concepts used to explain the correlation of gender and religious identities with relational well-being. Both identities become elements of citizenship, which is the primary concept, whereas social well-being is specifically focused on relational well-being, which includes the following three dimensions: perception/trust, participation, and interaction.

1.1.1 Citizenship and Politics of Belonging

In the context of related literature from the past few decades, the citizenship discourse includes political aspects, comprising legal status, rights, and memberships in a nation-state (Isin & Turner, 2002; Lukose, 2005), as well as discourses on the social and cultural power of citizenship that works on individuals as members of society (Kipnis, 2004). Yuval-Davis and Werbner (1999: 4) presented a similar perspective toward the notion of citizenship by defining citizenship as a relation influenced by "identity, social position, cultural assumption, institutional practice, and a sense of belonging," because citizenship determines the status and position of an individual, as well as their access and participation in resources. Therefore, citizenship is a key concept for showing the individual's sense of belonging toward a political collectivity (Cooper, 2018).

Jónsdóttir (2016) quoted Gellner (1983), who explained that the state is an institution exercising order in society. Jónsdóttir emphasized that a group of elites run this political institution. In an effort to protect their own interests and power, this elite group exercises its domination over other groups by legitimizing their group and cultural values as the basis order applied in the social, economic, and political domains of society. This is where the politics of belonging occurs. The dominant group determines the ideas of membership in the country—who receives priority and who does not. Politics of belonging is related to building boundaries in the community regarding "who is in and who is out" (Abdou, 2017: 84). Through this mechanism, the line that separates "us" and "them" is planted and cultivated (Yuval-Davis, 2006: 204). As a result, the "minority" groups are often discriminated against by the "majority" (Rizman, 2000). Groups categorized as "minority" in the stratification of society include women, ethnic groups, religious groups, and poor people.

According to feminist perspectives, citizenship is not a neutral concept. This conception is instead constructed based on men's frame of mind, which is integrated into the theory and practice of citizenship, among others, through the dichotomy of public and private spheres as a basis of the sexual division of labor that often occurs in many societies (Lister, 2007: 52).

Gender is a key element in politics of belonging because women are considered the "symbolic border guards of the nation" (Yuval-Davis, 2011: 11). This implies that politics of belonging can lead to the exclusion and inclusion of individuals or groups because politics of belonging does not only address the question "What is the nation?" but also "Who is the nation?" (Yuval-Davis, 2011).

In the notion of identity, religion is a "cultural identity marker" (Watzlawik, 2012). Religion constructs boundaries among collective groups and determines people who are defined as the in-group ("us") and out group ("them"). Accordingly, in this context, religion works as social capital that provides members of religious groups with networking and supports their daily life with emotional and spiritual needs. In a diverse community, religious groups serve as a significant factor for their members, provide trust, and create cohesiveness among those in the in-group. The association between the politics of belonging and religion is related to the use of religious identity to determine an individual or a group's belonging to the community, society, and nation-state levels. Belonging produces stratification through which the positions of individuals and groups are determined, thereby having implications on social relations in the community. Religion is a social capital; thus, dominant or majority religious groups have gained privilege from their association and network with their religious group.

1.1.2 Social Well-Being in Association with Gender and Religious Identities

Social well-being is defined as the subjective perceptions of an individual with relation to three issues: their living conditions, quality of relationships with other people at the community level, and the condition of their community. This definition was elaborated through three dimensions, namely personal, relational, and societal well-being (Koo et al., 2016).

Diversity does not necessarily correlate positively with social well-being (Putnam, 2007; Tsai et al., 2011). On the contrary, diversity can suppress social solidarity (Putnam, 2007) because gender, social class, and religious identities affect the establishment and development of social trust. In addition, identities influence individual participation and interaction in the community, because identities work in both political and social contexts. In Indonesia, religious capital is important for social well-being at the community level, as indicated by the higher score of relational well-being among the majority of Muslims, compared to those who are not Muslim (Seda et al., 2018).

Intersectionality in the study of discrimination and social exclusion experienced by individuals or groups due to their social and cultural identities is an analytical framework employed in feminism and other research (Crenshaw, 1989; Yuval-Davis, 2011). As described by Crenshaw (1989), who initiated the tools of analysis, multidimensional experiences of discrimination or disadvantages of individuals or groups can be uncovered through intersectionality. Intersectionality serves as a lens to examine the complex oppression and discrimination caused by a combination of individual social and cultural backgrounds.

In this chapter, the intersection between gender and religious identities serves as a combination contributing to the level of social well-being. Women and people of minority religions are the most vulnerable groups. In Indonesia, religion is a key identity and although gender inequality persists in society, the hypothesis of this study is that non-Muslim women occupy the lowest rank in terms of well-being. Meanwhile, in South Korea, although gender continues to significantly contribute to the status and social position of citizens, religion is not a prime identity. However, considering that citizens with religious affiliation constitute majority of the population, those who are not affiliated with a specific religion are a minority. Accordingly, the most vulnerable and marginal positions in South Korea, with relation to happiness and well-being, are women who are not affiliated to any religion.

The intersection between religion and gender serves as a source of oppression in Indonesian society, as noted by many scholars (Robinson, 2016; Wierienga, 2015). Robinson (2016) noted that "religious identity and gender relations are integral to women's experiences of citizenship in Indonesia," and this is indicated in religious norms that arrange women's rights and duties, particularly in the family. This is reflected in marriage law.

In addition, the Indonesian historical context shows a problematic relationship between them (Qibtiyah, 2019). Particularly among Muslim, since the independence movement era, a contradiction has existed in positions between religion and gender equality. According to Qibtiyah (2019: 168), "the opposition of Muslim women and gender equality activists to the dominant culture and state policy derives from a wide variety of positions." For example, the opposite position in the discussion of polygamy occurred in the 1928 Indonesian Women's Congress. Women represented religious organizations, such as Aisyah, and supported polygamy, whereas more "liberal" women's groups rejected it. Likewise, during the New Order government, religious values influenced various gender policies promoted by the state, including marriage laws, which positioned men as breadwinners and women as homemakers. After the Indonesian reformation, marriage between religious and patriarchal values remains persistent. For instance, in several provinces and districts, the adoption and implementation of Sharia law places women in subordinate positions (Brenner, 2011; Rinaldo, 2008).

Intersectionality analysis for social divisions in South Korea, which is based on religion and gender values, differs from that of Indonesia. The intersection between religion and gender can be problematic in South Korea, as noted by Koh (2008) regarding the relationship between Korean Confucianism and gender equality. She emphasized that "the idea of men's superiority to women is embedded in Confucian philosophy." However, in South Korea, the intersection between the two is not institutionalized by the state through policies and regulations. Especially in this country, religion is not a key identity in the public sphere. However, a higher proportion of the population is affiliated with a specific religion. Therefore, the intersection between religion and gender does not appear to be significant in South Korean society.

2 Data and Method

This chapter utilizes the 2015–2017 dataset from the SoWSA in Asia, which was conducted by the International Consortium for Social Well-being Studies in seven participating consortium countries, namely, Japan, South Korea, Taiwan, Indonesia, Vietnam, Thailand, and the Philippines. However, we focus on datasets from Indonesia and South Korea in this chapter. The Indonesian survey was conducted in 2017 and covered seven provinces, including Jakarta, Banten, West Java, Yogyakarta, Central Java, East Java, and Bali; 1248 samples were considered using a multistage random sampling method to represent the population conditions in Indonesia. The South Korean survey was conducted in seven regions: Seoul, Inchon/Kyeonggi, Daejeon/Chungcheong, Kwangju/Jeonla, Daegu/Keongbuk, Busan/Ulsan/Kyeongnam, and Kangwon/Jeju. The total sample comprised 2000 respondents.

We employed a quantitative approach and method; thus, the process was stated by establishing conceptual and operational definitions for relational well-being as the dependent variable, and gender and religious identities as independent variables. We defined three indicators of relational well-being: perception, interaction, and participation. "Perception" is measured by the level of trust among respondents in their interactions within their own communities, such as family, neighbors, friends, and colleagues. "Interaction" is measured by the level of intensity and frequency of interaction and the number of people interacting with the respondents within their own communities. "Participation" is measured by the level of intensity and frequency of respondents' participation in common activities within their communities. These indicators are statistically analyzed to measure the composite index of relational well-being.

Gender identity as an independent variable is measured by perceptions of amenity based on gender, satisfaction with their married life, and equal treatment received due to their gender identity. Time spent on domestic activities—preparing meals, washing clothes, and clearing houses—and reproductive activities, such as taking care of children and other household members, is used to describe the gender division of labor. Religious identity is measured by individuals' subjective perceptions of their life experiences of equal treatment and amenity due to their religious identity. To describe religious activities and associations, we refer to religious memorials and services activities, and reliance on religious institutions/organizations, both in coping with problems in daily life and in special circumstances (such as natural disasters and grieves). These activities and trust are important for indicating how religious institutions and organizations at the community level transform into social capital that contributes to an individual's well-being.

Subsequently, based on the related items available in the questionnaire, we determined the appropriate items to measure these variables. The items are as follows (Table 1):

The indexation process was run by measuring every variable based on data from the appropriate items in the questionnaire to measure every variable. Recategorization data were used to increase the ease of interpreting and inferring data. To examine the correlation between the independent and dependent variables, we applied bivariate and multivariate regression analyses.

Table 1 Items in questionnaire used in this study

Variable	Items in the questionnaire
Gender identity	F16, F01, F05, W0206, W0201, W0301, W0401, F2311, F2321, F2331, F2341, F2351
Religious identity	C07, C0701_ID, F29, R0209, R0609, W0311, W0411
Relational well-being	C0102, C0103, C0104, C0105, C0106, C0201, C0202, C0301, C0302, C0402, C0403, C0404, C0407, C05

Reliability analysis results show that all indicators are constructed using valid and reliable variables, with a Cronbach's alpha value of 0.792 for perception, 0.758 for interaction, and 0.868 for participation.

3 Result

This section focuses on relational well-being in Indonesia and South Korea. Several studies on social well-being have shown a tendency for a correlation that is not always positive between the level of national social welfare, their degree of happiness, and life satisfaction in society (Easterlin, 1995, 2001; Seda et al., 2018). The comparison between East Asian countries, such as Japan, South Korea, and Taiwan, with good economic growth and Southeast Asian countries, such as Vietnam, Indonesia, the Philippines, and Thailand, with lower economic status, demonstrates that Southeast Asian countries have a better degree of social well-being. Various gap scores are noted while reviewing data from each country (Seda et al., 2018).

This condition is also observed in the relational well-being data for both Indonesia and South Korea, wherein Indonesia has a relatively higher relational well-being index than South Korea. Based on the indicators of relational well-being, composed of perception, participation, and interaction, the index of each indicator in Indonesia still showed a higher index score. Detailed data are presented in Fig. 2.

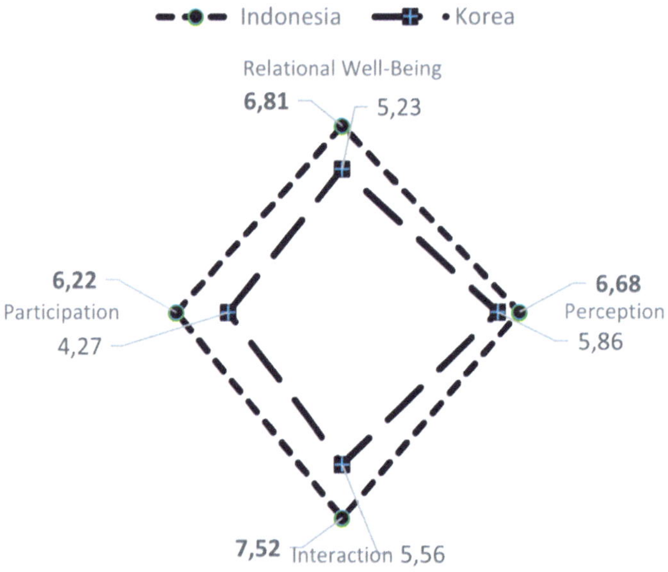

Fig. 2 Relational well-being Index in Indonesia and South Korea

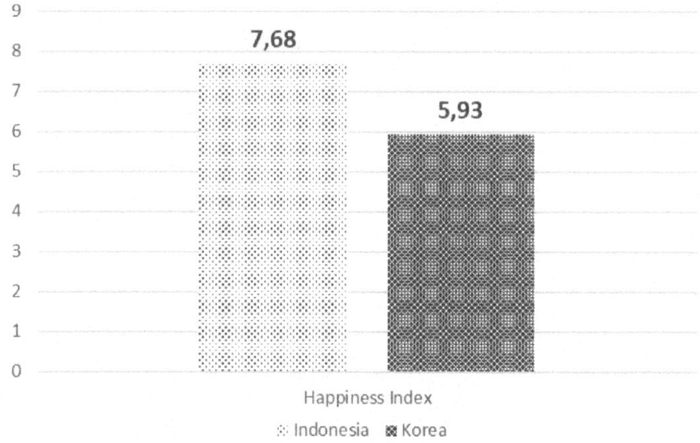

Fig. 3 Happiness Index in Indonesia and South Korea

Figure 2 shows that the relational well-being index score in Indonesia is 6.81, with a participation score of 6.22, interaction score of 7.52, and perception score of 6.68. In South Korea, the relational well-being index score is 5.23, the participation score is 4.27, the interaction score is 5.56, and the perception score is 5.86.

Both Indonesia and South Korea show no difference between male and female respondents. Similar results are also shown for the index scores between respondents from the religious majority group and minority groups.

Figure 3 shows that the index of happiness of survey respondents in Indonesia is 7.68. For South Korea, this score is 5.93. The happiness index is an individual's subjective perception, although this element is crucial for measuring an individual's quality of life outside of their objective economic condition. This result emphasizes the previous discussion about the correlation between economic welfare and social well-being.

3.1 Gender Identity and Relational Well-Being

Figure 4 presents data regarding happiness and fair treatment based on gender and shows that in Indonesia, with relation to Amenity, men scored 6.99, higher than women who scored 6.63. In terms of fairness, Indonesian men scored 7.21 and women scored 6.85. Regarding satisfaction with relation to married life, Indonesian men scored 8.62 and women scored 8.51. Interestingly, the happiness level shows that Indonesian men are less happy, compared with Indonesian women (men 7.63; women 7.74). This figure shows that in terms of amenity, fairness, and satisfaction with married life, Indonesian men scored higher than Indonesian women. Indonesian women scored higher than Indonesian men only at the current level of happiness.

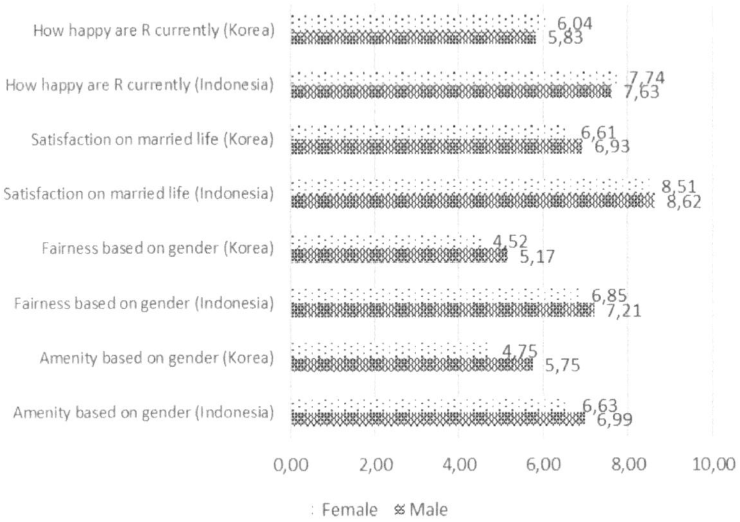

Fig. 4 Happiness and fair treatment based on gender

Figure 4 also shows that in South Korea, with relation to Amenity, men scored 5.75 and women scored 4.75. In terms of fairness, South Korean men scored 5.17 whereas women scored 4.52. Regarding satisfaction with married life, South Korean men scored 6.93, whereas women scored 6.61. Interestingly, the happiness level shows that South Korean men scored 5.83 and women scored 6.04. For South Korea, with relation to amenity, fairness, and satisfaction with married life, men scored higher than women. The sole exception is the current happiness level, wherein South Korean women scored higher than men.

Table 2 shows that according to the time spent for domestic work in Indonesia, women spend more time than men. For preparing meals, Indonesian men (79.1%) spent less than 30 min preparing meals, compared with Indonesian women (58.7%) who spent 30 min to 1 h. Similar results also show that for washing clothes and cleaning the house, Indonesian women spent significantly more time on domestic work than Indonesian men.

In South Korea, in terms of preparing meals, South Korean men (29.2%) spent less than 30 min, compared with South Korean women (65.0%), who spent 30 min to 1 h. Consistently, with washing clothes and cleaning the house, South Korean women spent significantly more time on domestic work than South Korean men.

Table 3 presents the time spent taking care of family members based on gender and shows that South Korean men (99.5%) take care of children less than 8 h, compared with South Korean women (93.0%). Moreover, Indonesian men (89.7%) take care of children for less than 8 h, compared with Indonesian women (66.6%).

Table 2 Time spent for domestic works based on gender in Indonesia and South Korea

Items	Category	Male (%)	Female (%)
Preparing meals (Indonesia)	Less than 30 min	79.1	15.6
	30 min—1 h	17.4	58.7
	More than 1 h	3.5	25.6
Preparing meals (Korea)	Less than 30 min	29.2	15.1
	30 min—1 h	63.0	65.0
	More than 1 h	7.9	20.0
Washing clothes (Indonesia)	Less than 30 min	66.8%	16.0
	30 min—1 h	25.9	58.5
	More than 1 h	7.3	25.5
Washing clothes (Korea)	Less than 30 min	55.6	23.3
	30 min—1 h	35.6	53.9
	More than 1 h	8.8	22.8
Clearing house (Indonesia)	Less than 30 min	67.1	21.8
	30 min—1 h	27.8	61.2
	More than 1 h	5.1	17.0
Clearing house (Korea)	Less than 30 min	48.9	22.7
	30 min—1 h	44.3	60.2
	More than 1 h	6.8	17.1

Table 3 Time spent for taking care family members based on gender in Indonesia and South Korea

Items	Category	Male (%)	Female (%)
Take care of children (Indonesia)	Less than 8 h	89.7	66.6
	8 h	2.5	5.0
	9–16 h	5.2	16.7
	More than 16 h	2.7	11.7
Take Care of Children (Korea)	Less than 8 h	99.5	93.0
	8 h	0.2	1.6
	9–16 h		3.9
	More than 16 h	0.2	1.6
Take Care of Others Household members (Indonesia)	Less than 8 h	80.3	78.5
	8 h	8.5	3.8
	9–16 h	5.6	11.5
	More than 16 h	5.6	6.2
Take Care of Others Household members (Korea)	Less than 8 h	99.5	99.3
	8 h	0.5	
	9–16 h		0.7

3.2 Religious Identity and Relational Well-Being

This section focuses on the correlation between religious identity and relational well-being in Indonesia and South Korea. In this chapter, religious identity is analyzed to examine the happiness level, which is measured based on an individual's subjective perception of equal treatment and amenity due to their religious identity. Individual perceptions of the roles of religious organizations are also described to show the contribution of religious organizations in coping with their daily and situational problems.

Figure 5 shows happiness and fair treatment based on religious identity. The description includes individuals' subjective perception on the amenity they experience based on their religious identity, and the fair treatment they receive due to their religious identity, and their overall happiness in life. For the data analysis, the case of Indonesia is emphasized because the Muslim population is the majority in Indonesia; thus, religious identity is categorized based on "Muslim" and "non-Muslim." However, for South Korea, majority of the population is people affiliated with a specific religion. Therefore, the categorization is divided into "Affiliated" and "Unaffiliated." The comparison of Indonesia and South Korea is presented in Fig. 5.

Figure 5 demonstrates that in Indonesia, no significant differences are noted between Muslims (7.69) and non-Muslims (7.67) groups on the overall happiness level. Regarding the elaboration of data based on amenity due to religious identity in Indonesia, the Muslim group experienced significantly higher level of amenity, as demonstrated by the score of 7.61, compared to 6.81, which is the average score for the non-Muslim group. A similar result is also indicated for fair treatment based on religious identity experienced by the Muslim group with a score of 7.37, as compared to 6.32 for the non-Muslim group. Religious identity provides a valuable contribution to the lives of individuals, although at the overall happiness level, no difference is

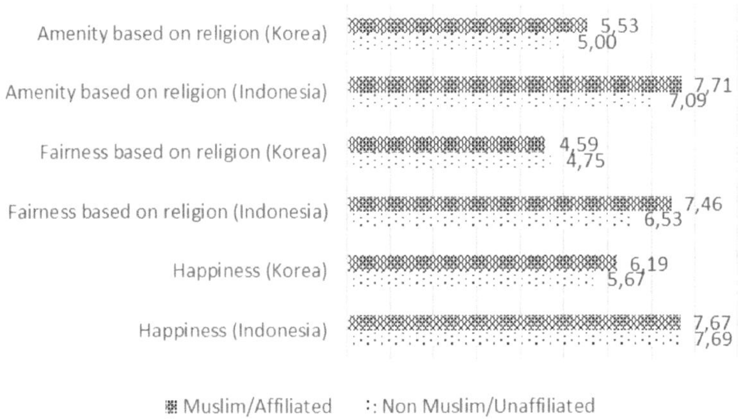

Fig. 5 Happiness and fair treatment based on religious identity

noted between the Muslim and non-Muslim groups. However, based on the perception of fair treatment and amenity they experienced, the Muslim group's score is higher. Being a member of the majority group seems to contribute to an individual's perception of fair treatment and amenity.

In South Korea, those in the affiliated group indicated higher happiness level (6.19), compared with the unaffiliated group (5.67). Similarly, the level of amenity based on religion was higher among the affiliated group (5.53), compared with that of the unaffiliated group (5.00). In contrast, the perception of fair treatment among the affiliated group (4.59) is lower than that of the unaffiliated group (4.75). In South Korea, religion contributes to the happiness level; however, the perception of fair treatment in the affiliated group is lower, compared to the unaffiliated group.

The following discussion describes individuals' perceptions regarding their reliance on religious organizations to cope with daily problems and difficulties in specific situations (such as natural disasters and major accidents) based on religion. Figure 6 presents the SoWSA data for Indonesia, and Fig. 7 presents the data overview for South Korea.

Figure 6 shows that in Indonesia, for both Muslim and non-Muslim groups, religious organizations are considered reliable particularly during having situational problems, such as disasters or major accidents, indicated by the score of 7.80 in the Muslim group and the score of 7.77 in the non-Muslim group. However, perception of the Muslim group regarding the roles of these organizations in overcoming their daily problems is higher, compared to the non-Muslim group (the score of the Muslim group is 7.25; the score of the non-Muslim group is 6.84). Figure 6 demonstrates that in both daily life and situational conditions, religious organizations perceived

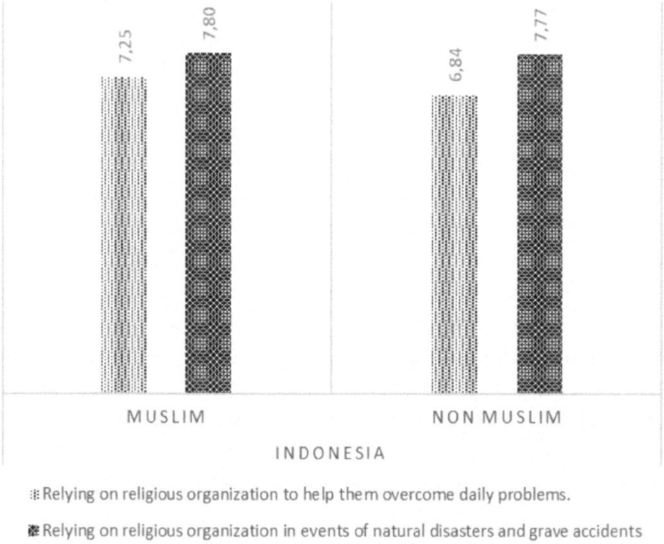

Fig. 6 Roles of religious organizations in Indonesia based on religion in Indonesia

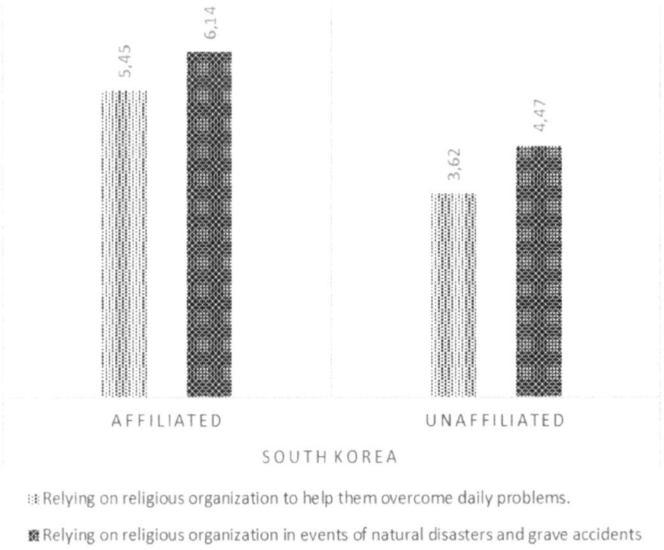

Fig. 7 Roles of religious organizations based on affiliation to a religion in South Korea

as reliable in each category of problems is above 6.50. This indicates that religious institutions are a key agent in society. In Indonesia, religious orientation and activities play an important role in communal life, and religious organizations thus become a source of moral and social support.

In South Korea, individuals' perceptions of the roles of religious organizations when experiencing difficulties in daily life and during disasters/major accidents are higher among affiliated groups than unaffiliated groups. However, both groups perceived religious organizations as reliable, particularly in coping with situational difficulties caused by natural disasters or major accidents. However, the score of the affiliated group (6.14) is significantly higher than that of the unaffiliated group (4.47). A similar result is also noted for the perception of the role of religious organizations in supporting individuals dealing with daily problems, as indicated by the score of 5.45 in the affiliated group, compared with 3.62 in the unaffiliated group.

Based on the descriptions in Figs. 6 and 7, in South Korea, perceptions of the roles of religious organizations for coping with difficulties in daily life and situational conditions are higher among the affiliated groups. In Indonesia, no difference is noted in perceptions of the reliability of religious organizations between Muslims and non-Muslims groups because both groups rely on organizations for handling problems and difficulties in any circumstances. The findings in Indonesia and South Korea indicate that religion is a form of social capital that contributes to the quality of life and social well-being of individuals. This finding is aligned with that of Hayward and Elliott (2014), with reference to Cohen (2004), who emphasized that religious-based support carried out by religious organizations provides social support that contributes to well-being.

3.3 Correlations of Gender and Religious Identities with Relational Well-Being

The correlations of gender and religious identities with relational well-being are shown in Table 4.

Table 4 shows the correlations of gender and religious identities with relational well-being in Indonesia and South Korea. The overall value of correlation between religious identity as independent variable and relational well-being as dependent variable in Indonesia is 0.241. A similar trend is noted in the correlation between gender identity and relational well-being, as indicated by the score of 0.244. The correlations between religious identity and each indicator of relational well-being is 0.153 for perception, 0.227 for interaction, and 0.135 for participation. Religious identity has the strongest correlation with interaction as the indicator of relational well-being, whereas participation has the lowest value of correlation. Different results are shown in the correlations between religious identity and each indicator of relational well-being. Perception has the highest value of 0.197, compared with 0.196 for interaction and 0.139 for participation.

In the case of South Korea, the overall value of correlation between religious identity and relational well-being is 0.328 and 0.38 of correlation value between gender identity and relational well-being. The figure for South Korea indicates a different pattern in the correlation between religious identity and each indicator of relational well-being, as shown by the value of each indicator, which is 0.315 for perception, 0.237 for interaction, and 0.215 for participation. Based on these values, religious identity had the strongest correlation with perception as an indicator of relational well-being. Compared to religious identity, gender identity has weaker correlation with each indicator of relational well-being (perception = 0.369, interaction = 0.277, and participation = 0.242). Among the other indicators, perception had the strongest correlation with gender identity.

Based on Table 4, religious identity and gender identity are correlated with relational well-being as separate independent variables. However, the correlation values

Table 4 Correlations of gender and religious identities with relational well-being

Independent variable	Dependent variable	Value (Correlation)	
		Indonesia	Korea
Religious identity	Relational well-being	0.241	0.328
Religious identity	Perception	0.153	0.315
Religious identity	Interaction	0.227	0.237
Religious identity	Participation	0.135	0.215
Gender identity	Relational well-being	0.244	0.38
Gender identity	Perception	0.197	0.369
Gender identity	Interaction	0.196	0.277
Gender identity	Participation	0.139	0.242

varied. The following discussion describes the intersection between gender and religious identities as independent variables, and their correlation with relational well-being. Based on the value of correlations, the argument of the study presented earlier is supported; the status and position of women as citizens in society contributes to their happiness and life satisfaction. According to Yuval-Davis (2011), politics of belonging shows how women as citizens have a more vulnerable position. In this context, gender identity is developed as the boundary to classify "who is in and who is out." However, in this study, the values of the correlations were not significantly high. This is related to relational well-being as the dependent variable. Further studies are necessary to determine whether the same results are presented for the relationship between gender identity and personal or societal well-being.

The second argument of this study regarding religious identity contributing to relational well-being is supported by the correlation results, although the value is relatively moderate. As described by Hayward and Elliott (2014), identification with a religious group provides a "positive sense of self" that plays a role in building relationships with other people in the community.

The intersection of religion and gender shows that in Indonesia, men are happier than women in both Muslim and non-Muslim groups (Muslim men's score is 7.07 and Muslim women's score is 6.61; non-Muslim men's score is 7.11 and non-Muslim women's score is 6.10). However, the results show no significant difference between Muslim and non-Muslim men in terms of relational well-being. On the contrary, there is a description of the intersection of gender and religious identity among women. The relational well-being score of Muslim women (6.61) is higher than that of non-Muslim women (6.10).

A similar description is presented for South Korea. Figure 8 shows that the affiliated group had a higher score of relational well-being than the unaffiliated group, as indicated by the men's score of 5.58 and women's score of 5.24 in the affiliated group, and the men's score of 5.15 and women's score of 4.95 in the unaffiliated group.

However, the two-way ANOVA tests show a similar pattern of differences in relational well-being based on gender differences in both South Korea and Indonesia. Gender contributes to relational well-being in Indonesia ($p. = 0.006$) as well as in South Korea ($p. < 0.01$). Regarding religious identity, different religious identities in Indonesia have no implications on relational well-being ($p. = 368$). Meanwhile, in South Korea, affiliation with a religion has implications on relational well-being ($p. < 0.01$). Based on a test of the relationship between the intersection of gender and religious identity and relational well-being, the results indicate that both variables work separately in influencing relational well-being.

The results of the correlation of gender and religious identity with relational well-being do not support the hypothesis proposed. Gender identity and religious identity separately showed a significant correlation with relational well-being, albeit as independent variables. In Indonesia, non-Muslim women as a minority group are not necessarily less happy and have lower life satisfaction than Muslim women. Furthermore, in South Korea, as a minority group, women who are unaffiliated with any

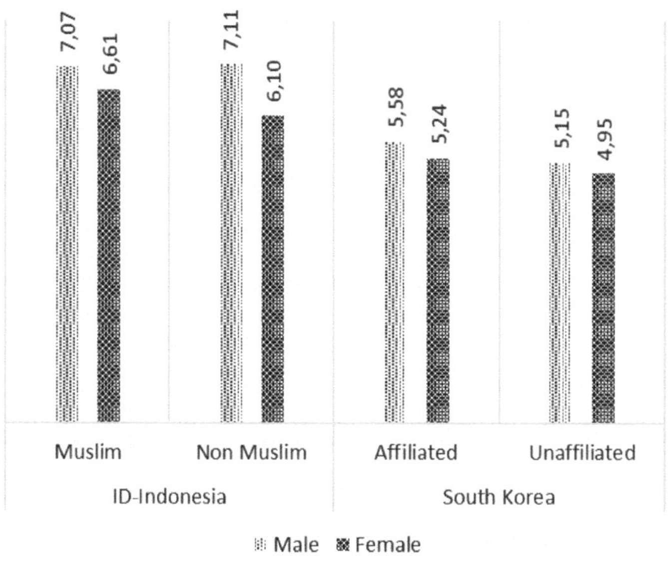

Fig. 8 Intersection of gender and religion identities toward the relational well-being

religion have low happiness and life satisfaction. Therefore, the case of South Korea supports the research hypothesis, whereas it is not proven in the case of Indonesia.

4 Conclusion

The findings of this research indicate that gender and religious identities influence relational well-being in both Indonesia and South Korea. However, in Indonesia, religious identity has higher influence, whereas in South Korea, gender identity has higher influence on relational well-being. The differences between Indonesia and South Korea are partially influenced by the political, social, cultural, and economic contexts of the two countries, including different relevant public state policies in post-war South Korea and independent Indonesia.

Both countries indicate that the horizontal dimension of social exclusion is based on social cleavages. In particular, gender and religious identities have a significant correlation with relational well-being, with the difference being related to the type of identity that is highly correlated depending on the country. These findings affirm and validate the intersectional theoretical analysis wherein discrimination and social exclusion experienced by individuals or groups are caused by their social and cultural identities in society. The intersection between gender and religious identities are combined in influencing the level of relational well-being in both South Korea and Indonesia.

The correlation between gender and religious identities with relational well-being shows relatively low significance, with Indonesia scoring higher significance in the correlation between religious identity and relational well-being than South Korea. Religion has a strong influence on relational well-being in Indonesia.

The correlation between gender identity and relational well-being shows that South Korea has a slightly higher score than Indonesia. Gender has a higher influence on relational well-being in South Korea.

This study shows that religious identity has a relatively higher correlation with relational well-being in Indonesia than in South Korea, and gender identity has a relatively higher correlation with relational well-being in South Korea than in Indonesia.

In the context of politics of belonging and citizenship, in the current political and cultural contexts of both South Korea and Indonesia, religion influences the relational well-being of Indonesian citizens, regardless of gender, compared to South Korean citizens. Belonging to a specific religion matters more for Indonesian citizens, compared with a particular gender. For South Korean citizens, a specific gender identity influences relational well-being more than belonging to a particular religion.

In Indonesia, compared with gender, religion becomes "the boundary marker" between who gets excluded and who gets included both by the state and by society. In South Korea, compared with religion, gender becomes "the boundary marker" of who belongs and who does not belong in the eyes of the state and of society.

A noteworthy aspect is that as separate independent variables, both gender and religious identity influence relational well-being in both Indonesia and South Korea. However, intersection analysis shows that the combination of gender and religious identities does not influence relational well-being. The research hypothesis is proven only in the context of South Korea, wherein women unaffiliated with any religion and in the minority group have low relational well-being. Furthermore, in Indonesia, non-Muslim women who are also a minority group, do not have low relational well-being.

Therefore, the results show how the politics of belonging and citizenship with particular political and cultural contexts in a specific period influence the relational well-being of both Indonesian and South Korean citizens.

References

Abdou, L. H. (2017). 'Gender Nationalism': The New (Old) Politics of Belonging. *Austrian Journal of Political Science I, Vol.46, issue 1*. Innsbruck University Press.

Abelmann, N. (1997). Women's Class mobility and identities in South Korea a gendered, transnational, narrative approach. *The Journal of Asian Studies, 56*(2), May 1997.

Brenner, S. (2011). Private moralities in the public sphere: Democratization, Islam, and gender in Indonesia. *American Anthropologist, 113*(3), 478–490, Sept 2011.

Cohen, S. (2004). Social relationships and health. *American Psychologist, 59*, 676–684. https://doi.org/10.1037/0003-066X.59.8.676

Cooper, F. (2018). *Citizenship, inequality, and difference: Historical perspectives*. Princeton University Press.

Crenshaw, K. (1989). Demarginalizing the intersection of race and sex: A black feminist critique of antidiscrimination doctrine, feminist theory and antiracist politics. *University of Chicago Legal Forum, 1989*(1), Article 8.

Easterlin, R. (1995). Will raising the incomes of all increase the happiness of all?. *Journal of Economic Behavior & Organization, 27*(1), 35–47.

Easterlin, R. (2001). Income and happiness: Towards a unified theory. *Economic Journal, 111*(473), 465–484.

Gellner, E. (1983). *Nations and nationalism*. Cornell University Press.

Hayward, R. D. & Elliott, M. (2014). Cross-national analysis of the influence of cultural norms and government restrictions on the relationship between religion and well-being. *Review of Religious Research, 56*(1), 23–43, Mar 2014.

Isin, E. F. & Turner, B. S. (2002). *Citizenship studies: an introduction*. In E. F. Isin & B. S. Turner (Eds.), *Handbook of citizenship studies*. Sage.

Jónsdóttir, E. B. (2016). *Political and cultural belonging: Anthropological perspectives on citizenship*. Final project for a BA-degree in anthropology. Faculty of Social and Human Sciences School of Social Sciences of University of Iceland

Kim, H.-K. (2009). Analyzing the gender division of labor: The cases of the United States and South Korea. *Asian Perspective, 33*(2), 181–229.

Kipnis, A. (2004). Anthropology and the theorization of citizenship. *The Asia Pacific Journal of Anthropology, 5*(3), 257–278.

Koh, E. (2008). Gender issues and confucian scriptures: Is confucianism incompatible with gender equality in South Korea? *Bulletin of the School of Oriental and African Studies, University of London, 71*(2), 345–362.

Koo, H., Yee, J., Nam, E. Y., Kim, & Ee, S. (2016). Dimensions of social well-being and determinants in Korea: Personal, relational, and societal aspects. *The Senshu Social Well-Being Review, 3*.

Lister, R. (2007). Inclusive citizenship: Realizing the potential. *Citizenship Studies, 11*(1), 49–61.

Lukose, R. (2005). Empty citizenship: Protesting politics in the era of globalization. *Cultural Anthropology, 20*(4), 506–533.

Nam, S. (2010). The Women's movement and the transformation of the family law in South Korea interactions between local, national and global structures., European. *Journal of East Asian Studies, 9*(1).

Park, C. M. (2009). The quality of life in South Korea. *Social Indicators Research, 92*(2), June 2009

Putnam R. D. (2007). E pluribus unum: Diversity and community in the twenty-first century the 2006 Johan Skytte prize lecture. *Scandinavian Political Studies, 30*(2). Nordic Political Science Association.

Qibtiyah, A. (2019). Indonesian muslim women and the gender equality movement. *Journal of Indonesian Islam, 3*(01), June 2009.

Rinaldo, R. 2008. Envisioning the nation: Women activists, religion and the public sphere in Indonesia. *Social Forces, 86*(4), 1781–1804.

Rizman, M. R. (2000). The relevance of nationalism for democratic citizenship. *The Public 7*, 1, 5–14,

Robinson, K. (2016). Religion, Gender and the State in Indonesia. In *East Asia forum June, 22. 2016*. https://www.eastasiaforum.org/2016/06/22/religion-gender-and-the-state-in-indonesia/

Seda et al. (2018). The paradox of relational well-being: A COMPARATIVE Study of South-East and East Asia Countries. *The Senshu Social Well-being Review*, No. 5. 2018. Senshu University.

Tsai, M. C., Laczko, L., & Bjornskov, C. (2011). Social diversity, institutions and trust: A cross-national analysis. *Social Indicators Research, 101*(3), 305–322, May 2011. Published by: Springer.

Vincent, J. (2002). *Introduction. The anthropology politics, a reader in ethnography, theory, and critique*. Blackwell Publisher Ltd.

Watzlawik, M. (2012). Cultural identity markers and identity as a whole: Some alternative solutions. *Culture & Psychology, 18*(2), 253–260. Sage Publication.

Wierienga, S. (2015). Gender harmony and the happy family: Islam, gender and sexuality in post-Reformasi Indonesia. *South East Asia Research, 23*(1), 27–44.

World Economy Forum. (2018). *The Global Gender Gap Report 2018*. WEF.

You, S. & Yoo, J. E. (2016). Prayer and subjective well-being: The moderating role of religious support. *Archive for the Psychology of Religion, 38*(3), 301–315. Koninklijke Brill NV.

Yuval-Davis, N., & Werbner, P. (Eds.). (1999). *Women, citizenship and difference. postcolonial encounters*. Zed Books.

Yuval-Davis, N. (2006) Belonging and the politics of belonging, *Journal Patterns of Prejudice, 40,* 3 Boundaries, Identities and Borders: Exploring the Cultural Production of Belonging, 197–214. Taylor and Francis.

Yuval-Davis, N. (2011). Power, intersectionality and the politics of belonging. In *FREIA Working Series no. 75*. Institut for Kultur og Globale Studier, Aalborg Universitet Globale Studier, Aalborg Universitet.

Lugina Setyawati is a lecturer and the Coordinator of Cultural Transformation and Digital Society Research Cluster at the Department of Sociology, Universitas Indonesia, and a research fellow at the Asia Research Centre, Universitas Indonesia. Since 2017 she is a member of Universitas Indonesia Team for the Asian Consortium on Social Well-being in Asia. Her research interests include youth activism, digital sociology, social inequality and social exclusion, gender relations, ethnic and cultural identity.

Francisia S. S. E. Seda is a Professor of Developmental Studies and senior lecturer and the Coordinator of Natural Resources Economics and Extractive Industries Research Cluster at the Department of Sociology, Universitas Indonesia. Since 2016 she is a member of the Universitas Indonesia Team for the Asian Consortium on Social Well-being in Asia. Her research interests include poverty and social exclusion, gender relations, environmental issues, and sociological theory.

Religious Association and Relational Well-Being a Comparative Study Between Indonesia and Japan

Muhammad R. Damm, Lugina Setyawati, and Ruzaki Hamda

Abstract The importance of religion in the discussion of social well-being lies in its role of facilitating the formation of association in society. The institutionalization of religion enables people to associate with each other in their social lives. In the context of resacralization in the modern world, this form of association contributes toward enhancing social well-being. This chapter uses a quantitative approach to discuss the significance of religious associations for improving social well-being, particularly in its relational dimension. Religious association was measured using three indicators: religious fairness, religious activities, and religious organizations, whereas relational well-being was measured using three indicators: perception, interaction, and participation. This chapter primarily uses 2015–2017 data from the Social Well-Being Survey in Asia. A comparison between the cases of Indonesia and Japan served to highlight the significance of religious association by showing the relationship between religious association and relational well-being in both countries. The quantitative analysis results show that religious association is positively correlated with relational well-being. However, our analysis based on secondary literature shows that the social and historical context of each country determines how the variables are connected, as well as the outcomes of their relation.

Keywords Indonesia · Japan · Relational well-being · Religious association

1 Introduction

In sociology, the concepts of modernization and secularization were developed simultaneously, particularly in the 1950s and 1960s. A mainstream perspective details that the advancement of modernity will inevitably cause the decline of religion until it loses all significance in the future (Berger, 1967; see also Berger & Luckmann, 1967; Shimazono, 2012, p. 5). However, Shimazono (2012) noted that in the 1980s and

M. R. Damm · L. Setyawati (✉) · R. Hamda
Department of Sociology, Universitas Indonesia, Depok, Indonesia
e-mail: lugina.setyawati09@ui.ac.id

J. Yee et al. (eds.), *Social Well-Being, Development, and Multiple Modernities in Asia*,
https://doi.org/10.1007/978-981-97-3866-3_17

1990s, the number of sociologists who continued to have this theoretical stance was decreasing. Most sociologists believed that the influence of religions may be weakened in an advanced modern world, but this does not indicate that modern society will become completely secularized. Berger and Hefner (2003) affirmed that religions maintain their importance in society. The modern world has witnessed a return of the sacred in a process called "resacralization" (Shimazono, 2012, p. 5).

Shimazono (2012) suggested that "resacralization" can be observed from three aspects: the revival of traditional religions, rise of spirituality, and realization of the limit of secularization. These three aspects may occur simultaneously in society. However, the prominence of the revival of traditional religions over the remaining two aspects is observed primarily in developing countries, whereas the rise of spirituality is prominent in developed and industrialized countries. Compared with the first two aspects, the contexts for the realization of the limit of secularization are increasingly specific. Shimazono (2012, p. 6) noted that realization of the limit of secularization is primarily observed among people who work in hospitals and schools and thus feel the need for religion and spirituality in their lives.

In this chapter, we explore how Shimazono's notion of the three aspects of resacralization is useful for understanding the significance of religious association for social well-being, particularly in its relational dimension, in Indonesian and Japanese society. Since the 1970s, Japan has been undergoing a process wherein spirituality has become increasingly crucial over time as a response to the limitations of secularism brought about by modernity. In this process, the return of sacred aspects in social life has been reliant on more introspection and highlighting individuality more than the sacralization offered by traditional religion. Shimazono (2012) characterized resacralization with two simultaneous processes, namely, transformations "from secularism to religion" and "from religion to spirituality." Unlike traditional religions that tend to be institutional and bind people in a collectivity, rising spirituality places increased emphasis on individual well-being and gathers numerous like-minded people with loose ties.

The rising new spirituality movement in Japan is indicated by the adoption of the term "*supirichuarity*" (spirituality) or "*supirichuaru*" (spiritual) in modern Japanese vocabulary (Nakayama, 2019). However, unlike the growth of the "New Age" movement in America or Europe, the spirituality movement in Japan is a revival of Japanese folk and traditional spirituality that was already present among them. The trend of rising spirituality and religiosity, as noted by Nakayama (2019, p. 4), was observed in the results of surveys conducted in 1998 and 2008 by the International Social Survey Program regarding religious views among Japanese people. Compared with the 1998 findings, the 2008 survey shows that an increasing number of people felt closer to religion.

A different process occurred in Indonesia. Instead of the rise of spirituality, the return of the sacred has taken the form of the revival of religion, particularly among Muslims, who represent majority of the Indonesian population. Since the 1980s, an inflow of revivalist ideas has been noted from transnational Islamic movements (Van Bruinessen, 2002). During the 1980s, this idea was brought about primarily by Indonesian Muslim scholars who studied in some Middle Eastern countries, particularly Saudi Arabia and Egypt. This process led to the emergence of Islamic movements that sprouted through many social and political organizations as post-Suharto Indonesia entered the new millennium. In politics, this so-called transnational Islamism manifested as a political party—the most notable is the Justice and Prosperity Party (*Partai Keadilan Sejahtera*/PKS) that was established in 1999 as Justice Party (*Partai Keadilan*/PK) and rooted in the *Tarbiyah* movement that has been active since the 1980s. Some other organizations were founded as social organizations (*organisasi kemasyarakatan/ormas*), such as the Front of Islamic Defenders (*Front Pembela Islam*/FPI).

As transnational Islamic movements emerged in the Indonesian social and political landscape after the fall of the New Order, some "local" Islamic organizations also took turns awakening. For decades, Islamic social and political forces have been repressed since the later period of Sukarno's regime and along the course of Suharto's New Order (Bertrand, 2004). Eventually, in the 2000s, Islamic movements, with their diversity and antagonism, became apparent in the public sphere. Islamic discourse has also become more common when discussing many topics concerning contemporary social and political development. One of the most notable manifestations of this condition is the strengthening of identity politics in recent years, particularly one based on religion.

Against this background, the current chapter discusses how religious association contributes to the development of relational well-being in Indonesia and Japan. Their contrasting historical and social backgrounds may provide a richer context for understanding the significance of religious association in enhancing relational well-being. In this chapter, we define religious association as individuals' perceptions of their ties to religion-based groups or communities. Through religious association, religion assumes a role in providing people with a set of norms, networks, and grounds to nurture trust, similar to Putnam's account (2000) on social capital. Religiosity also works as a meaningful system that provides a foundation for people's coping strategies with their problems in life.

Religious association in the context of this chapter, covers several aspects of social life, and at least three of them are identified. The first aspect is called religious fairness and can be considered a condition wherein people can freely express their religious identification and derive opportunities to mingle with like-minded others, especially to practice religious activities. Hayward and Elliot (2013) noted that this condition determines the positive association between religion and well-being. The second aspect is called religious activities. VanderWeele (2017) noted that participation in communal religious practices is strongly associated with human flourishing. The third aspect is called religious organization and can be understood as a group or community tied with a relatively strong religious identity, whether or not it takes the form of a formal organization. Lim and Putnam (2010) noted that people's involvement in religious congregations positively affects their life satisfaction. These three aspects are combined to form the concept of religious association.

Furthermore, social well-being is defined as a combination of people's perceptions of their living conditions, the quality of their relationships with others at the community level, and the condition of the community (Koo et al., 2016). Accordingly, social well-being is a multidimensional concept because it has various levels of analysis, including personal, relational, and societal well-being (Seda et al., 2018, p. 86). This chapter, however, focuses on relational well-being, which primarily discusses individuals' subjective perceptions of their social relations at the community level.

This chapter aims to understand the relationship between religious association and social well-being in its relational dimension (or simply, relational well-being). In this chapter, we attempt to prove that they supposedly have a close relationship and show that their connections are determined by particular social and historical contexts that are unique to certain societies.

2 Method

This chapter uses a quantitative method for data collection and analysis. The deductive process of quantitative data collection was conducted by establishing conceptual and operational definitions for relational well-being as the dependent variable and religious association as the independent variable.

The relational well-being variable comprises three indicators: perception, interaction, and participation (Seda et al., 2018, p. 86). Perception indicators were measured based on respondents' trust toward their family, neighbors, friends, and colleagues in their interactions. Interaction indicators were measured based on the intensity and frequency of our respondents' interactions with others, as well as the number of people our respondents interacted with. Participation indicators were measured based on the intensity and frequency of the respondents' participation in public activities in their communities. These indicators were statistically analyzed to measure the composite index of RWB.

The variable of religious association comprises three indicators: religious fairness, activities, and organizations. Examining these indicators is a necessary task. Membership of a religious organization is an expression wherein a person associates themselves with a certain religion. However, more than just membership, the religious organizations indicator also indicates how reliable a religious community or institution is, according to people's perceptions in helping them cope with real-life problems. Likewise, people express their associations with certain religious groups by engaging in religious activities. Religious fairness must be considered because it determines people's freedom to grasp religious identity and express it without concerns about being discriminated against and treated unfairly. Moreover, the questionnaire used to collect quantitative data was designed to understand perceptions toward these indicators.

Indicators of the dependent and independent variables were identified, thus the availability of relevant items in the questionnaire of the 2015–2017 Social Well-Being Survey in Asia (SoWSA) can be used to measure them. Table 1 lists these items.

Data from the questionnaire for measuring each variable were subsequently processed by indexation (combining their scores) and re-categorization to increase

Table 1 Items in the SoWSA questionnaire

Variable	Items in SWB Survey's questionnaire
Relational Well-being	C0102, C0103, C0104, C0105, C0106, C0201, C0202, C0301, C0302, C0402, C0403, C0404, C0407, C05
Religious association	F29, W0311, W0411, C07, R0209, R0609

the ease of data interpretation and inference. Bivariate and multivariate regression analyses were conducted. The purpose of this analysis is to examine the relationship between religious association variables and relational well-being. The analytical model can be illustrated as follows.

The analysis model in Fig. 1 shows that to enrich our understanding of how religious associations contribute to relational well-being, we analyze its influence, as well as the influence of its three indicators, on each indicator of relational well-being—namely, perception, interaction, and participation. Hopefully, we will gain an improved understanding of which aspect of relational well-being significantly contributes to religious association, as well as which aspect of religious association significantly contributes to relational well-being.

Reliability analysis results show that all indicators were constructed using valid and reliable variables, with a Cronbach's alpha value of 0.825 for perception, 0.728 for interaction, and 0.857 for participation.

In line with the analysis model, the hypothesis to be tested in this chapter can be formulated as follows: higher religious association leads to higher relational well-being. Accordingly, the hypothesis is also applicable for predicting the relationship between the three indicators of religious association and the three indicators of relational well-being. This hypothesis aligns with the finding of Lim and Putnam (2010) that regular attendance in religious services (or activities) and the presence of social networks among members of a religious association contribute to people's satisfaction in their life.

However, testing and proving the hypothesis does not necessarily provide a sufficient explanation of the relationship between religious association and relational well-being. Both religious association and relational well-being comprise several components. Therefore, a detailed discussion must be conducted about how each indicator of religious association contributes to relational well-being and each of its

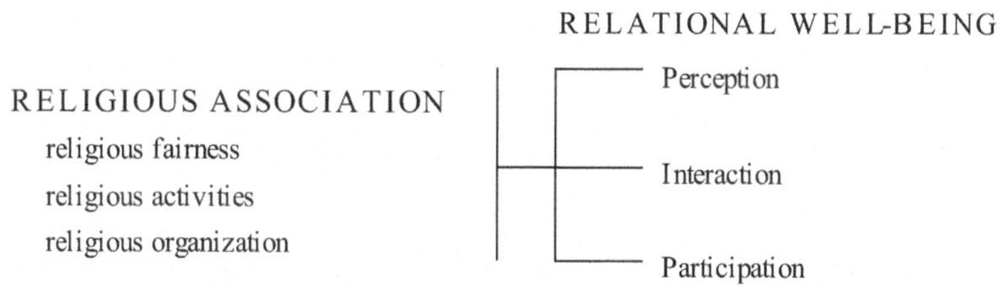

Fig. 1 Model of analysis

indicators. By discussing the relationship between the two variables in the historical and social contexts of Indonesia and Japan, we aim to derive an understanding of the social mechanisms that enable the two variables to be connected.

3 An Overview of Relational Well-Being Through Religion

This section provides a brief overview of relational well-being in Indonesia and Japan. Based on the analysis of the quantitative data from the questionnaire, we assigned scores in the range of 0–10 for every variable (relational well-being and religious association) and their respective indicators. The overall score of relational well-being in Indonesia is significantly higher than that of Japan, as indicated by their scores: 6.70 and 4.68, respectively. This indicates that the individual's subjective perception of relational well-being is higher in Indonesia than in Japan. In a more specific description, based on the score per indicator, the results show a similar trend. Table 2 provides detailed scores for each indicator in both countries:

Table 2 demonstrates that among the indicators of relational well-being in Indonesia, the indicator of interaction has the highest score (7.86), followed by participation (6.18) and perception (6.05). Meanwhile, in Japan, the perception indicator has the highest score (5.54), followed by interaction (5.11), and participation (3.27). It is also apparent that in both countries, the participation indicator has the lowest score among the relational well-being indicators.

However, we can delve deeper into the score of relational well-being in Indonesia and Japan to establish improved understanding and richer interpretation by identifying the different scores between different religion-based groups in each country. Therefore, the categorization of "majority" and "minority" is useful for classifying the population based on groups' size relative to total population of each country. The term "majority" refers to a group with the highest number of members in the population, whereas "minority" refers to groups with lower numbers of members in the population. However, in this chapter, the use of both terms is not intended to discuss their broader social and political meanings, because neither our theoretical framework nor analysis model includes any analytical tool to problematize power relations within society. The categorization aims solely to enable a simple analysis without making misleading or generalized claims.

Table 2 Comparison of relational well-being in Indonesia and Japan

		Indonesia		Japan	
		Overall	Std	Overall	Std
Dependent Variable	Relational Well-Being	6.70	1.11	4.68	1.02
Indicators	Perception	6.05	1.22	5.54	1.25
	Interaction	7.86	1.26	5.11	1.35
	Participation	6.18	2.07	3.27	1.48

According to data from Pew-Templeton's Global Religious Futures Project, Muslims comprise the largest population group in Indonesia. According to 2010 census, Muslims (87.2%) were the majority, thereby outnumbering adherents of other religions, such as Protestantism (6.9%), Catholicism (2.9%), and other religions whose adherents are less than 1 percent of the total population (Pew Research Center, 2015). The projection for 2020 shows a relatively similar composition as the Muslim population insignificantly decreased, that is, 87.0%. For Japan, the majority of its population consists of people who are unaffiliated with any particular religion, whereas its minority comprises groups of people affiliated with certain religions. According to the 2010 census, Buddhists comprise the largest portion of Japan's minority population, accounting for 36.2% of the total population (Pew Research Center, 2015). Regarding the unaffiliated group, although we can characterize it as the majority, its number is slightly higher than half of Japan's population, that is, 57.0% (Pew Research Center, 2015). Interestingly, the projection for 2020 shows that the number of unaffiliated people increased to 60.0 percent, whereas the number of Buddhists decreased to 33.2%. Table 3 provides detailed information about population by religion in Japan and Indonesia.

Although the general picture of relational well-being, as presented in Table 2, shows a significant gap in overall scores between Indonesia and Japan, the difference in the perception of relational well-being between the majority and minority groups in each country is insignificant. In Indonesia, the score for relational well-being among Muslims was 6.76, whereas that of other religious groups was 6.49. Likewise, in Japan, the group unaffiliated with any particular religion has a relational well-being score of 4.68, whereas the group with religious affiliation has a score of 5.44. For each indicator of relational well-being, the scores by religion in both countries are shown in Table 4.

Although no significant difference was noted in scores between the majority and minority groups in each country, the results show a different trend between the two groups in Indonesia and Japan. In Indonesia, the majority group had a higher score, whereas in Japan, the minority group had a higher score. Although the scores of the majority and minority groups were slightly discrepant, differences in trends may indicate a different condition that shapes the relationship between religion and relational well-being in both countries. The high score of relational well-being in Indonesia for both the majority and minority groups may indicate the contribution of religion to relational well-being. However, the score of the Muslim population, as the majority, is higher than that of others, thereby indicating that the status of being the majority has its own significance.

Contrarily, the case of Japan shows that majority status does not contribute positively to relational well-being. The score of the religion-affiliated group is likely to be higher than that of the unaffiliated group because the former is affiliated with a specific religion and its community that facilitates the formation of relational well-being. Furthermore, it is understandable that the so-called group of unaffiliated people is not actually a group in a proper sense. In this context, they are grouped only because they are not tied to a certain group.

Table 3 Population by religion in Japan and Indonesia (2010)

Country	Buddhists	Catholics	Protestants	Folk religions	Hindus	Jews	Muslims	Other religions	Unaffiliated
Japan	45,820,000	379,620	337,260	450,000	30,000	< 10,000	200,000	5,890,000	72,120,000
	36.2%	0.3%	0.7%	< 1%	< 1%	< 1%	< 1%	4.7%	57.0%
Indonesia	1,720,000	7,196,100	13,912,460	750,000	4,050,000	< 10,000	209,120,000	340,000	240,000
	< 1%	2.9%	6.9%	< 1%	< 1%	< 1%	87.2%	< 1%	< 1%

Sources Pew Research Center (2015)

Table 4 Comparison of relational well-being by religious affiliation in Indonesia and Japan

		Indonesia				Japan			
		Muslims		Others		Unaffiliated		Affiliated	
		Mean	Std	Mean	Std	Mean	Std	Mean	Std
Dependent Variable	Relational Well-Being	6.76	1.07	6.49	1.22	4.68	1.02	5.44	1.48
Indicator	Perception	6.09	1.19	5.89	1.30	5.54	1.25	5.39	1.59
	Interaction	7.93	1.25	7.62	1.26	5.11	1.35	6.25	1.48
	Participation	6.25	2.00	5.97	2.28	3.26	1.48	4.69	1.96

At this point, two interesting findings led to our hypothesis. First, in the case of Indonesia, the score of relational well-being was relatively high, both among the majority and minority religions. Second, in the case of Japan, the score of relational well-being was higher among religion-affiliated groups, compared with religion-unaffiliated groups, despite the latter comprising the majority of Japanese society. Based on these findings, it was intriguing that religion, especially at the mezzo level in its form as a religious association, seemingly contributes to the relational well-being of each country. In the next section, we discuss how religious association contributes to relational well-being.

4 Religious Association in Indonesia and Japan

As discussed in the previous section, religious associations as an independent variable in this chapter are stipulated to have three indicators: religious fairness, activities, and organization. However, it is important to emphasize that they were measured by surveying respondents, because they perceived these indicators. In other words, the operational definitions of these indicators are based on the perspective of individuals who perceive the existence of religious associations in their daily lives. To complement this "subjective" construction of religious association, our discussion on the topic utilizes explanations based on our literature study. These are primarily explanations at the mezzo and macro levels.

Based on the quantitative data provided by the SoWSA, Indonesia has a higher score for religious association than Japan. Their gap is also significant: Indonesia's score is 6.90, whereas Japan's score is 4.71. For each indicator of religious association, the trend was similar. Indonesia scored significantly higher than Japan, in terms of religious fairness, activities, and organizations. Detailed descriptions of this finding are presented in Table 5:

In subsequent sections, we discuss each indicator of religious association and their correlation with each indicator of relational well-being. We also simultaneously attempt to compare the context and conditions of the topic in both countries.

Table 5 Comparison of religious association in Indonesia and Japan

		Indonesia	Japan
Independent variable	Religious association	6.90	4.71
Indicators	Religious fairness	7.41	5.18
	Religious activities	5.85	4.89
	Religious organization	7.44	4.06

4.1 Religious Fairness in Indonesia and Japan

We compare the situations related to religious fairness in Indonesia and Japan. As an indicator of religious association, the scoring of religious fairness in this chapter was drawn from survey data about two issues: the fairness of the treatments experienced by individuals based on their religious affiliation, and the benefits of religion in their social life. Based on overall scores of the indicator, individual perceptions of religious fairness were higher in Indonesia than in Japan. The score for religious fairness in Indonesia is 7.41, whereas in Japan it is 5.18. Regarding the two aforementioned issues of religious fairness, the trend is similar. Indonesia has a significantly higher score for respondents' perception regarding fairness in the treatments people receive based on their religion, as well as for their perception of the benefits gained throughout their lives due to their religion.

Table 6 provides the overall score for religious fairness in Indonesia and Japan.

Indonesia's religious fairness score is higher than that of Japan. However, if we look at the data by considering the distinction between the majority and minority groups, as shown in Table 6, we see that the cases of both countries tell quite different stories.

For Indonesia, the scores presented in Table 6 clarify the importance of religion to the perception of religious fairness and show that affiliation with the religion of the majority positively contributes to such perceptions. The Muslim majority group had a higher score (7.59) for religious fairness than the non-Muslim minority group (6.80). The gap between their scores was significant. In this context, it is interesting to compare the results with the report from Pew-Templeton's Global Religious Futures Project (Pew Research Center, 2015) that places Indonesia in the "high" category for social hostilities (with an index score of 5.5 in the range of 0–10) and in the

Table 6 Comparison of religious fairness in Indonesia and Japan

	Overall	Std	By Religion			
			Mean	Std	Mean	Std
Indonesia			Muslims		Others	
Religious fairness	7.41	1.82	7.59	1.66	6.80	2.17
Japan			Unaffiliated		Affiliated	
Religious Fairness	5.18	1.32	5.18	1.32	4.47	1.50

"very high" category for government restrictions (with an index score of 8.5). The high index score was mainly caused by rising religious intolerance in Indonesia, particularly toward religious minorities. This indicates that being in the majority group helps people receive fair treatment and more benefits in their social life. In Indonesia, the discourse of majority and minority groups is intertwined with religious association in influencing how people perceive religious fairness in their social life.

In the context of Japan, the score of religious fairness of the majority group unaffiliated with any religion and the minority group affiliated with a certain religion is 5.18 and 4.47, respectively. Compared to Indonesia, wherein contrasts in identity, especially based on ethnicity and religion, can be a determinant in one's social life, it seems that a lower score of religious fairness in Japan is not an indication of the presence of unfairness but instead indicates that religion is less influential in shaping power relations between different social groups in terms of social matters. This result is likely due to the characteristics of the population, which are more homogenous. It can be said that in Japan, religious affiliation is insignificant for people's perception of fairness in their social lives.

Indonesia is well-known as an extremely diverse country, where religion, among many categories, contributes to its multifaceted diversity. This extreme diversity demands religious fairness, so people with various religious identities can express their own beliefs without being worried about facing discrimination or unfair treatment. In this context, the discourse of majority–minority plays an influential role. Those affiliated with the dominant religion or religion adhered to by the majority population will find it easier to receive fair treatment, compared to those affiliated with non-dominant religious groups because the use of religion as a reference is not limited to individuals' personal lives in the private domain. Religious identity and affiliation have also become a part of social relations. On the contrary, in addition to the Japanese society's characteristics of being homogenous, the demise of institutional religion, as indicated by the high numbers of religion-unaffiliated people, and the rise of spirituality that places increased emphasis on private individual spiritual life (Shimazono, 2012), may contribute to the condition wherein religious affiliation is less significant than fairness or unfairness that people experienced in their social lives.

When we measured the correlation between religious fairness and relational well-being, the resulting score for their correlation value in Japan indicates that their correlation was not significant (<0.05, i.e., 0.046 to be exact). For Indonesia, the correlation value is 0.197; therefore, religious fairness is positively correlated with relational well-being. However, when we conducted a one-way analysis of variance (ANOVA) between these two variables, the results showed a p-value of 0.000 in both Japan and Indonesia. This implies that religious fairness is significantly related to relational well-being. We will return to this aspect in the final section of this chapter.

4.2 Religious Activities in Indonesia and Japan

The indicator of religious activities was measured by the frequency of memorial services for ancestors or deceased relatives attended by respondents. This type of service is crucial for many religions in both countries. In addition to its ritualistic value, memorial services usually play an important role in creating or strengthening social ties, especially among the relatives of deceased individuals. In a memorial service, the ancestor or the deceased plays a constitutive role, in which their absence brings together relatives and other people who have close relationships.

The scores for this indicator in Indonesia and Japan are presented in Table 7.

Table 7 shows that Indonesia has a higher score than Japan in religious activities for overall categories of respondents. The gap between the two is quite significant—Indonesia's score is 5.85, whereas Japan's score is 4.89. This result is understandable, because the majority of Japanese respondents identify themselves as unaffiliated with any religion so that they are unlikely to regularly attend or engage in any religious activities, including memorial services. The comparison of scores between those unaffiliated and affiliated with a religion confirms this explanation, because their gap is quite significant.

A significant difference was also observed between Muslim and other adherents in Indonesia. Interestingly, although Indonesia is known as a country with a Muslim majority, the score among Muslims is lower than that among other adherents. We can find one explanation for this result by observing the diversity in practicing and interpreting Islamic teachings among Indonesian Muslims.

Memorial services are prominent among the traditional Muslims. They usually hold memorial services for deceased relatives several times, namely, seven days, forty days, hundred days, and a thousand days after death. In some places, especially among the Javanese, a kind of memorial service known as *haul* is also administered regularly for a late religious figure or *kiai*, usually annually on the day of their death. This is one of the most significant practices that serves to distinguish between traditional and modernist Muslims in Indonesia. Modernist Muslims view this type of religious ceremonial as a ritual with no foundational basis in Islamic teaching and instead being rooted in tradition inherited from Indonesian Buddhism-Hinduism. In recent years, this growing modernist perspective has challenged many memorial services considered essential for religious practices by traditional Muslims.

Table 7 Comparison of religious activities in Indonesia and Japan

	Overall	Std	By Religion			
			Mean	Std	Mean	Std
Indonesia			Muslims		Others	
Religious activities	5.85	2.12	5.75	1.91	6.19	2.69
Japan			Unaffiliated		Affiliated	
Religious activities	4.89	2.14	4.89	2.14	3.98	1.91

When we measured the correlation between religious activities and relational well-being, the resulting score for their correlation value in both Japan and Indonesia indicated that religious activities positively contribute to relational well-being. The value of the correlation between them in Japan is 0.276, whereas in Indonesia, it is 0.216. We also conducted an ANOVA to determine the relationship between religious activities and relational well-being. One-way ANOVA test resulted in a p-value of 0.000. This implies that religious activities are significantly related to relational well-being. We will return to this topic in the final section of this chapter.

4.3 Religious Organization in Indonesia and Japan

In this chapter, the indicator of religious organization was defined neither from the perspective of the organizations themselves nor by objective measurements, such as the number of religion-based social organizations in both countries. Quantitative data for scoring religious organization indicators were collected from items in the SoWSA questionnaire regarding two issues: respondents' reliance on temples, churches, or other religious groups for dealing with personal problems and for help when natural disasters occurred in respondents' residential areas. Therefore, the indicator of religious organization was defined based on people's perspectives of the existence and importance of religious groups or organizations around them.

With regard to religious organizations, Indonesia had a significantly higher score than Japan. The overall score for Indonesia was 7.44, whereas that of Japan was 4.06. This indicates that religious groups or organizations play a significant role as a kind of safety net for Indonesians, either for coping with problems in their daily lives or for surviving a natural disaster. More detailed scores for religious organizations in both countries are available in Table 8.

In Indonesia, the gap between the scores of Muslims and other religious groups was insignificant. Both categories had high religious organization scores. A different situation has been observed in Japan. Unsurprisingly, the score for the religion-affiliated group was significantly higher than that for the religion-unaffiliated group. This finding indicates that those who tend to rely on religious organizations are those who have affiliations with such organizations.

Table 8 Comparison of religious organization in Indonesia and Japan

	Overall	Std	By Religion			
			Mean	Std	Mean	Std
Indonesia			Muslims		Others	
Religious organization	7.44	1.71	7.46	1.70	7.35	1.74
Japan			Unaffiliated		Affiliated	
Religious organization	4.06	1.75	4.05	1.75	5.94	1.76

Rituals and religious ceremonials contribute to public festivities in Indonesia and Japan. Indonesia has several public holidays sanctioned by the government based on the holidays of its six officially acknowledged religions: Islam, Protestant, Catholic, Hindu, Buddha, and Confucianism. The ruling of a religious holiday as a national public holiday has become a way for the government to express official recognition of religion. As Bertrand (2004) noted, in a diverse society, the government's recognition of religious groups and their representation in governmental institutions are crucial for Indonesian people. For example, the enactment of the Presidential Instruction to confirm the Chinese New Year (*Imlek*) as a national public holiday in 2002 signified an official recognition of Confucianism as a religion acknowledged by the Indonesian government. It also signified the end of a long state's discrimination toward ethnic Chinese people in Indonesia.

In the context of Indonesia, where a state's recognition is crucial for the well-being of religious groups, it is also important for them to establish an organization as a vehicle to access many forms of resources; in particular, when the relationship between the state and religious organizations and communities took the form of patronage during the course of the New Order. This patronage tendency has been occurring since, until contemporary post-Suharto Indonesia. Therefore, it is unsurprising if religious organizations (usually in the form of social organizations) play roles in distributing resources to people (particularly those affiliated with them), especially when natural disasters occur.

When we measure the correlation between religious organizations and relational well-being, the resulting value of their correlation in both Japan and Indonesia indicates that religious organizations positively contribute to relational well-being. Their correlation value in Japan is 0.301, whereas in Indonesia it is 0.207. We ensured the relationship between religious organization and relational well-being by conducting a one-way ANOVA, which resulted in a p-value of 0.000. This implies that religious organizations, such as religious fairness and activities, are also significantly related to relational well-being. This is discussed in the next section.

5 The Contribution of Religious Association to Relational Well-Being in Indonesia and Japan

To examine the relationship between religious association as an independent variable and relational well-being as a dependent variable, we conducted a quantitative analysis to verify their correlation. The results of the analysis show that in both countries, the value of the correlation is significant (>0.05); the overall score of Indonesia and Japan is 0.531. This finding indicates that in both Indonesia and Japan, religious association has influenced relational well-being. Accordingly, the hypotheses of this chapter were confirmed, namely, that there is a positive correlation between religious association as an independent variable and relational well-being as a dependent variable. However, the scores of the correlation coefficient between religious associations and each indicator of relational well-being varied. Among the three indicators of relational well-being (perception, interaction, and participation), religious association had the strongest correlation with interaction, at 0.512. Meanwhile, the lowest score was for the correlation between religious association and perception (0.286). The correlation between religious associations and participation was 0.452.

When the value of the correlation is elaborated based on the country, the overall score for Japan is higher than that of Indonesia (0.372 and 0.337, respectively). Table 9 provides a detailed description of the correlation between religious associations and relational well-being in Indonesia and Japan, including the correlation between each indicator of both variables.

From Table 9, we observe that in Indonesia, religious association has utmost significance for participation, whereas in Japan, it has utmost significance for interaction. Although religious association correlates with relational well-being in both countries, its indicator of religious fairness has an insignificant score in Japan (<0.05). This indicates that only the other two indicators, religious activities and religious organizations, contribute to relational well-being in Japan. However, for Indonesia, all three indicators of religious associations have a strong correlation with relational well-being. Among the indicators, religious activities had the highest score in Indonesia (0.216), whereas Japan's score for this indicator was higher (0.276). Meanwhile, the religious organization indicator has the highest score in Japan, with a score of 0.301, whereas Indonesia's score for the same indicator is 0.207.

Table 9 Correlation between religious association and relational well-being in Indonesia and Japan

Independent variable	Dependent variable	Value (Correlation)	
		Indonesia	Japan
Religious association	Relational Well-Being	0.337	0.372
Religious association	Perception	0.195	0.272
Religious association	Interaction	0.263	0.342
Religious association	Participation	0.266	0.260
Religious fairness	Relational Well-Being	0.197	0.046
Religious fairness	Perception	0.133	0.085
Religious fairness	Interaction	0.202	0.032
Religious fairness	Participation	0.115	-0.012
Religious activities	Relational Well-Being	0.216	0.276
Religious activities	Perception	0.087	0.140
Religious activities	Interaction	0.129	0.311
Religious activities	Participation	0.217	0.209
Religious organization	Relational Well-Being	0.207	0.301
Religious organization	Perception	0.146	0.258
Religious organization	Interaction	0.158	0.216
Religious organization	Participation	0.151	0.223

Although we found that a correlation exists, we still need to understand *how* religious associations correlate with relational well-being. Considering that our strategy of analysis uses the contrast between religion-based majority and minority in each country as a tool to capture the nuance of the relationship between the two measured variables, we need to measure the value of their correlation along the line of this contrast. In the last section of our discussion, we will also try to situate this quantitative finding in the larger context of Indonesia and Japan, so that we can understand how religious association contributes to relational well-being in both countries. Table 10 provides the detailed scores for the correlation.

Table 10 informs us that among all categories of the sample in both Indonesia and Japan, religious association has a significant correlation with relational well-being, as well as with each of its indicators. The strongest correlation between religious association and relational well-being manifests in Japan's religion-affiliated group, with a value of 0.679. A similar result is also apparent regarding the correlation between religious association and the three indictors of relational well-being: Japan's religion-affiliated group has the highest score for each correlation. For Indonesia, no significant difference was noted between Muslims and those of other religions. There is a tendency for religious associations to be as influential for relational well-being among Muslim majorities as among non-Muslim minorities.

Table 10 Correlation between religious association and relational well-being by religious affiliation in Indonesia and Japan

Independent variable	Dependent variable	Indonesia		Japan	
		Muslim	Others	Affiliated	Unaffiliated
Religious association	Relational Well-Being	0.329	0.344	0.679	0.371
Religious association	Perception	0.164	0.266	0.723	0.272
Religious association	Interaction	0.252	0.281	0.458	0.342
Religious association	Participation	0.272	0.243	0.626	0.259
Religious fairness	Relational Well-Being	0.151	0.257	0.020	0.046
Religious fairness	Perception	0.071	0.245	0.114	0.085
Religious fairness	Interaction	0.167	0.247	-0.196	0.033
Religious fairness	Participation	0.096	0.133	0.129	-0.011
Religious activities	Relational Well-Being	0.254	0.169	0.608	0.277
Religious activities	Perception	0.111	0.057	0.571	0.139
Religious activities	Interaction	0.156	0.103	0.496	0.311
Religious activities	Participation	0.244	0.182	0.571	0.209
Religious organization	Relational Well-Being	0.219	0.168	0.618	0.299
Religious organization	Perception	0.130	0.188	0.663	0.258
Religious organization	Interaction	0.160	0.142	0.502	0.214
Religious organization	Participation	0.173	0.082	0.499	0.221

Interestingly, among religion-affiliated groups in Japan, religious fairness tends to have a notably weaker correlation with both relational well-being (0.020) and all its indicators. We found a negative correlation between religious fairness and interaction (− 0.196). An interesting finding was also observed in Indonesia, where the correlation between religious fairness and relational well-being, as well as its correlation with each indicator of relational well-being, is stronger among non-Muslim minorities than among Muslim majorities.

Regarding the correlation between religious activities and relational well-being as well as the correlation between religious activities and each of the three indicators of relational well-being, the strongest correlation manifests among Japan's religion-affiliated group, followed by Japan's unaffiliated group. Meanwhile, in Indonesia, the correlation among Muslim majorities was slightly higher than that among non-Muslim minorities.

There is also a positive correlation between religious organization and relational well-being among religion-unaffiliated groups in Japan, but this correlation is notably stronger among religion-affiliated groups. In Indonesia, the value of the correlation between the Muslim majority and non-Muslim minority is slightly different.

The results of the quantitative analysis indicate that religious association with all of their indicators contribute to relational well-being in Indonesia, but in Japan, only the indicators of religious activities and religious organizations contribute to the significance of religious association for relational well-being. We must understand this by placing them in each country's sociopolitical context. As discussed in the earlier part of this chapter, there are different trends in both countries in how religiosity develops as a response to the trajectory of modernity that brings secularism and secularization. In Indonesia, it has been taking place as a revival of traditional religion, particularly among Muslims, since the 1980s. Furthermore, in Japan, the return of religion to modern Japanese life has assumed a form of the rise of spirituality since the 1970s.

Indonesia's democratization after the collapse of the New Order in 1998 provides fertile ground for the public expression of diverse identities. Considering that this development is necessary for understanding the contribution of religious associations to Indonesians' relational well-being, Hayward and Elliot (2013) suggested that the positive association between religion and well-being depends on religious freedom and the opportunity to congregate (Hayward & Elliot, 2013).

During the course of the New Order, there was a code of conduct that limited freedom of expression, including the expression of identity. Some primordial identifications were considered "too sensitive" to be expressed publicly—these identifications were commonly labeled as "SARA" (an acronym for *suku, agama, ras, dan antargolongan*, i.e., ethnicity, religion, race, and intergroup) and rendered as a taboo for public sphere due to its potential to threat national unity. The minority groups experienced oppression and discrimination and had virtually no freedom to express their cultural uniqueness in the public sphere. A well-known example is the case of ethnic Chinese people, who were prohibited from public celebrations for their holidays, such as the Chinese New Year (*Imlek*). However, oppression and discrimination were not limited to minorities, and even Muslims, who comprise the majority of the Indonesian population, have experienced these. For example, until the early 1990s, female Muslim students were prohibited from wearing a scarf (*hijab*) while attending public schools.

However, with the demise of the New Order's oppressive legacy, the recent wave of democratization has developed on the basis that everyone is free to be different and has the right to express their difference. One notable unintended consequence of this process of democratization is the growing identity politics in Indonesian social and political life. Many scholars have noted the importance of "representation" in understanding the dynamics of Indonesian diversity in their social lives. It is crucial for Indonesians that their social identity is represented in public life, either through the presence of their representatives in public institutions, especially in the legislative and executive branches of the government, or through regulations issued by the government. Along with the advancement of democratization, identity politics have proven to be effective in facilitating the struggle for this representation. The 2017 Jakarta gubernatorial election and the 2019 Indonesian presidential election are the most notable cases to illustrate the recent rise of identity politics in Indonesian public life. Within this context, religious association and its three indicators play a significant role in Indonesians' perceptions of relational well-being.

This finding reminds us of a statement by Berger and Luckmann (1967) on their account that living in a religious world, as shown by the case of Indonesia, requires affiliation with the religious community. However, affiliation with the religious community, as we argue in this chapter, not only helps people to *survive*; it also helps people to *flourish*—to be happy and satisfied with their life, maintaining mental and physical health, as well as having meaning and purpose, character and virtue, and close social relationships (VanderWeele, 2017). Moreover, VanderWeele's findings (2017) show that the association of communal religious participation with human flourishing is notably stronger than that of spiritual-religious identity or private religious practices. These findings align with that of Lim and Putnam (2010), who found little evidence that private or subjective aspects of religiosity affect life satisfaction independent of attendance and congregational friendship.

In the context of the discussion in this chapter, a comparison between Indonesia and Japan also produces similar results. In contemporary Indonesia, where the return of the sacred takes a path into a more public and outward-looking religiosity, its religious association (see Table 5) and relational well-being (see Table 2) tend to be higher than that of Japan, wherein the current development of religiosity is primarily oriented toward a more private and inward-looking spirituality. However, both cases maintain that religious associations contribute significantly to relational well-being (see Table 9).

6 Conclusion

The findings discussed in this chapter demonstrate that religious association contributes to relational well-being. The cases of Indonesia and Japan confirm this finding, as indicated by the value of the correlation between those variables in Indonesia, both among Muslims and other groups, and among religion-affiliated groups in Japan.

The overall score for each indicator of religious associations—fairness, activities, and organization—among Indonesians was higher than that of Japanese respondents. However, the analysis of each indicator based on religious groups found no specific trend or pattern. In Indonesia, the score of religious fairness among Muslims, that is, individuals' perception of fairness treatment based on religion, is the highest. A similar result was also indicated in the score of religious organizations, that is, individuals' perceptions of the role of religious organizations in coping with various problems in life. However, the score for religious activities is higher among non-Muslim people; they have a higher frequency of religious activities compared to that of Muslims. The analysis results show that Japan has experienced different trends regarding religious associations. The unaffiliated group scored higher for religious fairness and religious activities than the affiliated group. However, the score for religious organizations among the affiliated group was higher than that of the unaffiliated group.

Furthermore, both countries have been experiencing different trajectories regarding the dynamics of religiosity of their people in response to the development of modernity that leads to secularism and secularization. Indonesia's recent condition is characterized by the revival of traditional religion, especially among Muslims. The spread of transnational Islamic movements and traditional Muslims' responses toward them contribute significantly to this development. The rise of identity politics following Indonesia's practice of direct elections in its national and regional politics as part of its democratization also promotes more public and outward-looking characteristics of its resacralization process. In Japan, the rise in spirituality has become increasingly prominent. In an industrialized society, the population of religiously unaffiliated people outnumbers those who maintain their affiliation, especially with Buddhism. In the absence of religious affiliation, private and personal practices of spirituality are likely to occur as a response to secular modernity. This promotes increased private and inward-looking spirituality. Moreover, this contrast helps us understand that the historical and social context of a society determines how religious association contributes to its relational well-being.

Appendix

See Table 11.

Table 11 List of questions used in this article

Variable	Dimension	Indicator	Question
Religious association	Religion as profile	Religion	F29
(Independent variable)	Religion as practice	Religious fairness	W0311 "Religion fairness"
			W0411 How much advantages or disadvantages in your life due to: Religion?
		Religious activities	C07 How frequently do you attend memorials or services for those close to you or ancestors who have already died?
		Religious organization	R0209 How much do you rely on for dealing with personal problems: temple, church, or other religious group?
			R0609 How much would you rely on if natural disasters occur in your residential area: temple, church, or other religious group?
Social Well-Being	Relational	Perception	C01 To what degree can you trust or not trust… ?
(Dependent variable)			C0101 most people
			C0102 family members
			C0103 your neighbors
			C0104 friends and acquaintances
			C0105 work colleagues
			C0106 unknown individuals
		Interaction	C02 How often do you interact with… ?
			C0201 family/relatives
			C0202 friends or acquaintances
			C0301 How do you describe your level of interaction with your neighbors?
			C0302 How many people do you interact with in your neighborhood?
		Participation	C04 How often do you participate in… ?
			C0401 sports or hobby
			C0402 community engagement
			C0403 helping the elderlies
			C0404 supporting children
			C0405 preventing criminal activities
			C0406 social support during disaster

(continued)

Table 11 (continued)

Variable	Dimension	Indicator	Question
			C0407 engage in other forms of neighborhood activities
			C05 How often do you participate in traditional/religious activities in your neighborhood?

References

Berger, P. L. (1967). *The sacred canopy: Elements of a sociological theory of religion*. Open Road.

Berger, P. L., & Luckmann, T. (1967). *The social construction of reality*. Penguin Books.

Berger, P. L., & Hefner, R. W. (2003). Spiritual capital in comparative perspective. *Paper prepared for the Spiritual Capital Planning Meeting*.

Bertrand, J. (2004). *Nationalism and ethnic conflict in Indonesia*. Cambridge University Press.

Hayward, R. D., & Elliot, M. (2013). Cross-national analysis of the influence of cultural norms and government restrictions on the relationship between religion and well-being. *Review of Religious Research, 56*, 23–43.

Koo, H., Yee, J., Nam, E. Y., & Kim, E. S. (2016). Dimensions of social well-being and determinants in Korea: Personal, relational, and societal aspects. *The Senshu Social Well-Being Review, 3*, 27–58.

Lim, C., & Putnam, R. D. (2010). Religion, social networks, and life satisfaction. *American Sociological Review, 75*(6), 914–933.

Nakayama, O. (2019). New spirituality in Japan and its place in the teaching of moral education. *Religions, 10*(4), 278.

Pew Research Center. (2015). *The future of world religions: population growth projections, 2010–2050*. Pew Research Center.

Putnam, R. (2000). *Bowling alone: The collapse and revival of American community*. Simon and Schuster.

Seda, F. S. S. E., Setiono, L. S., Pera, Y. H. T., Febriani, R., Damm, M. R., & Kurniawan, K. N. (2018). The paradox of relational well-being: A comparative study of South-East and East Asian countries. *The Senshu Social Well-Being Review, 5*, 83–91.

Shimazono, S. (2012). From salvation to spirituality: The contemporary transformation of religions viewed from East Asia. *Religious Studies in Japan, 1*, 3–23.

Van Bruinessen, M. (2002). Genealogies of Islamic radicalism in post-Soeharto Indonesia. *South East Asia Research, 10*(2), 117–154.

Van Bruinessen, M. (2018). Indonesian muslims in a globalising world: westernisation, arabisation, and indigenising responses. *RSIS Working Paper No.311*.

VanderWeele, T. J. (2017). Religious communities and human flourishing. *Current Directions in Psychological Science, 26*(5), 476–481.

Muhammad R. Damm is a lecturer at Universitas Indraprasta PGRI, a research fellow at the Asia Research Centre, Universitas Indonesia, and a PhD student at the University of Gothenburg. He has been a member of Universitas Indonesia Team for the Asian Consortium on Social Well-being in Asia in 2017–2020. His research interests include urban water governance and social inequality.

Lugina Setyawati is a lecturer and the Coordinator of Cultural Transformation and Digital Society Research Cluster at the Department of Sociology, Universitas Indonesia, and a research fellow at the Asia Research Centre, Universitas Indonesia. Since 2017 she is a member of Universitas Indonesia Team for the Asian Consortium on Social Well-being in Asia. Her research interests include youth activism, digital sociology, social inequality and social exclusion, gender relations, ethnic and cultural identity.

Ruzaki Hamda graduated from the Department of Sociology, Universitas Indonesia. He currently works as a staff in the Research and Development Planning Agency at Sub-National Level, Padang Panjang City, West Sumatera Province, Indonesia. He has been a member of Universitas Indonesia Team for the Asian Consortium on Social Well-being in Asia in 2017–2020.

Multiple Ways to Improve Life Satisfaction in Asian Countries

Dong-Kyun Im, Hearan Koo, and Sang-Hee Park

Abstract This study examines the pathways by which individuals' well-being and life satisfaction are shaped by employing social surveys conducted in three East Asian and four Southeast Asian countries, and makes a cross-regional comparison. Previous studies on well-being and life satisfaction have largely neglected the complex interdependencies and chain of effects between the components of well-being and their determinants from a holistic standpoint. Taking advantage of the relatively novel empirical strategy of Bayesian network analysis, this study uncovers the conditional dependency structure of multidimensional social well-being and its regional heterogeneity with regard to how well-being is determined in a processual manner. The results show that regions in East and Southeast Asia share some commonalities, such as the importance of economic and social capital; however, there are key differences as to how individuals' well-being is determined. The most notable difference is that the entire dependency structure is denser in East Asia, that reveals a strong correlational structure. We also found that income had a much higher differential effect on life satisfaction in East Asia. Hence, we propose a compensatory mechanism

This chapter is based on Im, Dong-Kyun, Hearan Koo, and Sang-Hee Park. 2020. "Similar but Different: Uncovering the Multiple Pathways to Life Satisfaction in Asia." *Journal of Asian Sociology* 49(2): 219–251. We thank the members of the editorial board of *Journal of Asian Sociology* for generously allowing us to revise the paper and publish it for this edited volume.

D.-K. Im (✉)
Department of Sociology, Seoul National University, Seoul, Republic of Korea
e-mail: dongkyunlm@snu.ac.kr

S.-H. Park
Division of Social Sciences, Sungkonghoe University, Seoul, Republic of Korea
e-mail: socialpark@skhu.ac.kr

H. Koo
Institute for Social Development and Policy Research, Seoul National University, Seoul, Republic of Korea

Korea Social Science Data Archive, Seoul National University, Seoul, Republic of Korea

H. Koo
e-mail: hrkoo@snu.ac.kr

J. Yee et al. (eds.), *Social Well-Being, Development, and Multiple Modernities in Asia*,
https://doi.org/10.1007/978-981-97-3866-3_18

hypothesis to explain the difference; various economic and relational mechanisms have been developed, and they effectively compensate for the low level of baseline life satisfaction in East Asia.

Keywords Well-being · East Asia · Southeast Asia · Bayesian network analysis

1 Introduction

For many years, pursuing the betterment of people's "well-being" has gained broad acceptance as a policy goal to replace the economy-centered model of social progress. Persistent efforts have been made to achieve this goal. Policymakers have attempted to construct well-being measures to investigate and monitor the social progress and to design relevant policies. National governments and international organizations have invested a significant amount of resources in developing the indicators of well-being that can be compared across different countries and at different periods of time.

Despite these efforts, we still lack sufficient knowledge regarding effective policy tools for improving the well-being of individuals and societies (Dolan et al., 2008; Duncan, 2010; Kenny, 2011). A major reason for this is that there are notable inconsistencies in the empirical findings regarding the factors that impact the well-being of people and societies. Over the last three decades, many studies have ascertained the determinants of well-being. However, the results demonstrate that the determinants of well-being are not considered equally important across countries or regions (Bonini, 2008; Fleche et al., 2011; Helliwell et al., 2009; Kroll, 2013) Stages of development, culture, religion, and other values, such as (post) materialism, are the significant factors that make a difference (Diener, 1995; Okulicz-Kozaryn, 2010). In this context, the widely held assumption that the better the economic conditions, the better the individual's well-being, also referred to as the homogeneity perspective, has been questioned in a number of studies (Delhey, 2010; Easterlin, 1995, etc.)

Although the understanding of the pathways to well-being has deepened with the knowledge of the effects of the contextual differences at the national or regional level, the debate regarding homogeneity versus heterogeneity is far from over. Helliwell et al. (2009) argue that there are key universal factors that eventually determine the level of life satisfaction, despite some minor differences across countries. It was found that several key variables, such as income, age, attainment of basic needs, having someone to count on, perceived corruption level, and a sense of freedom, work in more or less the same way. They concluded: "the same factors come into play in much the same way and to much the same degree," after applying identical well-being predictors to analyze the life satisfaction in 105 different societies, (Helliwell et al., 2009: 10). In contrast, Kroll (2013) showed that the heterogeneity in the relationship between the components of life satisfaction and human development is considerable according to the stages of development and the goals of individual countries. Adopting the human development approach, he revealed that the impact of material conditions, health, and education on life satisfaction varies not only across countries, but also across different sub-groups within each country.

How can these contradictions between the homogeneity and heterogeneity perspectives and their implications be resolved? In this chapter, we provide empirical evidence that contributes to such a discourse and our understanding of the generalizability of the models of well-being, particularly by examining the cross-regional patterns of relationships among the components of well-being. As revealed by the literature, well-being is a multidimensional and complex concept. Multidimensionality is often addressed by highlighting the multiple dimensions, such as subjective and objective, micro and macro, and economic and social. The complexity of well-being is also captured as an aggregate of various life domains, such as health, job, family, income, housing, and social relations, among others, in the metrics of well-being. It should be noted, however, that the multidimensionality of well-being not only refers to the fact that well-being is multi-dimensional but also implies that those multiple dimensions interact together and jointly determine an individuals' well-being as an outcome. We argue that while previous studies have focused on the former, they overlooked the latter.

The above-mentioned reasons helped in ascertaining the purpose of this study. This study intends to investigate the overall patterns of interrelationships between the determinants of well-being to achieve a clear understanding of the multidimensional nature of social well-being and yield implications for policy development. We examined the structure of multiple pathways to life satisfaction in a holistic manner rather than focusing on binary associations between the variables. For the purpose of empirical analysis, we employed the Bayesian network analysis, modeling well-being as a complex system made up of chains of dependencies among the numerous components of well-being. This allowed us to explore the holistic and systematic interrelations among the various components of well-being.

Our empirical investigation focused on the Eastern and Southeast Asia, in particular, employing a cross-national survey that was conducted in seven Asian countries (i.e., Japan, Korea, Taiwan, Indonesia, the Philippines, Thailand, and Vietnam). We were interested in exploring life satisfaction in Asia because it has undergone rapid economic growth and social transformation over the past few decades. As the economy develops, people become concerned about whether the rising economic prosperity which they are likely to experience will be able to enrich their lives and improve their social well-being. This clearly highlights the idea of pursuing multifaceted well-being, as well as the question of Easterlin's paradox. Nevertheless, previous studies on social well-being have predominantly focused on Western countries and relatively few studies have been conducted to explore individuals' well-being in Asia. This study has the potential to add important empirical evidence to our understanding of well-being of the Asians.

We compared the two Asian regions: East Asia and Southeast Asia. While these two regions share similar historical and cultural characteristics, there are marked differences in terms of the population structure, developmental stage of the economy, and socio-cultural and political systems. With respect to the two regions, we were interested in revealing how the components of well-being are linked in the two regions, and the similarities and differences in determining the level of subjective well-being. By examining these non-western regions, we attempted to gain a more comprehensive understanding of the social well-being and develop more appropriate policy tools for improving individuals' well-being.

This study intends to focus our attention toward exploration of the additional influencers of well-being and life satisfaction to analyze the structure of interdependence between the determinants of well-being across heterogeneous regional contexts. The empirical findings have been illustrated and discussed in the following sections.

2 Data and Methods

2.1 Data and Variables

We used the data[1] from the Social Well-Being Survey in Asia (SoWSA), that was conducted in seven Asian countries (International Consortium for Social Well-Being Studies, 2018). We focused on the respondents aged 20–69 years. Before we conducted the Bayesian network analysis (BNA), we selected the variables of interest from the SoWSA. Following the definition of social well-being based on Koo et al., (2016, p.45), we define social well-being as the joint configuration of the three dimensions: personal, relational, and societal well-being. Personal well-being is defined as a positive evaluation of one's life. Relational well-being refers to the state of having rich and meaningful relationships with others, and trusting and embracing attitudes toward others. Societal well-being is shaped by the quality of institutions and their positive perceptions regarding the functioning of a society (Koo et al., 2016, p. 45). This definition implies that individuals as a part of a trusting and inclusive society and those who form rich and meaningful relationships with others are likely to enjoy a high level of life satisfaction and happiness.

The variables used in the analysis can be categorized into the following five groups: socioeconomic variables, subjective life conditions, relational well-being, societal well-being (i.e., perceptions of the functioning of society), and overall personal well-being (i.e., life satisfaction). The following list shows the variables used in the analysis and the labels attached to the nodes in the Bayesian network DAG (directed acyclic graph).

Socioeconomic Variables

- AGE: Respondents' age
- EDU: Level of education
- INC: Household income
- JOB: Work status
- FAM: The number of household members

[1] The data that we analyzed is the integrated SoWSA data set version 0.5 which was prepared by KOSSDA and shared between the ICSWB members.

Subjective Life Conditions

- INC_SAT: Satisfaction with family income
- EMPL_SAT: Satisfaction with the state or security of employment
- LEI_SAT: Satisfaction with the amount of leisure time

Relational Well-Being

- NEIGHBOR: Degree of participation in neighborhood activities and frequency of interaction with neighbors
- SUPPORT: Respondents' reliance on family, relatives, friends, regional groups, and neighbors.
- RF_INT: The frequency of interaction with relatives and friends
- TRUST: General trust

Societal Well-Being

- FAIR_DIS: Perceptions of how fairly people are treated on the basis of their gender, age, education, occupation, income, assets, or family background
- INC_GAP: Opinions about whether the income gap is too large

Overall Personal Well-Being

- LIFE_SAT: Life satisfaction

It should be noted that the EDU (education) and (INC) income variables were standardized, and other variables, except JOB, were mean-centered for each country before the country-level data were merged and utilized for further analysis.

2.2 Methods

In this section, we introduce the results of the BNA to explore the multiple and heterogeneous pathways of well-being in Eastern and Southeast Asia. BNA is a statistical method that can reveal the structure of the probabilistic dependencies in the given set of variables. It uncovers the conditional independent relationships among the variables and visualizes them as a directed acyclic graph (DAG). For instance, when there are three variables X, Y, and Z, and if Y is conditionally dependent on X, Z is conditionally dependent on Y, but Z is not dependent on X, their probabilistic causal relationships can be shown as a DAG of $X \rightarrow Y \rightarrow Z$. The links in the graph are directed, and there are no circular loops (*acyclic*). The presence of directed links represents the structure of probabilistic dependence, and the absence of such a link between two variables indicates statistical independence. Compared to more conventional regression-based methods such as ordinary least squares, BNA, in particular, has an advantage because it can illustrate the *social processes* that determine well-being more clearly. Thus, it can provide a more holistic picture than the approaches based on regression analysis.

When applied to a large set of variables, BNA can effectively exhibit the complex relationships and probabilistic dependencies among them. The causal structure is represented by a graphical structure (G), which consists of vertices (nodes) and edges (arcs or links). Bayesian network analysis produces a DAG of the joint probability structure distribution induced by the model, which can encode various states of well-being of individuals and their background information.

To summarize, this graphical representation does not reveal the structure of deterministic relationships but rather the probability structure as a probabilistic model. This implies that the Bayesian network model constructs a joint distribution structure over every combination of responses of N variables, according to which one can estimate a posterior distribution of any X_j when the value of X_i is specified. Thus, analyzing individuals' requirements for well-being with Bayesian networks means treating multidimensional elements as complex probability distributions, thereby unearthing the diverse pathways to life satisfaction. Assigning a probability structure (or stochastic structure) to such an analysis reveals the extent of uncertainty in the formation of individuals' well-being and life satisfaction (Im, 2014).[2]

Determining the knowledge structure by factoring a distribution using a graphical representation (network) is usually performed by determining the conditionally independent relationships among the variables. Hence, the concept of d-separation (direction-dependent separation; Pearl, 1988) is used. Simply speaking, the two nodes (X and Y) in the network are conditionally independent, or "d-separated" in graphical tests, if every path from X to Y is blocked by a set of random variables Z in the DAG.[3] As mentioned earlier, conditional independence between the two variables is represented as a graphical segregation (i.e., no edge) in the visualized output, whereas an arrow (directed edge) from node A to node B indicates that B is dependent on A. Conditional independence tests using d-separations are used in various types of structure-learning algorithms built on constraint-based algorithms, which are used in this study (see Scrutari, 2010).[4]

Although Bayesian network analysis is often used for determining the "causal" relational patterns by using DAGs and testing the conditional independencies between the variables, we did not use Bayesian networks in this study for illustrating the "causal" relationships, but to reveal and project a holistic picture of the embeddedness of individuals' well-being. The cross-sectional nature of our data, the

---

[2] Although this analysis is called "Bayesian" network analysis, it does not mean that Bayesian analysis was used to explore the structure of the network. The Bayesian part becomes relevant when a researcher, by taking advantage of the relational structure of random variables (i.e., nodes) of a Bayesian network (DAG), computes conditional probabilities and uses such probabilities, for example, to analyze the reasons for a specific outcome. Prior information is required to construct such conditional probabilities. "Bayesian network" should be understood in this context as a specific term that indicates a probabilistic DAG model.

[3] More specifically, X and Y are d-separated given Z when their connective structures are either serial (X→Z→Y; X←Z←Y) or diverging (X←Z→Y), or when the structure is converging and Z (X→Z←Y) is not conditioned. See Pearl (2000) for a more detailed explanation.

[4] There are other kinds of structure learning algorithms such as score-based algorithms that do not use conditional independence tests.

possibility of occurrence of the omitted-variable bias problem, and mutual feedback that arises among a given set of variables preclude us from interpreting the results in highly causal terms. Therefore, the results of the BNA presented in this chapter should be interpreted as patterns of interrelationships rather than causal relationships. More information on the BNA can be found in Darwiche (2009), Koller and Friedman (2009), Lopez et al. (2012); and Ceriani and Gigliarano (2016).

We used various Bayesian network learning algorithms and compared their goodness-of-fit scores to evaluate their fit and determine the choice of algorithm. We found that the Grow-Shrink algorithm, which is a constraint-based structure-learning algorithm, produced the best results by showing the lowest BIC values. All the procedures were conducted using the *bnlearn* package in *R*.

To compute the fit statistics, all edges in the Bayesian network need to be directed. To create a directed network and ease the identification process, we eliminated some possible directed relationships in advance. There were two kinds of relationships that we eliminated: the first was those that contradicted common sense, the arcs from the subjective variables to sociodemographic variables (e.g., any subjective attitude → age) or to relatively objective variables (e.g., employment satisfaction → frequency of interaction with neighbors). Second, the arcs were less convincing than their counterparts (e.g., life satisfaction → and social support). While most of the second type of blacklists appealed to our common sense, some of them needed further discussion, which will be taken up in the results section (see footnote 5). This process was performed using a blacklist setting in the *bnlearn* package in R. It should be noted that BNA often relies on expert knowledge so that researchers can effectively engage in the identification process (e.g., blacklisting arcs) (Lee & Kim, 2019).

3 Results

3.1 Correlational Analysis

Before introducing the results of the BNA, we first explored the correlation between our selected variables in order to check how the variables presumably related to individuals' well-being are associated with one another. As the first step, we show the interrelationships and dependencies among the variables. Denser and tighter relationships among the variables are likely to suggest that more various pathways to life satisfaction and well-being are socially developed, and individuals tend to make efforts to take advantage of these channels.

The tables in Appendix 1 are correlation matrices that are statistically significant ($p < 0.05$) Pearson's correlation coefficients. Although the correlation matrices illustrate some differences between the East and Southeast Asian countries, concrete patterns from the seven matrices cannot be easily detected. Therefore, we visualized the correlational patterns as network plots, as shown in Fig. 1. To ensure comparability of the statistical significance tests across countries, approximately 1000 cases were randomly selected from the sample of each country. The sample sizes of East Asian countries were particularly large; therefore, we randomly selected 1000 cases from each of the sample.

Each link in the figure indicates a statistically significant correlation between the two variables. The absence of a link between the two variables implies that the relationship between them is not significant. The thickness of the link is proportional to the correlation coefficient. The "life satisfaction" variable, the item of focus in this study, is indicated in gray so that its relationship with other variables can be easily identified.

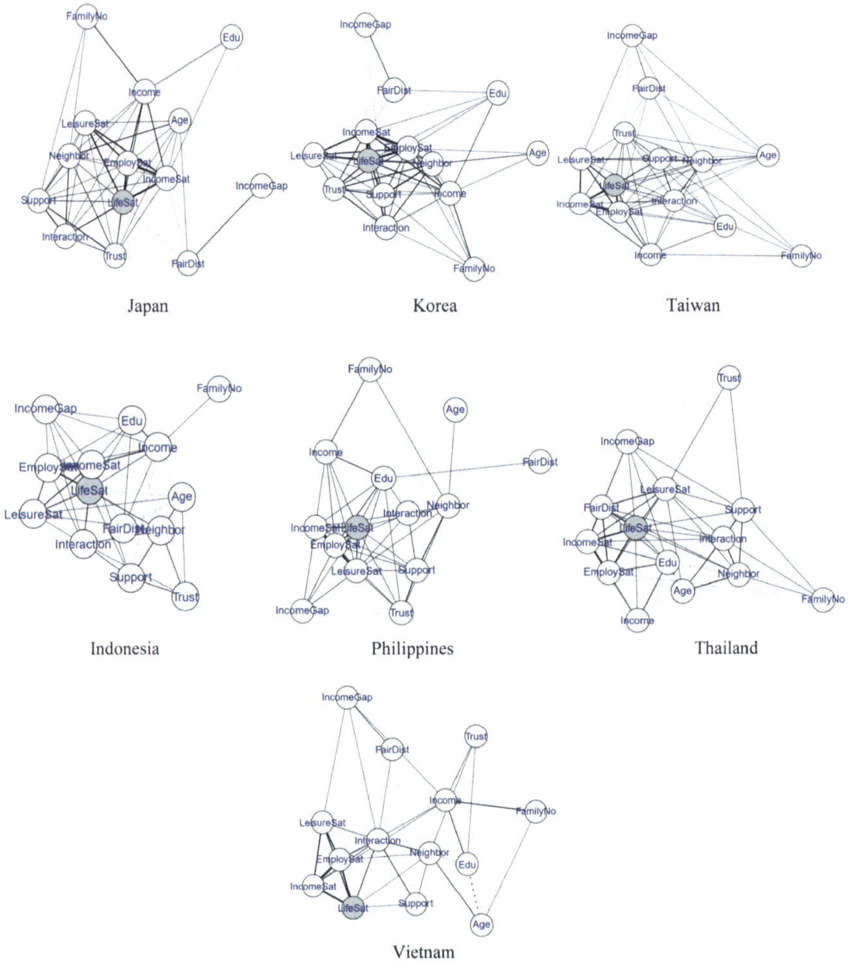

Fig. 1 Correlations of items by country

Since we focused on examining the difference between the two Asian regions, we analyzed the quantitative information for the purpose of comparison. First, the network density of each network plot was determined which was as follows: Japan (0.73), South Korea (0.63), Taiwan (0.75), Indonesia (0.63), Philippines (0.51), Thailand (0.64), and Vietnam (0.48). The values reveal that Taiwan and Japan have denser networks than others. Overall, the network density of East Asian countries is somewhat higher than that of Southeast Asian countries. The next question that we intended to explore was: how many variables does the "life satisfaction" variable have significant relationships with? This question pertains to how strongly individuals' well-being is embedded in various social, institutional, and individual-level factors.

This question was answered on the basis of the degree centrality of the life satisfaction variable in the network. The results pertaining to degree centrality were as follows: Japan (11), South Korea (10), Taiwan (11), Indonesia (11), the Philippines (9), Thailand (11), and Vietnam (7). This result suggests that the number of variables associated with the life satisfaction variables, and not much regional difference, seems to exist, although the degree centrality score was found to be somewhat lower in the Philippines and Vietnam.

This comparison based on the correlational analysis was informative, but had two clear limitations. Although the regional difference was not very large with a cutoff p-value of 0.05, the difference became larger and more inherent when a much lower p-value (e.g., $p < 0.001$) was considered. When the results were analyzed considering the p-value 0.001, denser and tighter interrelationships were revealed among the variables in the East Asian sample. It was found that there existed various channels and pathways for attainment of life satisfaction in East Asia. This pattern was more clearly confirmed by the results of the Bayesian network analysis. Of course, this does not mean that the East Asian citizens are in a better condition to seek their well-being. Our findings suggest that the situation is actually the opposite, which will be discussed later in this chapter.

The second limitation was that the correlations were determined on the basis of the bivariate relationships, and hence they failed to consider the effects of all other variables, such as the confounding and the mediating variables. Therefore, a more methodological approach needs to be employed that can reveal the dependency structure closer to causal relations, which can be better achieved by the BNA.

3.2 Bayesian Network Analysis

Figure 2 shows the Bayesian network of the aforementioned list of variables using an East Asian sample. It shows a large dependency structure where the sociodemographic variables and the various dimensions of the well-being variables yield complex pathways to life satisfaction. The presence of an edge between any two variables indicates that the relationship is conditional. Because the large sample size enabled the significance test to detect even minimally meaningful relationships as significant, the threshold of statistical significance was lowered to $p < 0.01$. The

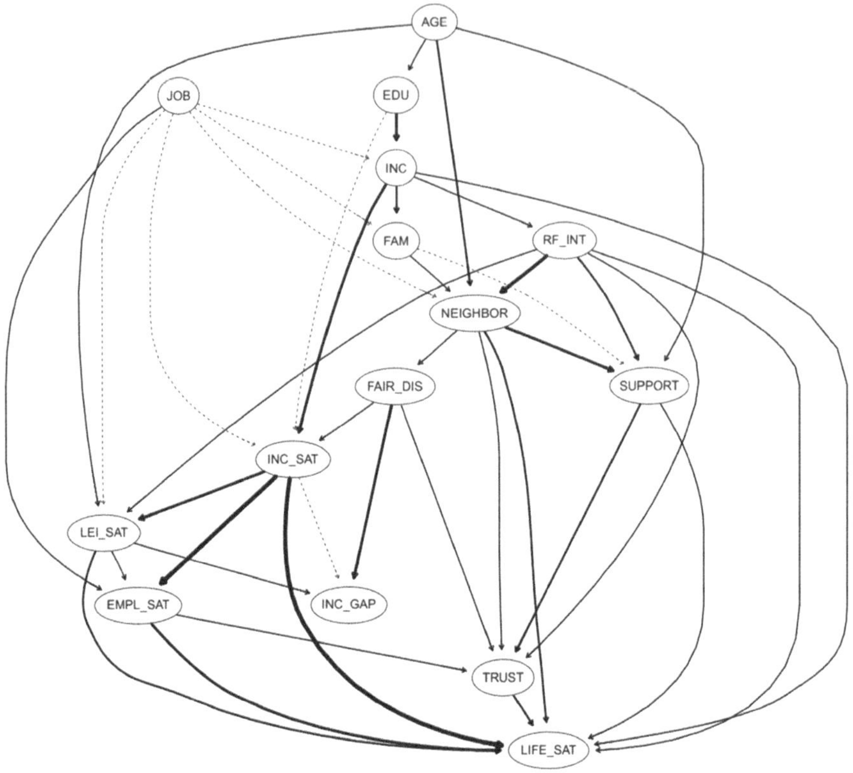

Fig. 2 A Bayesian network plot for East Asian countries (Japan, South Korea, and Taiwan)

arc thickness is proportional to the probability that the arc is significant in bootstrap replicates. The probabilities were derived by calculating the frequency with which the arc was found to be significant in bootstrapped samples. We generated 100 nonparametric bootstrapped samples, each having a sample size equal to 100. The arc thickness represents the confidence in each arc.

The points which need to be noted are as follows: first, an individual's life satisfaction is affected by various factors, including economic well-being (e.g., family income, satisfaction with income, and employment), relational well-being (e.g., trust, social support, interaction with neighbors, and interaction with family and friends), and other kinds of personal well-being (i.e., satisfaction with leisure). One important caveat here is that the directions of some of the arcs in the Bayesian network were predetermined in the BNA procedure (see footnote 5 for details).[5] The results

[5] By using the 'blacklist' option in the *bnlearn* package, we forced the arcs from life satisfaction to leisure satisfaction and employment satisfaction to be excluded. Despite the possibility that life satisfaction can affect the two satisfaction variables, we hypothesized that the two variables can be conceptualized as the determinants of life satisfaction which is regarded as the final destination and the most inclusive concept in our multidimensional well-being model. There were two other

showed that people's satisfaction with their lives in East Asia can be determined through various channels and is dependent on multiple processes. An increase in the household income may not affect life satisfaction only due to satisfaction with one's income; it can also influence social capital, which can consequently lead to improvement in life satisfaction.

Second, Fig. 2 clearly shows that satisfaction with one's income (INC_SAT) plays a prominent role throughout the network. The importance of this variable is particularly due to its strong mediator position. INC_SAT affected the satisfaction with leisure, employment, and life, all of which were the key variables of well-being considered in the BNA. The fact that income satisfaction is strongly affected by the household income and that the level of income is affected by the level of education shows why education is often heavily emphasized in East Asia.

Third, the roles of relational well-being variables (i.e., NEIGHBOR, SUPPORT, RF_INT, and TRUST) need close attention. They occupy significant positions within the network that connects socioeconomic variables with subjective attitudes and well-being. These factors influence life satisfaction through diverse channels or pathways. Sometimes, they are directly linked to life satisfaction, which means that life satisfaction is conditionally dependent on them (e.g., NEIGHBOR, SUPPORT, and RF_INT → LIFE_SAT). Sometimes, they affect other kinds of well-being and satisfaction, which subsequently affects the life satisfaction. For example, they can increase their leisure satisfaction, which can subsequently increases their life satisfaction. They can also enhance individuals' social trust, leading to higher life satisfaction. Among the relational well-being variables, TRUST showed a particularly interesting characteristic. This will be discussed when we examine the results for the Southeast Asian region.

In summary, with regard to the East Asian samples, it was found that there are two distinct pathways to life satisfaction. In other words, there are two prominent mediators. The two major mediators with the highest degree centrality in the network are income satisfaction (INC_SAT) and interaction with neighbors (NEIGHBOR). It is noteworthy that these two main channels are not heavily intertwined; therefore,

---

kinds of blacklisted arcs that required clarification. One of them was the arc from life satisfaction to trust. Again, although it was possible that the level of life satisfaction changed the level of trust, previous studies, such as Elgar et al., Helliwell and Huang (2011) and Kroll (2008), suggested that possessing a high level of trust toward other people or living in an environment where a high level of generalized trust is nurtured tends to generate higher levels of happiness and life satisfaction. The other blacklisted arc which was relatively less important in the network but still needed explanation was the arc from life satisfaction to perceptions of income inequality in society (INC_GAP). Considering the possibility that the perceptions of inequality affect one's life satisfaction, we excluded such a directed arc for two reasons. First, it is difficult to imagine that an ordinary person's evaluation of inequality in society would have a great impact on the overall life satisfaction even after the person's income, income satisfaction, and other characteristics are controlled for. Second, studying the relationship between inequality and happiness is usually meaningful at the cross-national level or by looking at the objective level of inequality and the associated changes in the levels of happiness, using panel data. Although our data was based on multiple countries, the INC_GAP variable was standardized so that we could ignore the effect of country-level differences in the level of inequality.

the two pathways based on economic and social capital remain relatively distinct and distinguishable. Nevertheless, the strength of the arcs shows that economic satisfaction is more important than social capital in determining life satisfaction.

On the other hand, Fig. 3 shows the Bayesian network produced with the Southeast Asian samples (i.e., Indonesia, the Philippines, Thailand, and Vietnam). The two regions, Eastern and Southeast Asia, display some commonalities in Bayesian networks. Both results show that two distinct pathways have been developed, that center around income satisfaction and social capital. As in the case of East Asia, the data pertaining to Southeast Asia also shows that these two paths are not very closely related to each other. In addition, similar to the case of East Asia, the most robust pathways in the case of Southeast Asia are those that radiate from income satisfaction and directly or indirectly reach life satisfaction. NEIGHBOR had the highest degree centrality in the network. A similar pattern was observed across Southeastern and East Asia.

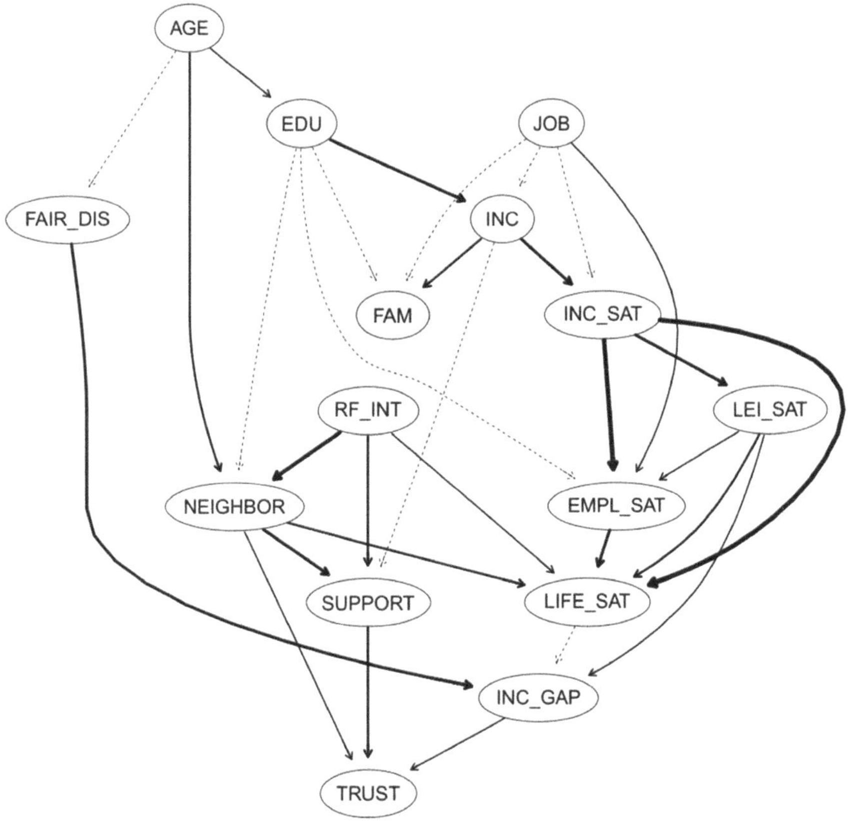

Fig. 3 A Bayesian network plot for Southeast Asian countries (Indonesia, Thailand, the Philippines, and Vietnam)

Despite these similarities, some significant differences between the two regions were also observed. First, the Bayesian network pertaining to East Asia has a relatively denser conditional dependency network than that of Southeast Asia. While both the networks have 15 nodes, the East Asian network has 42 edges (density = 0.400) and the Southeast Asian network has 31 edges (density = 0.295). The nodes with the highest degree centrality in East Asia are income satisfaction, life satisfaction, and neighbors, which have a degree centrality of 8. Several other variables had degree centralities of 6. In Southeast Asia, only life satisfaction and NEIGHBOR had the highest degree centrality of 6. When the BNA was applied to each country to examine the country-level heterogeneity, the results revealed similar differences between the two regions. The network density scores of the Bayesian networks were as follows: Korea (0.33), Japan (0.31), Taiwan (0.32), Indonesia (0.16), the Philippines (0.22), Thailand (0.18), and Vietnam (0.21). The overall configuration of the BNA plots for each country confirm the regional-level differences (see Appendix 2).

Such a difference in network density and the overall level of connectedness suggests that, in Southeast Asia, the paths to life satisfaction are less structured or solidified than in East Asia. Another important factor related to the difference in network density is the role of income. Household income directly affects life satisfaction and social capital in East Asia. In Southeast Asia, household income is not directly associated with life satisfaction and has a relatively limited role in influencing social capital. The relative impacts of the income satisfaction on the life satisfaction also differed. The conditional density computed by the Bayesian networks shows that income satisfaction has an effect of 0.320 on life satisfaction in East Asia, while its effect is 0.240 in Southeast Asia. When all other direct and indirect paths are considered together, the effect of income on life satisfaction is much less on Bayesian networks. To confirm these differences, we examined the conditional probability distribution of life satisfaction that was computed using Bayesian networks.

Figure 4 shows the probability distribution of the life satisfaction conditional variable on household income level. The solid line indicates the conditional probability distribution when an individual's household income is equal to or less than 1 standard deviation from the mean. The dashed line depicts the same type of distribution when the income is equal to or greater than one standard deviation. The figure clearly shows that the effect of income on life satisfaction in Bayesian networks is far greater in East Asia than in Southeast Asia.

In general, the entire Southeast Asian dependency network shows a weaker correlational structure than that in East Asia. Satisfaction with one's income, interactions with neighbors and friends, social support, and life satisfaction are linked to relatively fewer other variables via conditional dependencies. Even the absolute size of the correlation coefficients was considerably lower in most cases in the Southeast Asian sample, which indicates that the pathways suggested by the network have much weaker differential effects on individuals' well-being.

In addition, the role of generalized trust (TRUST) was markedly different as indicated in the two graphs. While a few paths are directed towards trust, they do not have any significance in relation to life satisfaction in Southeast Asia. In contrast,

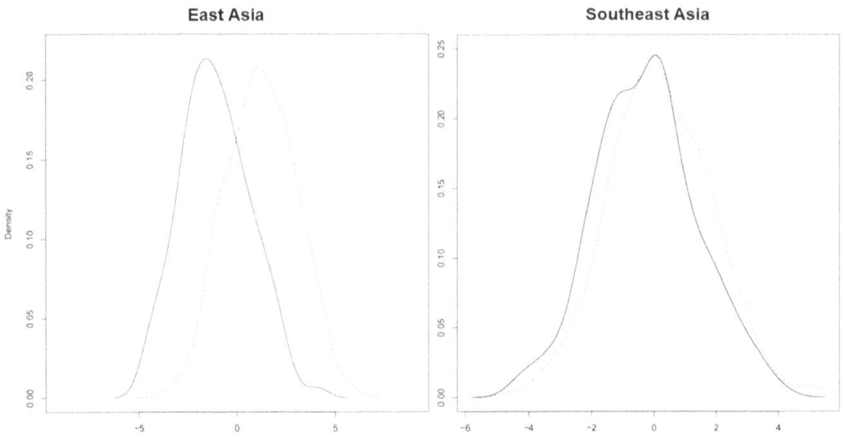

Solid line: household income <= -1 s.d.
Dashed line: household income => 1 s.d.

Fig. 4 Probability distribution of life satisfaction conditional on household income. Solid line: household income $< \; = -1$ s.d., Dashed line: household income $= \; > 1$ s.d.

trust is one of the most important nodes in the entire dependency network in East Asia, grouping the five edges together and sending them on the pathway to life satisfaction. This result illustrates that the sociological implications and importance of trust in people's lives can differ remarkably depending on the sociocultural context.

The difference in the importance of other relational well-being indicators needs to be focused on. The three indicators that measure individuals' interpersonal embeddedness (i.e., NEIGHBOR, RF_INT, and SUPPORT) were associated with a larger number of variables related to satisfaction in East Asia. Hence, the results collectively suggest that relational well-being has a larger differential effect on well-being and life satisfaction in East Asia than it does in Southeast Asia.

To summarize, we found striking similarities as well as commonalities between the two Asian regions with regard to big-picture comparisons. However, a close examination of the two dependency networks clearly reveals that there are a great number of channels and pathways in East Asia through which the level of individuals' well-being and life satisfaction is shaped. Individuals' economic and relational conditions and resources have large differential effects on the life satisfaction in East Asia. In the following section, we discuss the probable reasons behind the regional differences.

4 Discussion

The results of the BNA revealed interesting differences between East Asian and Southeast Asian societies and confirmed the heterogeneity in the social processes involved in determination of individuals' well-being. Why do we observe such differences between the two regions? How do we explain these major differences?

One possible explanation is the diversity in the structural and societal contexts of the two regions. It is worth noting that all the four Southeast Asian countries in our sample reported significantly higher levels of life satisfaction than the three East Asian countries. Specifically, the mean life satisfaction scores of the countries, based on an 11-point scale, were as follows: Thailand (7.29), Vietnam (7.02), Indonesia (6.92), the Philippines (6.67), Japan (5.65), South Korea (5.54), and Taiwan (5.54). Even the standard deviation of life satisfaction was larger in the case of East Asia, reflecting a higher level of inequality in life satisfaction in the region.

The lower levels and larger standard deviations on life satisfaction in East Asia indicate that there is more room for various factors to affect individuals' well-being in the region. To delve deeper into this problem, we examined the relationship between life satisfaction and the other key variables in Eastern and Southeast Asia. The results are illustrated in Fig. 5.

The results displayed a consistent pattern with regard to the differences between Eastern and Southeast Asia. In East Asian societies, the average level of life satisfaction is low, especially when economic and relational conditions are poor. However, the satisfaction gap shrinks and eventually becomes negligible once such conditions improve. In other words, the differential effects of economic and relational factors are greater in East Asia, where the baseline life satisfaction is low. Such a powerful differential effect was reflected in the additional conditional dependencies in the Bayesian network model of East Asian cases.

Based on this observation, we posit that *compensatory mechanisms* are one of the main operating mechanisms that result in patterns depicted in Fig. 5 and through Bayesian networks. This implies that, due to the mix of cultural and structural forces, the overall level of life satisfaction is low in East Asia, and some social pathways have been developed to compensate for such a low level of satisfaction. Within a societal context that suppresses life satisfaction, East Asians strive to attain resources to bolster their happiness. Our results revealed that economic conditions and interpersonal relationships play an important compensatory role in determining life satisfaction of individuals. Furthermore, at least for individuals who enjoy such resources, life satisfaction improves significantly and reaches the level of life satisfaction experienced by Southeast Asians. However, for East Asians who fail to accumulate such resources, their life satisfaction is likely to remain considerably low, as is evident from the conditional dependency structure from the BNA.

In summary, in order to account for the differences displayed in the BNA that compared the two Asian societies, we focused on the lower mean score and higher variance of life satisfaction in East Asian societies. It is our view that, in the East Asian

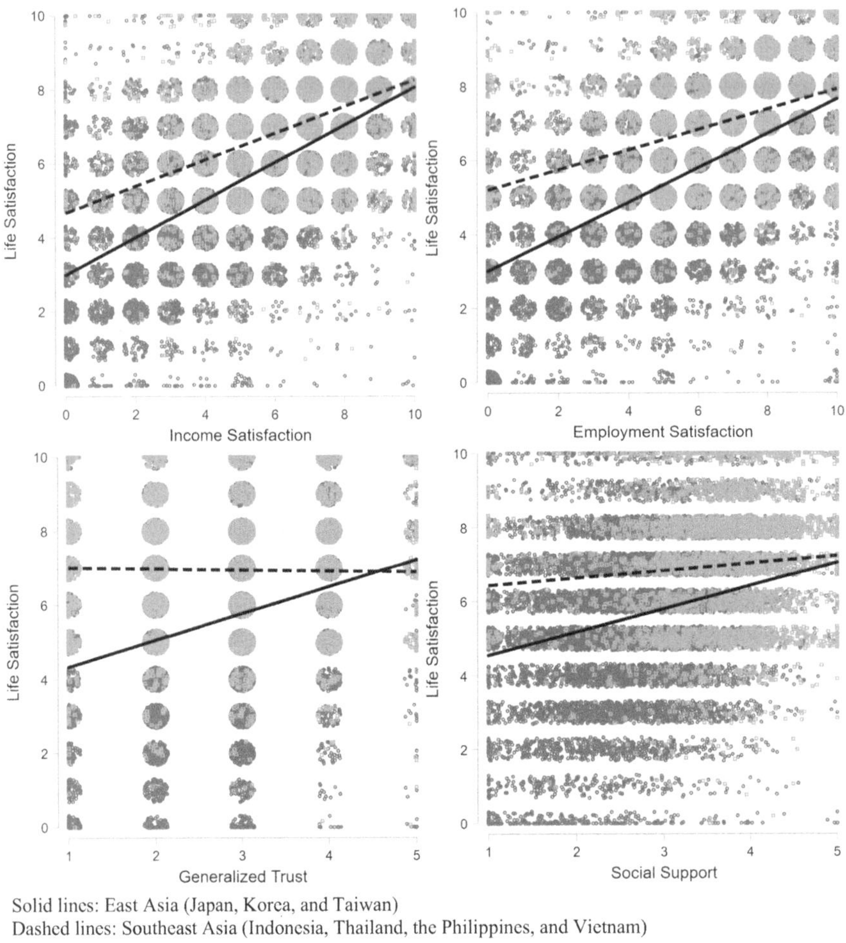

Fig. 5 Relationship between life satisfaction and other well-being indicators in East and Southeast Asia. Solid lines: East Asia (Japan, Korea, and Taiwan). Dashed lines: Southeast Asia (Indonesia, Thailand, the Philippines, and Vietnam).

context, compensatory mechanisms are developed for individuals to compensate for their low baseline life satisfaction.

5 Conclusion

In this chapter, we argue that the inter-connectedness of the determinants of well-being should be examined to develop a deeper understanding of the role of each determinant in improving individuals' well-being in society. We hypothesized that the structures and dynamics of interconnected determinants of well-being are likely to vary depending on the societal context.

We investigated the similarities and differences in the pathways to well-being and life satisfaction in affluent East Asian (AEA) and developing Southeast Asian (DSA) countries, using Bayesian networks. We found that economic elements such as satisfaction with one's income play a pivotal role in improving the life satisfaction of individuals in both the regions. We also found that two distinct routes that developed around both income satisfaction and social capital, serve as prominent pathways to life satisfaction in the two regions.

However, the results showed that there were significant differences between the pathways of the two regions. The most notable difference was that the entire dependency structure was denser in East Asia, showing a stronger correlational structure. We also found that household income had a much higher differential effect on life satisfaction in East Asia. Social trust also had differential role; in East Asian countries, various well-being factors influence life satisfaction via general trust, whereas in Southeast Asian countries, the route from TRUST to life satisfaction is disconnected. In the Discussion section, we propose a compensatory mechanism hypothesis to account for such regional differences.

In this study, we demonstrated that the Bayesian network approach can prove to be a useful tool to examine the conditional dependencies of various dimensions of well-being and for effectively identifying structures of diverse pathways across societies with different social and institutional environments. The network approach to explore the determinants of well-being has great potential to improve our understanding of the complex relationships between the determinants, and also for guiding research in contemporary well-being. In particular, it can be used to provide an integrated model for public policy decision-making because it can identify, and thereby prioritize, key elements to target and find efficient pathways to develop synergies between the determinants of well-being.

Acknowledgements This work used the data version 0.5 (May 5, 2018) of the Social Well-Being Survey in Asia (SoWSA) which was formerly called as International Comparative Surveys on Lifestyle and Values (ICSLV). The survey was supported by the MEXT-Supported Program for the Strategic Research Foundation at Private Universities of Japan, 2014-18 (S1491003), Senshu University, LabSosio Department of Sociology—Universitas Indonesia, and ROIS-DS-JOINT, 2017-18 (002RP2017 and 003RP2018).

Appendix 1

Tables 1, 2,3, 4, 5, 6 and 7.

Table 1 Pairwise correlations: Japan ($p < 0.05$ only)

Variables	(1)	(2)	(3)	(4)	(5)	(6)	(7)	(8)	(9)	(10)	(11)	(12)	(13)	(14)
(1) AGE	1													
(2) EDU	− 0.107	1												
(3) INC		0.186	1											
(4) FAM	− 0.105	− 0.079	0.298	1										
(5) TRUST	0.135				1									
(6) NEIGHBOR	0.280	− 0.080	0.080	0.113	0.233	1								
(7) SUPPORT			0.091	0.062	0.318	0.322	1							
(8) RF_INT	− 0.075		0.100		0.213	0.308	0.355	1						
(9) FAIR_DIS	0.064				− 0.170	− 0.077	− 0.119	− 0.111	1					
(10) INC_GAP		− 0.100	− 0.156		− 0.076				0.246	1				
(11) LEI_SAT	0.176			− 0.142	0.127	0.085	0.104	0.142			1			
(12) LIFE_SAT	0.090		0.249		0.200	0.166	0.199	0.214	− 0.139	− 0.073	0.437	1		
(13) INC_SAT	0.062	0.093	0.330		0.154	0.104	0.173	0.165	− 0.214	− 0.161	0.430	0.589	1	
(14) EMPL_SAT	0.065		0.317		0.126	0.099	0.145	0.150	− 0.117	− 0.077	0.415	0.589	0.672	1

Table 2 Pairwise correlations: South Korea ($p < 0.05$ only)

Variables	(1)	(2)	(3)	(4)	(5)	(6)	(7)	(8)	(9)	(10)	(11)	(12)	(13)	(14)
(1) AGE	1													
(2) EDU	– 0.067	1												
(3) INC	0.069	0.205	1											
(4) FAM			0.277	1										
(5) TRUST			0.109		1									
(6) NEIGHBOR	0.214		0.119	0.127	0.295	1								
(7) SUPPORT			0.115	0.129	0.284	0.392	1							
(8) RF_INT	– 0.064		0.174	0.104	0.319	0.293	0.338	1						
(9) FAIR_DIS	– 0.082	0.091			– 0.228	– 0.182	– 0.117		1					
(10) INC_GAP						– 0.107	– 0.064		0.211	1				
(11) LEI_SAT			0.104		0.221	0.124	0.141	0.184	– 0.073		1			
(12) LIFE_SAT		0.108	0.305		0.332	0.267	0.282	0.219	– 0.169		0.432	1		
(13) INC_SAT		0.079	0.326		0.246	0.205	0.240	0.194	– 0.150	– 0.067	0.416	0.691	1	
(14) EMPL_SAT	0.133	0.099	0.287	0.063	0.242	0.243	0.236	0.193	– 0.107		0.339	0.597	0.629	1

Table 3 Pairwise correlations: Taiwan ($p < 0.05$ only)

Variables	(1)	(2)	(3)	(4)	(5)	(6)	(7)	(8)	(9)	(10)	(11)	(12)	(13)	(14)
(1) AGE	1													
(2) EDU	– 0.151	1												
(3) INC		0.185	1											
(4) FAM	– 0.075		0.149	1										
(5) TRUST	0.056	0.024	0.055		1									
(6) NEIGHBOR	0.213	– 0.084	0.024	0.059	0.175	1								
(7) SUPPORT		– 0.039		0.040	0.188	0.269	1							
(8) RF_INT	– 0.028	– 0.032	0.052	0.029	0.123	0.265	0.261	1						
(9) FAIR_DIS	– 0.026	0.022			– 0.113	– 0.091	– 0.069		1					
(10) INC_GAP	0.031				– 0.061	– 0.028			0.178	1				
(11) LEI_SAT	0.087		0.048		0.116	0.109	0.106	0.135		0.075	1			
(12) LIFE_SAT	0.024	0.077	0.206		0.156	0.171	0.185	0.186	– 0.070		0.364	1		
(13) INC_SAT		0.098	0.251		0.106	0.107	0.147	0.171	– 0.059		0.398	0.565	1	
(14) EMPL_SAT	0.047	0.110	0.220		0.124	0.132	0.127	0.154	– 0.034		0.346	0.504	0.642	1

Table 4 Pairwise correlations: Indonesia ($p < 0.05$ only)

Variables	(1)	(2)	(3)	(4)	(5)	(6)	(7)	(8)	(9)	(10)	(11)	(12)	(13)	(14)
(1) AGE	1													
(2) EDU	– 0.089	1												
(3) INC	– 0.131	0.251	1											
(4) FAM			0.060	1										
(5) TRUST	0.087				1									
(6) NEIGHBOR	0.216	– 0.096	– 0.138		0.201	1								
(7) SUPPORT			– 0.070		0.202	0.231	1							
(8) RF_INT	– 0.112				0.132	0.186	0.173	1						
(9) FAIR_DIS	– 0.091	0.062	0.075		– 0.124	– 0.136	– 0.123	– 0.078	1					
(10) INC_GAP		0.065	0.105					0.066		1				
(11) LEI_SAT	0.067					0.093		0.068	– 0.103		1			
(12) LIFE_SAT	– 0.058	0.132	0.174			0.089	0.102	0.112	– 0.171	0.125	0.230	1		
(13) INC_SAT	– 0.137	0.141	0.272				0.076	0.144	– 0.071	0.137	0.260	0.479	1	
(14) EMPL_SAT		0.079	0.155			0.069		0.141	– 0.071	0.080	0.249	0.318	0.498	1

Table 5 Pairwise correlations: The Philippines ($p < 0.05$ only)

Variables	(1)	(2)	(3)	(4)	(5)	(6)	(7)	(8)	(9)	(10)	(11)	(12)	(13)	(14)
(1) AGE	1													
(2) EDU	− 0.172	1												
(3) INC		0.237	1											
(4) FAM			0.210	1										
(5) TRUST		0.092			1									
(6) NEIGHBOR	0.069			0.108	0.128	1								
(7) SUPPORT					0.313	0.286	1							
(8) RF_INT	− 0.104	0.137				0.158	0.228	1						
(9) FAIR_DIS		0.061				− 0.111			1					
(10) INC_GAP					− 0.078					1				
(11) LEI_SAT		0.119	0.070		0.062	0.109	0.117	0.115		0.196	1			
(12) LIFE_SAT		0.118	0.172		0.085	0.073	0.157			0.107	0.250	1		
(13) INC_SAT		0.178	0.157				0.065	0.124		0.184	0.393	0.324	1	
(14) EMPL_SAT		0.239	0.191		0.074		0.132	0.164		0.193	0.322	0.308	0.642	1

Table 6 Pairwise correlations: Thailand ($p < 0.05$ only)

Variables	(1)	(2)	(3)	(4)	(5)	(6)	(7)	(8)	(9)	(10)	(11)	(12)	(13)	(14)
(1) AGE	1													
(2) EDU	– 0.566	1												
(3) INC	– 0.128	0.277	1											
(4) FAM				1										
(5) TRUST					1									
(6) NEIGHBOR	0.278	– 0.274	– 0.107	0.097		1								
(7) SUPPORT	0.140	– 0.201	– 0.091	0.083	0.089	0.266	1							
(8) RF_INT	0.101	– 0.199		0.091		0.304	0.195	1						
(9) FAIR_DIS	– 0.110	0.079				0.063		0.109	1					
(10) INC_GAP		0.072			– 0.097		0.067		0.130	1				
(11) LEI_SAT	0.067				0.081	0.110	0.168	0.140	0.281	0.152	1			
(12) LIFE_SAT	– 0.075	0.129	0.110			0.081	0.075	0.134	0.344	0.155	0.211	1		
(13) INC_SAT	– 0.120	0.197	0.152					0.085	0.349	0.119	0.224	0.428	1	
(14) EMPL_SAT	– 0.114	0.242	0.141	– 0.070					0.314		0.162	0.368	0.556	1

Table 7 Pairwise correlations: Vietnam ($p < 0.05$ only)

Variables	(1)	(2)	(3)	(4)	(5)	(6)	(7)	(8)	(9)	(10)	(11)	(12)	(13)	(14)
(1) AGE	1													
(2) EDU	− 0.488	1												
(3) INC		0.260	1											
(4) FAM	0.082		0.299	1										
(5) TRUST		0.107	0.157		1									
(6) NEIGHBOR	0.238	− 0.134			0.142	1								
(7) SUPPORT		− 0.131	− 0.166			0.145	1							
(8) RF_INT		− 0.107	− 0.102			0.229	0.256	1						
(9) FAIR_DIS			− 0.083		− 0.123	− 0.100	− 0.072	0.108	1					
(10) INC_GAP			0.075					0.086	0.186	1				
(11) LEI_SAT		− 0.063						0.145	− 0.076	0.087	1			
(12) LIFE_SAT	− 0.092					0.107	0.084	0.259			0.322	1		
(13) INC_SAT			0.064					0.190			0.394	0.532	1	
(14) EMPL_SAT			0.091			0.076		0.175	− 0.065		0.395	0.498	0.687	1

Appendix 2

See Figs. 6 and 7.

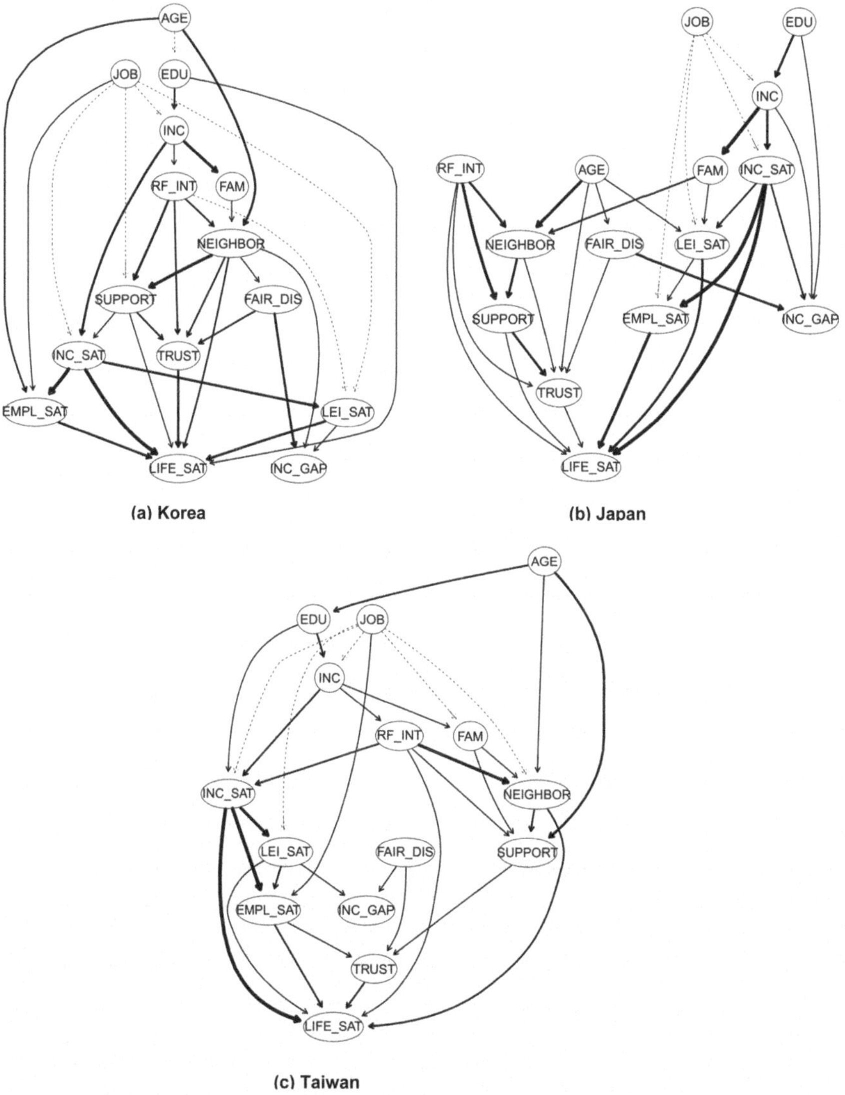

Fig. 6 Results of Bayesian network analysis: East Asia

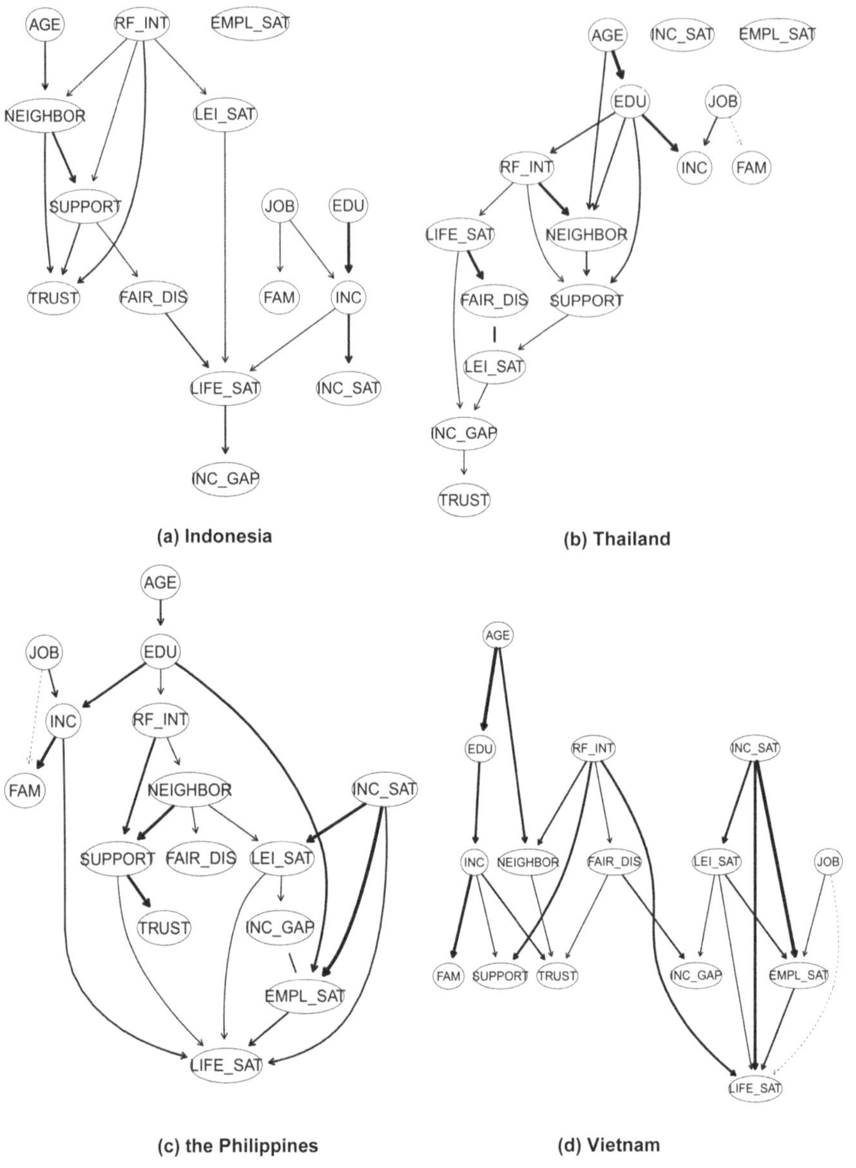

Fig. 7 Results of Bayesian network analysis: Southeast Asia

References

Bonini, N. A. (2008). Cross-national variation in individual life satisfaction: effects of national wealth, human development, and environmental conditions. *Social Indicators Research, 87*, 223–236. https://doi.org/10.1007/s11205-007-9167-6

Ceriani, L., & Gigliarano, C. (2016). Multidimensional well-being: A Bayesian Networks approach. Working Papers 399, ECINEQ, *Society for the Study of Economic Inequality*.

Darwiche, A. (2009). *Modeling and reasoning with Bayesian networks*. Cambridge University Press.

Delhey. (2010). From materialist to post-materialist happiness? National affluence and determinants of life satisfaction in cross-national perspective. *Social Indicators Research, 97*(1), 65–84.

Diener, E., & Diener, M. (1995). Cross-cultural correlates of life satisfaction and self-esteem. *Journal of Personality and Social Psychology, 68*(4), 653–663.

Dolan, P., Peasgood, T., & White, M. (2008). Do we really know what makes us happy? A review of the economic literature on the factors associated with subjective well-being. *Journal of Economic Psychology, 29*(1), 94–122.

Duncan, G. (2010). Should happiness-maximization be the goal of government? *Journal of Happiness Studies, 11*(2), 163–178. https://doi.org/10.1007/s10902-008-9129-y

Easterlin, R. A. (1995). Will raising the incomes of all increase the happiness of all? *Journal of Economic Behavior & Organization, 27*(1), 35–47.

Fleche, S., Smith, C., & Sorsa, P. (2011). *Exploring determinants of subjective wellbeing in OECD countries: Evidence from the world value survey*. OECD Economics Department Working Papers 921, OECD Publishing.

Helliwell, J. F., Huang, H., & Harris, A. (2009). International differences in the determinants of life satisfaction. In Ray, T., Somanathan, E., & Dutta, B. (Eds.), *New and enduring themes in development economics* (pp. 3–40). World Scientific.

Helliwell, J. F., & Huang, H. (2011). Well-being and trust in the workplace. *Journal of Happiness Studies, 12*(5), 747–767.

Im, D. -K. (2014). *Beliefs and attitudes about distributive justice in China*. (Unpublished Doctoral Dissertation) Harvard University.

International Consortium for Social Well-Being Studies. (2018). Social well-being survey in Asia, 2015–2017: Data Version 0.5 (May 5, 2018).

Kenny, C. (2011). Bentham from the crypt once more: politicians in pursuit of happiness. *Center for Global Development Essay*, June 2011. Available online at: https://www.cgdev.org/publication/bentham-crypt-once-more-politicians-pursuit-happiness

Koller, D., & Friedman, N. (2009). *Probabilistic graphical models: Principles and techniques*. MIT Press.

Koo, H., Yee, J., Nam, E. Y., & Kim, E. S. (2016). Dimensions of social well-being and determinants in Korea: Personal, relational and societal aspects. *The Senshu Social Well-Being Review, 3*, 37–58.

Kroll, C. (2008). *Social capital and the happiness of nations: The importance of trust and networks for life satisfaction in a cross-national perspective*. Peter Lang.

Kroll, C. (2013). Global development and happiness: How can data on subjective well-being inform development theory and practice? *IDS Working Papers, 2013*(432), 1–36.

Lee, S. M., & Kim, S. B. (2019). Identification of I-equivalent subnetworks in Bayesian networks to incorporate experts' knowledge. *Expert Systems, 36*(1), 1–13.

Lopez, J., Ramirez, A., & Casado, P. (2012). Modelling entrepreneurial attitudes in women entrepreneurs with bayesian networks. *Psychology, 3*(3), 265–271.

Okulicz-Kozaryn, A. (2010). Religiosity and life satisfaction across nations. *Mental Health, Religion & Culture, 13*(2), 155–169.

Pearl, J. (1988). *Probabilistic reasoning in intelligent systems: networks of plausible inference*. Morgan Kaufman Publishers Inc.

Pearl, J. (2000). *Causality: Models, reasoning, and inference*. Cambridge University Press.

Scutari, M. (2010). Learning Bayesian networks with the bnlearn R package. *Journal of Statistical Software, 35*(3), 1–22.

Dong-Kyun Im is an associate professor in sociology at Seoul National University. His research interests include social psychology, cognitive sociology, individuals and communities, social theory, and sociological methods.

Hearan Koo is a senior researcher at the Korean Social Science Data Archive, Seoul National University. Her research interests are social well-being, mental health, and comparative sociological methods.

Sang-Hee Park is an assistant professor in sociology at SungKongHoe University. Her research interests include refugees, migration, and well-being.

Correction to: Data Harmonization of Social Well-Being Survey in Asia

Hearan Koo, Hye-ok Heo, Yi-Fu Chen, and Tadahiko Maeda

Correction to:
Chapter 3 in: J. Yee et al. (eds.), *Social Well-Being, Development, and Multiple Modernities in Asia*, https://doi.org/10.1007/978-981-97-3866-3_3

The original version of the book was inadvertently published with an incorrect affiliation of the second author "Hye-ok Heo" in Chapter 3, which has now been removed. The book and the chapter have been updated with the changes.

The updated version of this chapter can be found at
https://doi.org/10.1007/978-981-97-3866-3_3

J. Yee et al. (eds.), *Social Well-Being, Development, and Multiple Modernities in Asia*,
https://doi.org/10.1007/978-981-97-3866-3_19

SPRINGER NATURE

GPSR Compliance

The European Union's (EU) General Product Safety Regulation (GPSR) is a set of rules that requires consumer products to be safe and our obligations to ensure this.

If you have any concerns about our products, you can contact us on ProductSafety@springernature.com

In case Publisher is established outside the EU, the EU authorized representative is:

Springer Nature Customer Service Center GmbH
Europaplatz 3
69115 Heidelberg, Germany

The manufacturer's authorised representative in the EU is Springer Nature Customer Service Centre GmbH, Europaplatz 3, 69115 Heidelberg, Germany. If you have any concerns regarding our products, please contact ProductSafety@springernature.com

Printed and bound by CPI Group (UK) Ltd, Croydon, CR0 4YY
01/10/2026
02225857-0010